Ambulatory Sleep Medicine

Editors

NICK A. ANTIC
TEOFILO LEE-CHIONG Jr

SLEEP MEDICINE CLINICS

www.sleep.theclinics.com

Consulting Editor
TEOFILO LEE-CHIONG Jr

September 2016 • Volume 11 • Number 3

ELSEVIER

1600 John F. Kennedy Boulevard • Suite 1800 • Philadelphia, Pennsylvania, 19103-2899

http://www.theclinics.com

SLEEP MEDICINE CLINICS Volume 11, Number 3
September 2016, ISSN 1556-407X, ISBN-13: 978-0-323-46267-9

Editor: Katie Pfaff
Developmental Editor: Donald Mumford

Sleep Medicine Clinics (ISSN 1556-407X) is published quarterly by Elsevier Inc., 360 Park Avenue South, New York, NY 10010-1710. Months of issue are March, June, September and December. Business and Editorial Offices: 1600 John F. Kennedy Blvd., Ste. 1800, Philadelphia, PA 19103-2899. Customer Service Office: 3251 Riverport Lane, Maryland Heights, MO 63043. Periodicals postage paid at New York, NY and additional mailing offices. Subscription prices are $195.00 per year (US individuals), $100.00 (US students), $458.00 (US institutions), $235.00 (Canadian and international individuals), $135.00 (Canadian and international students), $519.00 (Canadian institutions) and $509.00 (International institutions). Foreign air speed delivery is included in all *Clinics* subscription prices. All prices are subject to change without notice. **POSTMASTER:** Send change of address to *Sleep Medicine Clinics*, Elsevier Health Sciences Division, Subscription Customer Service, 3251 Riverport Lane, Maryland Heights, MO 63043. Customer Service: **Tel: 1-800-654-2452 (U.S. and Canada); 314-447-8871 (outside U.S. and Canada). Fax: 314-447-8029. E-mail: journalscustomerservice-usa@elsevier.com (for print support); journalsonline support-usa@elsevier.com (for online support).**

Reprints. For copies of 100 or more of articles in this publication, please contact the Commercial Reprints Department, Elsevier Inc., 360 Park Avenue South, New York, NY 10010-1710. Tel.: 212-633-3874; Fax: 212-633-3820; E-mail: reprints@elsevier.com.

Sleep Medicine Clinics is covered in *MEDLINE/PubMed (Index Medicus)*.

PROGRAM OBJECTIVE

The goal of *Sleep Clinics of North America* is to keep practicing physicians up to date with current clinical practice by providing timely articles reviewing the state of the art in patient care.

TARGET AUDIENCE

All practicing physicians and other healthcare professionals.

LEARNING OBJECTIVES

Upon completion of this activity, participants will be able to:
1. Review therapy and treatment options for obstructive sleep apnea.
2. Discuss comorbid illnesses, management, and consequences of obstructive sleep apnea.
3. Recognize management techniques of other disorders of excessive daytime sleepiness such as idiopathic hypersomnia and narcolepsy.

ACCREDITATION

The Elsevier Office of Continuing Medical Education (EOCME) is accredited by the Accreditation Council for Continuing Medical Education (ACCME) to provide continuing medical education for physicians.

The EOCME designates this enduring material for a maximum of 15 *AMA PRA Category 1 Credit*(s)™. Physicians should claim only the credit commensurate with the extent of their participation in the activity.

All other health care professionals requesting continuing education credit for this enduring material will be issued a certificate of participation.

DISCLOSURE OF CONFLICTS OF INTEREST

The EOCME assesses conflict of interest with its instructors, faculty, planners, and other individuals who are in a position to control the content of CME activities. All relevant conflicts of interest that are identified are thoroughly vetted by EOCME for fair balance, scientific objectivity, and patient care recommendations. EOCME is committed to providing its learners with CME activities that promote improvements or quality in healthcare and not a specific proprietary business or a commercial interest.

The planning committee, staff, authors and editors listed below have identified no financial relationships or relationships to products or devices they or their spouse/life partner have with commercial interest related to the content of this CME activity:

Nick A. Antic, MBBS, FRACP, PhD; Joseph Andrew Berkowski, MD; Josiane L. Broussard, PhD; Ching Li Chai-Coetzer, MBBS, FRACP, PhD; Lyndon Chan, MBBS, FRACS; Julia L. Chapman, BSc, BA, MHSc; Walter D. Conwell, MD; Charles R. Davies, MD, PhD, FAASM; Bradley A. Edwards, PhD; Anjali Fortna; Garun S. Hamilton, MBBS, FRACP, PhD; John J. Harrington, MD, MPH, FAASM; Bretton Hevener, BS, RPSGT; William Hevener, RPSGT; Simon A. Joosten, MBBS, BMedSc, FRACP, PhD; Shane Landry, PhD; Stuart G. MacKay, BSc(Med), MBBS(Hons), FRACS; Michelle Magee, PhD; Patrick Manley; Emily M. Marbas, BA; R. Doug McEvoy, MBBS, FRACP, MD; Adam Pleister, MD; Erin Scheckenbach; Yasmina Serinel, BSc, MBBS, FRACP; Anita Valanju Shelgikar, MD; Kate Sutherland, PhD; Alexander Sweetman, BPsych(Hons); Sheila C. Tsai, MD; Rajakumar Venkatesan.

The planning committee, staff, authors and editors listed below have identified financial relationships or relationships to products or devices they or their spouse/life partner have with commercial interest related to the content of this CME activity:

Ahmad A. Bamagoos, MBBS, MSc has an employment affiliation with the government of Saudi Arabia, and NeuroSleep, the Centre for Translational Sleep and Circadian Neurobiology.

Peter A. Cistulli, MBBS, PhD, MBA, FRACP is on the speakers' bureau for ResMed, is a consultant/advisor for Zephyr Sleep Technologies, Inc.; Fisher & Paykel Appliances Ltd; and Novo Nordisk A/S, has research support from SomnoMed, and receives royalties/patents from Quintessence Publishing Co, Inc. and UpToDate, Inc. His spouse/partner has stock ownership in SomnoMed.

Ronald R. Grunstein, MBBS, MD, PhD, FRACP is on the speakers' bureau for Merck & Co., Inc, with research supoprt from Koninklijke Philips N.V.

Rami Khayat, MD has research support from Koninklijke Philips N.V.

Leon Lack, PhD has stock ownserhip in, research support from, and receives royalties/patents from Re-Time Pty Ltd.

Teofilo Lee-Chiong Jr, MD is a consultant/advisor for Elsevier and CareCore International, has stock ownsership in and an employment affiliation with Elsevier, and receieves royalties/patents from Lippincott; Oxford University Press; CreateSpace; and Wiley.

Nathaniel S. Marshall, BSc, BCom, PGDipHealSc, PhD has an employment affiliation with Medtronic.

Shantha M.W. Rajaratnam, PhD is a consultant/advisor for Teva Pharmaceutical Industries Ltd., and Alertness CRC, has stock ownership from Telstra, research support from Shell; Koninklijke Philips N.V.; and Rio Tinto, and has an employment affiliation with Alertness CRC.

Kenneth P. Wright Jr, PhD is on the speakers' bureau for American College of Chest Physicians; The Obesity Society; and Obesity Medicine Association, has research support from Koninklijke Philips N.V.; the National Institutes of Health; and Office of Naval Research, and is a consultant/advisor for, with stock ownership in, and research support from, Torvec, Inc.

UNAPPROVED/OFF-LABEL USE DISCLOSURE

The EOCME requires CME faculty to disclose to the participants:

1. When products or procedures being discussed are off-label, unlabelled, experimental, and/or investigational (not US Food and Drug Administration [FDA] approved); and
2. Any limitations on the information presented, such as data that are preliminary or that represent ongoing research, interim analyses, and/or unsupported opinions. Faculty may discuss information about pharmaceutical agents that is outside of FDA-approved labelling. This information is intended solely for CME and is not intended to promote off-label use of these medications. If you have any questions, contact the medical affairs department of the manufacturer for the most recent prescribing information.

TO ENROLL

To enroll in the Sleep Medicines Clinic Continuing Medical Education program, call customer service at 1-800-654-2452 or sign up online at http://www.theclinics.com/home/cme. The CME program is available to subscribers for an additional annual fee of USD $140.

METHOD OF PARTICIPATION

In order to claim credit, participants must complete the following:

1. Complete enrolment as indicated above.
2. Read the activity.
3. Complete the CME Test and Evaluation. Participants must achieve a score of 70% on the test. All CME Tests and Evaluations must be completed online.

CME INQUIRIES/SPECIAL NEEDS

For all CME inquiries or special needs, please contact elsevierCME@elsevier.com.

SLEEP MEDICINE CLINICS

Contributors

CONSULTING EDITOR

TEOFILO LEE-CHIONG Jr, MD
Professor of Medicine, National Jewish Health;
Professor of Medicine, School of Medicine,
University of Colorado Denver, Denver,
Colorado; Chief Medical Liaison, Philips
Respironics, Pennsylvania

EDITORS

NICK A. ANTIC, MBBS, FRACP, PhD
Adelaide Institute for Sleep Health, A Flinders
Centre of Research Excellence, School of
Medicine, Flinders University, Adelaide, South
Australia, Australia; Sleep Health Service,
Respiratory and Sleep Services, Repatriation
General Hospital, Southern Adelaide Local
Health Network, Daw Park, South Australia,
Australia

TEOFILO LEE-CHIONG Jr, MD
Professor of Medicine, National Jewish Health;
Professor of Medicine, School of Medicine,
University of Colorado Denver, Denver,
Colorado; Chief Medical Liaison, Philips
Respironics, Pennsylvania

AUTHORS

NICK A. ANTIC, MBBS, FRACP, PhD
Adelaide Institute for Sleep Health, A Flinders
Centre of Research Excellence, School of
Medicine, Flinders University, Adelaide, South
Australia, Australia; Sleep Health Service,
Respiratory and Sleep Services, Repatriation
General Hospital, Southern Adelaide Local
Health Network, Daw Park, South Australia,
Australia

AHMAD A. BAMAGOOS, MBBS, MSc
Department of Respiratory and Sleep
Medicine, Royal North Shore Hospital,
St Leonards, New South Wales, Australia;
Sleep Group, Charles Perkins Centre,
Northern Clinical School, University of Sydney,
Camperdown, New South Wales, Australia;
Department of Physiology, Faculty of Medicine
in Rabigh, King Abdulaziz University, Jeddah,
Kingdom of Saudi Arabia

JOSEPH ANDREW BERKOWSKI, MD
Clinical Assistant Professor; Michael S. Aldrich
Sleep Disorders Laboratory, Department of
Neurology, University of Michigan, Ann Arbor,
Michigan

JOSIANE L. BROUSSARD, PhD
Assistant Research Professor, Sleep and
Chronobiology Laboratory, Department of
Integrative Physiology, University of Colorado,
Boulder, Colorado

**CHING LI CHAI-COETZER, MBBS,
FRACP, PhD**
Adelaide Institute for Sleep Health, A Flinders
Centre of Research Excellence, School of
Medicine, Flinders University, Adelaide, South
Australia, Australia; Sleep Health Service,
Respiratory and Sleep Services, Repatriation
General Hospital, Southern Adelaide Local
Health Network, Daw Park, South Australia,
Australia

LYNDON CHAN, MBBS, FRACS
Department of ENT Surgery, Illawarra ENT
Head and Neck Clinic, Wollongong, New South
Wales, Australia

JULIA L. CHAPMAN, BSc, BA, MHSc
NeuroSleep Centre of Research Excellence,
Woolcock Institute of Medical Research, Sleep
and Circadian Research Group, University of
Sydney; Respiratory and Sleep Department,
Royal Prince Alfred Hospital, Sydney Local
Health District, Sydney, New South Wales,
Australia

**PETER A. CISTULLI, MBBS, PhD,
MBA, FRACP**
Professor, Department of Respiratory and
Sleep Medicine, Royal North Shore Hospital,
St Leonards, New South Wales, Australia;
Sleep Group, Charles Perkins Centre, Sydney
Medical School, University of Sydney,
Camperdown, New South Wales,
Australia

WALTER D. CONWELL, MD
Sleep Medicine Fellow, Department of
Medicine, University of Colorado Denver
School of Medicine, Aurora, Colorado

CHARLES R. DAVIES, MD, PhD, FAASM
Clinical Instructor, Carle Neuroscience
Institute, Carle Foundation Hospital, College of
Medicine, University of Illinois at Urbana-
Champaign, Urbana, Illinois

BRADLEY A. EDWARDS, PhD
Senior Research Fellow, Sleep and Circadian
Medicine Laboratory, Department of
Physiology, School of Psychological Sciences
and Monash Institute of Cognitive and Clinical
Neurosciences, Monash University, Notting
Hill, Australia

**RONALD R. GRUNSTEIN, MBBS, MD,
PhD, FRACP**
Professor, NeuroSleep Centre of Research
Excellence, Woolcock Institute of Medical
Research, Sleep and Circadian Research
Group, University of Sydney; Respiratory and
Sleep Department, Royal Prince Alfred
Hospital, Sydney Local Health District, Sydney,
New South Wales, Australia

GARUN S. HAMILTON, MBBS, FRACP, PhD
Director of Sleep Research, Monash Lung and
Sleep, Monash Medical Centre; Department of
Medicine, School of Clinical Sciences, Faculty
of Medicine, Nursing and Health Sciences,
Monash University, Clayton, Victoria,
Australia

JOHN J. HARRINGTON, MD, MPH, FAASM
Associate Professor, Division of Pulmonary,
Critical Care, Sleep and Allergy, Department of
Medicine, Omaha, Nebraska

BRETTON HEVENER, BS, RPSGT
Sleep Data Services LLC, Sleep Data
Diagnostics Inc, San Diego, California

WILLIAM HEVENER, RPSGT
Sleep Data Services LLC, Sleep Data
Diagnostics Inc, San Diego, California

**SIMON A. JOOSTEN, MBBS, BMedSc,
FRACP, PhD**
Adult Respiratory Physician, Monash Lung
and Sleep, Monash Medical Centre;
Department of Medicine, School of Clinical
Sciences, Faculty of Medicine, Nursing and
Health Sciences, Monash University, Clayton,
Victoria, Australia

RAMI KHAYAT, MD
Associate Professor, Internal Medicine-
Pulmonary, Allergy, Critical Care, and Sleep
Medicine, Wexner Medical Center, The Ohio
State University, Columbus, Ohio

LEON LACK, PhD
Emeritus Professor in Psychology, School of
Psychology, Flinders University of South
Australia, Adelaide, South Australia,
Australia

SHANE LANDRY, PhD
Postdoctoral Research Fellow, Sleep and
Circadian Medicine Laboratory, Department of
Physiology, School of Psychological Sciences
and Monash Institute of Cognitive and Clinical
Neurosciences, Monash University, Notting
Hill, Australia

**STUART G. MacKAY, BSc(Med),
MBBS(Hons), FRACS**
Clinical Associate Professor, Department of
ENT Surgery, Illawarra ENT Head and Neck
Clinic, Wollongong, New South Wales,
Australia

MICHELLE MAGEE, PhD
Postdoctoral Research Fellow, Cooperative
Research Centre for Alertness, Safety and
Productivity, School of Psychological
Sciences, Notting Hill, Victoria, Australia;
Monash Institute of Cognitive and Clinical
Neurosciences, Monash University, Clayton,
Victoria, Australia

EMILY M. MARBAS, BA
Professional Research Assistant, Sleep and
Chronobiology Laboratory, Department of
Integrative Physiology, University of Colorado,
Boulder, Colorado

**NATHANIEL S. MARSHALL, BSc, BCom,
PGDipHealSc, PhD**
Associate Professor, Sydney Nursing School,
The University of Sydney, Sydney, New South
Wales, Australia

R. DOUG McEVOY, MBBS, FRACP, MD
Adelaide Institute for Sleep Health, A Flinders
Centre of Research Excellence, School of
Medicine, Flinders University, Adelaide, South
Australia, Australia; Sleep Health Service,
Respiratory and Sleep Services, Repatriation
General Hospital, Southern Adelaide Local
Health Network, Daw Park, South Australia,
Australia

ADAM PLEISTER, MD
Assistant Professor of Clinical Medicine,
Division of Cardiovascular Medicine (Advanced
Heart Failure and Cardiac Transplant) and
Division of Pulmonary, Allergy, Critical Care,
and Sleep Medicine (Sleep Medicine),
Department of Internal Medicine, Wexner
Medical Center, Davis Heart and Lung
Research Institute, The Ohio State University,
Columbus, Ohio

SHANTHA M.W. RAJARATNAM, PhD
Program Leader, Cooperative Research
Centre for Alertness, Safety and Productivity,
School of Psychological Sciences; Professor,
Monash Institute of Cognitive and Clinical
Neurosciences, Monash University, Clayton,

Victoria, Australia; Lecturer and Associate
Neuroscientist, Division of Sleep and Circadian
Disorders, Departments of Medicine and
Neurology, Brigham and Women's Hospital;
Division of Sleep Medicine, Harvard
Medical School, Boston,
Massachusetts

YASMINA SERINEL, BSc, MBBS, FRACP
NeuroSleep Centre of Research Excellence,
Woolcock Institute of Medical Research, Sleep
and Circadian Research Group, University of
Sydney, Sydney, New South Wales,
Australia

ANITA VALANJU SHELGIKAR, MD
Clinical Assistant Professor; Michael S. Aldrich
Sleep Disorders Laboratory, Department of
Neurology, University of Michigan, Ann Arbor,
Michigan

KATE SUTHERLAND, PhD
Department of Respiratory and Sleep
Medicine, Royal North Shore Hospital,
St Leonards, New South Wales, Australia;
Sleep Group, Charles Perkins Centre, Sydney
Medical School, University of Sydney,
Camperdown, New South Wales, Australia

ALEXANDER SWEETMAN, BPsych(Hons)
School of Psychology, Flinders University of
South Australia, Adelaide, South Australia,
Australia

SHEILA C. TSAI, MD
Associate Professor, Department of Medicine,
National Jewish Health, Denver, Colorado;
Department of Medicine, University of
Colorado Denver School of Medicine, Aurora,
Colorado

KENNETH P. WRIGHT Jr, PhD
Director, Sleep and Chronobiology Laboratory;
Professor, Department of Integrative
Physiology, Center for Neuroscience,
University of Colorado, Boulder, Colorado

Contents

Obstructive sleep apnea has increased in prevalence in recent years and despite the expansion in sleep medicine services there is a significant unmet burden of disease. This burden presents a challenge to specialists and requires a reappraisal of service delivery, including a move toward lower-cost, simplified methods of diagnosis and treatment, an expansion of the sleep apnea workforce to include suitably trained and equipped primary care physicians and nurses, and the incorporation of chronic disease management principles that link patients to relevant community resources and empower them through new technologies to engage more fully in their own care.

Obstructive sleep apnea (OSA) is present in up to 25% of otherwise healthy individuals. OSA is associated with intermittent hypoxia, oxidative stress, sympathetic activation, and an inflammatory response. These perturbations mediate the role of OSA as an independent and modifiable risk factor for cardiovascular disease (CVD). OSA can induce CVD or accelerate the progression of CVD into an end-stage disorder, including heart failure and stroke. Current clinical recommendations are based on existing clinical trial data and the clinical experience of our program; current and future clinical trials will help to optimize management of OSA in the setting of CVD.

There is evidence that obstructive sleep apnea (OSA) can negatively impact attention, memory, learning, executive function, and overall intellectual function in adults and children. Imaging techniques, including MRI, MR diffusion tensor imaging, MR spectroscopy, and fMRI, have provided additional insight into the anatomic and functional underpinnings of OSA-related cognitive impairment. Both animal and human studies have looked to elucidate the separate effects of oxygen desaturation and sleep fragmentation on independent aspects of cognition. Data from animal models point to neuro-inflammation and oxidative stress as driving factors of cognitive impairment.

Currently there is no method to predict which treatments for obstructive sleep apnea will have the best outcomes in individual patients. Given that there is increasing interest in a personalized medicine approach to the treatment of a variety of disorders, this review describes the personalized approaches that are currently available for the treatment of obstructive sleep apnea as well as future directions for individualized obstructive sleep apnea treatment.

Obstructive sleep apnea (OSA) is associated with numerous comorbid medical conditions. Symptoms of OSA may mimic those of comorbid conditions. The presence of OSA may worsen outcomes from the primary condition. Conversely, OSA treatment may benefit both sleep symptomatology and comorbid illness. Because of potential significant benefit, it is important to screen for sleep apnea symptoms, to have a low threshold to perform diagnostic testing, to treat OSA if present, and to closely monitor symptoms. OSA management does not necessarily replace, but rather, should be performed in conjunction with primary therapy for comorbid conditions.

Sleep apnea is a form of sleep-disordered breathing that is associated with an increase in disease comorbidities, mortality risks, health care costs, and traffic accidents. Sleep apnea is most commonly treated with positive airway pressure (PAP). PAP can be difficult for patients to tolerate. This leads to initial and long-term noncompliance. Most insurance companies require compliance with PAP treatment to cover ongoing reimbursements for the device and related disposable supplies. Therefore, there are both clinical and financial incentives to a sleep apneic patient's compliance with PAP therapy.

Surgery in adult obstructive sleep apnea (OSA) has undergone significant advancement in recent years and continues to evolve. It is a modality of treatment used in the context of failed device use, specifically, failed continuous positive airway pressure or mandibular advancement splint. In this context, the role of surgery is either as salvage therapy or to facilitate better tolerance of device use. Other treatments such as weight loss, adjuvant nasal therapy (medical ± prephase nasal surgery) and positional devices may be combined with airway surgery. In general, patients with OSA are managed with in-hospital monitoring perioperatively.

Although mandibular advancement splints (MAS) are not as efficacious as continuous positive airway pressure (CPAP) in reducing obstructive respiratory events, patient adherence and preference are greater than CPAP. Additionally, the effectiveness of both treatments on general health outcomes, cognitive function, and quality of life appears to be equivalent. The main barrier for the implementation of MAS treatment in clinical practice is the interindividual variability in response to MAS treatment. Several prediction tools have been proposed to enhance patient selection for MAS treatment. Phenotyping obstructive sleep apnea patients may reveal patient characteristics that enable the prediction of response to MAS treatment.

Excessive daytime sleepiness (EDS) is common in obstructive sleep apnea (OSA), but it is also common in the general population. When sleepiness remains after continuous positive airway pressure (CPAP) treatment of OSA, comorbid conditions or permanent brain injury before CPAP therapy may be the cause of the residual sleepiness. There is currently no broad approach to treating residual EDS in patients with OSA. Individual assessment must be made of comorbid conditions and medications, and of lifestyle factors that may be contributing to the sleepiness. Modafinil and armodafinil are the only pharmacologic agents indicated for residual sleepiness in these patients.

Central disorders of hypersomnolence are rare conditions with a poorly understood pathophysiology, making the identification and management challenging for sleep clinicians. Clinical history is essential for ruling out secondary causes of hypersomnolence and distinguishing among diagnoses. Current diagnostic criteria rely heavily on the polysomnogram and multiple sleep latency test. The current focus of treatment of hypersomnolence is on drugs that promote alertness. Additionally, in the case of narcolepsy type 1, medication management addresses control of cataplexy, the hallmark symptom of this disorder. Elucidation of pathophysiology of these disorders in the future will be essential to better categorization and management.

Insomnia is often comorbid with obstructive sleep apnea. It reduces positive airway pressure (PAP) therapy acceptance and adherence. Comorbid patients show greater daytime impairments and poorer health outcomes. The insomnia often goes undiagnosed, undertreated, or untreated. Pharmacotherapy is not recommended for long-term treatment. Although care should be taken administering behavioral therapies to patients with elevated sleepiness, cognitive behavior therapy for insomnia (CBTi) is an effective and durable nondrug therapy that reduces symptoms and may increase the effectiveness of PAP therapy. Sleep clinics should be alert to comorbid insomnia and provide adequate diagnostic tools and clinicians with CBTi expertise.

Delayed sleep-wake phase disorder (DSWPD) is commonly defined as an inability to fall asleep and wake at societal times resulting in excessive daytime sleepiness. Although the cause is multifaceted, delays in sleep time are largely driven by misalignment between the circadian pacemaker and the desired sleep-wake timing schedule. Current treatment approaches focus on correcting the circadian delay; however, there is a lack of data investigating combined therapies for treatment of DSWPD.

Ambulatory Diagnosis and Management of Obstructive Sleep Apnea
Screening Questionnaires, Diagnostic Tests, and the Care Team

R. Doug McEvoy, MBBS, FRACP, MD[a,b,*],
Ching Li Chai-Coetzer, MBBS, FRACP, PhD[a,b],
Nick A. Antic, MBBS, FRACP, PhD[a,b]

KEYWORDS

- Obstructive sleep apnea • Ambulatory care • Self-care

KEY POINTS

- The prevalence of obstructive sleep apnea (OSA) is increasing, and there is currently a large, unmet community burden of disease.
- There is a need to involve a wider range of health professionals in the identification and care of patients with OSA, using simplified diagnostic and treatment systems.
- With the appropriate sleep training, nurses and primary care physicians can achieve patient outcomes that are comparable with those of sleep physicians.
- An integrated multidisciplinary approach to care is needed and patients with OSA should be empowered to engage more actively in their own care.

Referral to specialist services for the diagnosis and management of obstructive sleep apnea (OSA) has increased markedly in the last 2 decades. This increase has been driven by increased public awareness and greater appreciation by health professionals of the importance of OSA (ie, its potential to negatively affect quality of life because of daytime fatigue and sleepiness and to increase the risk of accidents and cardiovascular disease) and by the increasing prevalence of the disease caused by the global obesity epidemic. In Australia, where almost all sleep apnea diagnostic tests are charged to the national insurer, Medicare, the number of polysomnography (PSG) tests increased by 150% more than population growth in the decade 1995 to 2004[1] and this growth trend has continued unabated since then.[2] Despite this increased clinical activity there is evidence of considerable residual undiagnosed symptomatic and/or severe OSA in the Australian community. For example, a recent community cohort study of adult men aged more than 45 years in South Australia showed that although 10% indicated they had been previously diagnosed with OSA by sleep study, PSG studies on the remaining participants uncovered 26% who had moderate to

Disclosure: The authors have nothing to disclose.
[a] Adelaide Institute for Sleep Health, A Flinders Centre of Research Excellence, School of Medicine, Flinders University, Bedford Park, Adelaide, South Australia 5042, Australia; [b] Sleep Health Service, Respiratory and Sleep Services, Repatriation General Hospital, Southern Adelaide Local Health Network, Daws Road, Daw Park, South Australia 5041, Australia
* Corresponding author. Sleep Health Service, Respiratory and Sleep Services, Repatriation General Hospital, Southern Adelaide Local Health Network, Daws Road, Daw Park, South Australia 5041, Australia.
E-mail address: doug.mcevoy@flinders.edu.au

Sleep Med Clin 11 (2016) 265–272
http://dx.doi.org/10.1016/j.jsmc.2016.05.001
1556-407X/16/$ – see front matter © 2016 Elsevier Inc. All rights reserved.

severe OSA (apnea-hypopnea index [AHI] $\geq$20).[3] This high, unmet burden of disease is unlikely to be limited to Australia. This observation, and the already rapidly increasing cost of sleep apnea investigations and treatment, has led to a reexamination of how patients might be more efficiently identified and managed.

Evidence-based sleep apnea practice guidelines have been produced in several countries.[4,5] These guidelines have helped establish evidence-based pathways for diagnosis and care in specialist practice, but the extent to which these have been promulgated and found to be useful in primary care is less certain.

With the community prevalence of moderate to severe OSA (defined as an AHI >15 events per hour of sleep) now reported to be as high as 10% to 25%,[6,7] sleep specialists alone are not able to assess and manage every case of OSA. The authors and others think that there is a need to involve primary care physicians (PCPs) and other health professionals in the care of patients, while facilitating connections to specialist sleep services in a hub-and-spoke fashion. It would also be advantageous if the large numbers of people with simple snoring or mild to moderate, minimally symptomatic OSA could be directed toward preventive and self-care programs that encourage lifestyle changes (eg, weight loss, alcohol avoidance) and simple treatment strategies (eg, avoidance of supine sleep), perhaps supported by nurses or other suitably trained professionals.

THE IMPORTANCE OF PATIENT HISTORY, EXAMINATION, AND CLINICAL JUDGEMENT

The identification of patients at high risk of OSA requires that an appropriate history and examination be undertaken and an assessment made as to the likelihood not only that the patient has OSA but of whether it is adversely affecting their daytime functioning and/or increasing their long-term risk of accidents or cardiovascular disease, and might therefore benefit from treatment. The initial clinical assessment is often followed by a diagnostic sleep study, either full PSG or a limited-channel overnight respiratory or cardiorespiratory recording. However, the clinical diagnosis and assessment of patients suspected of OSA is imprecise. For example, a great deal of weight is often placed on a single-night measurement of the AHI and a specific AHI diagnostic cut-point value, but there is significant night-to-night variability in the severity of OSA, such that, when patients are retested, 20% or more move from one diagnostic category to another.[8]

Also, assessing the degree of daytime sleepiness and the extent to which OSA is the cause of the sleepiness, and advising on long-term accident and cardiovascular risk, is not straightforward. Although OSA is associated with a 2.5-fold increased risk of accidents,[9] many patients with OSA, even those with severe OSA (AHI>30), do not report excessive daytime sleepiness, and do not show hypersomnolence on objective testing, including during driving simulation.[10] In contrast, in some patients with OSA who report daytime sleepiness, alternative causes of sleepiness can be identified (eg, chronic sleep restriction caused by lifestyle factors, co-occurring medical disorders, or concomitant use of sedating medication). Observational studies point to a strong association between severe OSA and increased risk of stroke and cardiovascular mortality, but weaker associations between OSA and ischemic heart disease.[11–13] Few studies support that mild or moderate OSA increases cardiovascular risk. At present there are no adequately powered randomized controlled studies showing that continuous positive airway pressure (CPAP) treatment reduces cardiovascular risk[14] and, with the exception of patients with OSA with resistant hypertension,[15] randomized controlled trials (RCTs) of CPAP treatment show only small reductions in blood pressure.[16] Thus, advising patients with OSA on the likelihood of long-term adverse sequelae can be difficult because of the marked phenotypic variation between patients with OSA and a scarcity of level 1 evidence supporting the role of treatment to influence long-term outcomes.

It is critically important therefore that attending health professionals have adequate training and knowledge of OSA, including the treatment options available to patients, how overlapping sleep disorders can affect patients' symptoms, the limitations of diagnostic sleep studies, and the evidence as it relates to the effects of OSA and its treatment on long-term health outcomes.

OBSTRUCTIVE SLEEP APNEA SCREENING QUESTIONNAIRES AND CLINICAL PREDICTION TOOLS

There has been considerable recent interest in the value of questionnaires and simple clinical prediction tools to assist PCPs and sleep specialists in the identification and management of OSA. Such tools also have the potential to be useful for occupational screening (eg, truck drivers) and to help people in the general community assess and manage their own risk.

The clinical usefulness of an OSA questionnaire or clinical prediction tool depends on (1) the extent to which it can distinguish between people with and without moderate to severe OSA (best quantified by the area under the questionnaire's receiver operating characteristic [ROC] curve), (2) the ease with which it can be applied by busy practitioners (and potentially members of the public), (3) the underlying prevalence of moderate to severe OSA in the population of interest, and (4) the purpose for which the questionnaire or screening procedure is to be used.

Most screening questionnaires and clinical prediction tools have been developed from sleep clinic populations. In a survey of patients referred to a sleep disorders clinic, the variables most predictive of OSA (AHI $\geq$ 10/h) were found by Flemons and colleagues[17] to be neck circumference, hypertension, habitual snoring, and partner reports of nocturnal choking or gasping, and were incorporated into a Sleep Apnea Clinical Score (SACS). The predictive factors in Multivariable Apnea Risk (MAP) Index developed by Maislin and colleagues[18] in a sleep clinic population are snorting and gasping, loud snoring, breathing cessation, body mass index (BMI), age, and sex. Rowley and colleagues[19] prospectively evaluated the utility of 4 previously published clinical prediction models,[17,18,20,21] including the SACS and MAP index, for detecting OSA and prioritizing patients for a split sleep study in a sleep disorders clinic. For an AHI greater than or equal to 10/h, the 4 models had generally high sensitivities but low specificity values.

The Berlin Questionnaire[22] is one of the most widely cited screening tools. It was developed to assist PCPs in identifying patients at risk of OSA. The STOP and STOP-BANG questionnaires have also been widely used and were developed initially for use by anesthetists to screen surgical patients preoperatively.[23] Less commonly deployed screening questionnaires include the Wisconsin[24] and 4-Variable questionnaires.[25]

A systematic review of questionnaires by Abrishami and colleagues[26] in 2010 found considerable variability between studies even when the same questionnaire was used in a similar population. However, studies of OSA questionnaires generally report higher sensitivity (70%–80%) than specificity (50%–60%) values and higher negative predictive than positive predictive values.

Researchers have also evaluated the role of anatomic measures of the upper airway and craniofacial structures to see whether they will improve the prediction of OSA risk. Kushida and colleagues[27] developed a predictive morphometric model for OSA syndrome (Epworth Sleepiness Score [ESS] $\geq$10 and PSG AHI $\geq$5/h), which consisted of mandibular size, palatal height, BMI,

and neck circumference, reporting a sensitivity of 98% and specificity of 100%. Tsai and colleagues[28] found that the presence of 3 anatomic variables (ie, cricomental space $\leq$1.5 cm, pharyngeal grade > II, and presence of overbite) had a specificity of 96% and positive predictive value of 95% for an AHI greater than or equal to 10/h. Although these studies have yielded promising results, the procedures and measurements involved are complicated, time consuming, and difficult to standardize. Their diagnostic accuracy awaits independent verification by other investigators and to date they have not been adopted in routine clinical practice.

The authors recently developed and validated the OSA50, a simple 4-item screening questionnaire for use in primary care.[29] It is arguably much easier to use than previous questionnaires and clinical prediction tools, taking less than 5 minutes for a nurse or general practitioner to administer. Scores are given for obesity (3), snoring (3), witnessed apneas (2), and age greater than or equal to 50 years (2) to give a possible total score of 10. The authors found similar results to other questionnaires, such as the Berlin and STOP-BANG: using a cutoff value of greater than or equal to 5 out of 10 the OSA50 questionnaire had an ROC area under the curve of 0.84 (95% confidence interval [CI], 0.75–0.94; $P<.001$) for detecting moderate to severe OSA (AHI $\geq$ 30/h, American Academy of Sleep Medicine [AASM] 1999 criteria). Sensitivity was 100% (95% CI, 86%–100%), negative predictive value 100% (95% CI, 73%–100%), specificity 29% (95% CI, 17%–44%), and positive predictive value 48% (95% CI, 35%–63%).

Thus, in the general population, primary care, or sleep clinics in which the prevalence of moderate to severe OSA is expected to be at least 20%, questionnaire screening may have utility as a means of identifying patients at low or very low risk of OSA, which may obviate further sleep testing in a significant proportion of patients, and it will increase the probability of disease in those who test positive. However, low specificity and positive predictive values mean that a positive questionnaire response cannot be relied on to definitively diagnose OSA. Screen-positive patients need to proceed to a diagnostic sleep study, although this need not necessarily be PSG. In a primary care setting in which patients with hypoxemic lung disease, morbid obesity, neuromuscular disease, and cardiac failure were excluded, the authors showed an overall diagnostic accuracy (sum of the true positive and true negative rates) for moderate to severe OSA of 90% using a 2-stage diagnostic model (OSA50 questionnaire followed by overnight home oximetry in OSA50-positive respondents).[29]

HOME SLEEP TESTS VERSUS IN-LABORATORY POLYSOMNOGRAPHY

In 2007, the Portable Monitoring Task Force of the AASM published clinical guidelines for the use of unattended portable monitors in the diagnosis of OSA based on a review of the literature.[30] It recommended that unattended, portable monitoring (recording a minimum of airflow, respiratory effort, and oximetry) may be used as an alternative to PSG for the diagnosis of OSA in patients with high pretest probability of moderate to severe OSA without significant medical comorbidities, in conjunction with comprehensive evaluation by a sleep specialist. Based on the recommendations of the 2007 AASM Task Force, the Centers for Medicare and Medicaid Services in the United States approved the use of a limited home sleep recording device with at least 3 channels to diagnose OSA for the purposes of reimbursement for CPAP treatment, and many health care providers not only in the United States but elsewhere have moved or are moving toward greater use of home sleep testing for OSA. The Australasian Sleep Association recently revised its guidelines for sleep studies and is in broad agreement with the AASM guidelines but has also drawn attention to the need to retain sleep laboratory beds and services to accommodate the significant numbers of patients who are not suitable for home testing because of frailty or severe comorbid physical and mental illness.[31]

HOME AUTO-ADJUSTING POSITIVE AIRWAY PRESSURE TREATMENT VERSUS IN-LABORATORY CONTINUOUS POSITIVE AIRWAY PRESSURE TITRATION

The invention of autoadjusting positive airway pressure (APAP) devices has reduced the reliance on sleep laboratories to establish the correct fixed CPAP level for patients with OSA proceeding to positive airway pressure treatment and facilitated the trend toward more ambulatory community-based care. A Cochrane systematic review by Smith and Lasserson,[32] which included a total of 30 studies assessing the effects of APAP versus fixed CPAP, showed no differences in the percentage of nights when CPAP was used, odds of withdrawal, arousals, or mean AHI. Treatment pressure was noted to be 1.6 to 2.0 cm H_2O less for APAP than for fixed CPAP. In the meta-analyses of parallel studies/first arm crossover studies, no differences were seen in the average nightly machine usage, change in subjective sleepiness as measured by the ESS, or quality of life as measured by the Short Form 36 (SF-36). However meta-analyses of crossover studies showed small but statistically significant differences in nightly machine usage, change in ESS, and the vitality domain of the SF-36 in favor of APAP. Seven out of 10 studies reported that patients preferred using APAP to either CPAP or no treatment.

An Australian study conducted by McArdle and colleagues[33] evaluated the clinical outcomes and costs in patients with moderate to severe OSA who were randomized to either manual titration, laboratory APAP, or home APAP titration. Following 4 weeks of treatment, no differences in clinical outcomes were found between the groups and the total direct costs for home APAP titration were much lower than the costs for laboratory APAP and manual titration.

In 2007, the AASM updated their 2002 practice parameter report for the use of APAP following a review of the literature to include the recommendation that certain APAP devices may be used in an unattended way to determine a fixed CPAP treatment pressure for patients with moderate to severe OSA without significant comorbidities (heart failure, chronic obstructive pulmonary disease [COPD], central sleep apnea syndromes, or hypoventilation syndromes).[34]

PRINCIPLES OF OBSTRUCTIVE SLEEP APNEA CARE

OSA fulfils the criteria for a chronic disease: an illness that is prolonged in duration, does not often resolve spontaneously, and is rarely cured completely.[35] Several modifiable lifestyle factors contribute to OSA, including obesity and excessive alcohol use, and patients with OSA frequently present with co-occurring chronic medical comorbidities, including depression, diabetes mellitus, hypertension, and cardiovascular disease. The authors therefore think[36] that OSA is ideally suited to the sort of patient-centered, comprehensive, integrated chronic disease management approach first described by Wagner and colleagues[37] in the mid-1990s and that has been used with considerable success in other diseases, such as COPD,[38] diabetes mellitus,[39] asthma,[40] and congestive cardiac failure.[41] Wagner and colleagues[37] proposed that effective chronic disease management requires a shift in focus away from reactive treatment of acute symptoms, short appointments, brief and didactic patient education, and patient-initiated follow-up toward a system of regular, planned reviews involving patients and their caregivers, systematic assessment of disease, development and use of evidence-based guidelines, involvement of nonphysician health providers, promotion of patient self-management designed to prevent disease exacerbations and/or complications, and the use of information systems to facilitate creation of disease registries and reminder systems to enable practice-initiated patient follow-up.[37] Although the 2009 AASM "Clinical Guideline for the Evaluation, Management and Long-term Care of Obstructive Sleep Apnea in Adults"[4] recommends that the condition "should be approached as a chronic disease requiring long-term, multidisciplinary management," research studies of chronic disease management programs for OSA are scarce.

Obesity is the leading cause of OSA and a potentially modifiable risk factor not only for OSA but for cardiometabolic disease. Strategies designed to achieve and maintain weight loss are therefore critically important in managing patients with OSA. Providing access to a multidisciplinary team of health professionals (eg, dieticians, exercise physiologists, psychologists, and surgeons specializing in bariatric surgery) and community resources for overweight and obese patients to assist in and provide support for their weight loss efforts should be a priority for all OSA services, but the authors suspect that this is often overlooked as efforts and resources are directed more toward mechanical treatments such as CPAP and oral devices.

Web-based and mobile technologies, such as the use of telemedicine monitoring systems in CPAP devices[42] and e-health interventions,[43] hold significant promise as a means for promoting patient self-management and facilitating communication between patients and health care providers. However, further research into their effectiveness in patients with OSA is needed.

THE OBSTRUCTIVE SLEEP APNEA CARE TEAM

Up to now OSA has been managed principally by sleep physicians. However, the increasing prevalence of OSA, scarcity of sleep-trained specialists,[44] increasing costs, longer waiting times, and the need for a more integrated multidisciplinary approach has led our group and others (eg, Spanish investigators) to consider a greater role for PCPs, nurses, and other health professionals in the clinical care of OSA.[45–47] Appropriate knowledge and training in OSA and other sleep disorders is required for the professionals involved in these new models of care to ensure success. The authors think that a hub-and-spoke model is ideal, in which OSA is managed predominantly in the community, with support and shared care for more complicated or treatment-resistant patients in a sleep medicine center.

The authors recently conducted a randomized trial that showed that such an approach can be successful.[45] PCPs identified patients with moderate to severe OSA using a validated, 2-step diagnostic strategy of the OSA50 screen followed by home oximetry[29] and patients who had at least moderate daytime sleepiness (ESS ≥ 8) or resistant hypertension were randomly assigned to either ambulatory management by the PCP and nurse or to usual laboratory-based care by a sleep specialist. Before the study, PCPs and community-based nurses were provided with 6 hours of training in the management of OSA. Nurses undertook an additional intensive in-service week of training on CPAP treatment. After 6 months, primary care management was found to be noninferior to specialist management in terms of improvement in ESS score and no differences were found between groups in quality of life, OSA symptoms, CPAP adherence, and overall patient satisfaction. Per-patient costs were 38% less in the primary care arm of the study. Other investigators[48–50] have studied the reliability of simple automated single-channel nasal pressure devices to identify OSA cases requiring CPAP treatment, with a view to their future deployment in primary care. Initial results indicate a high degree of diagnostic reliability for identifying moderate to severe symptomatic OSA, with significant cost savings compared with traditional in-laboratory specialist center diagnosis. In another study,[47] newly diagnosed patients in a specialist center with OSA were randomized to primary care versus specialist sleep center for CPAP treatment follow-up. After 6 months, the primary care–managed group was not inferior to the specialist group in terms of CPAP compliance, although there were greater improvements in ESS scores and patient satisfaction in the specialist arm. Within-trial costs were lower in the primary care group. Other researchers have reported that the identification of OSA can be enhanced when community pharmacists screen for OSA by questionnaire and simple home sleep monitoring[51,52] and send the results to patients' PCPs. These various research studies provide proof-of-concept evidence that PCPs, practice nurses, and potentially pharmacists can assist in the diagnosis and management of OSA if they are adequately trained and resourced. The authors think that more active engagement of primary care professionals in OSA management will ultimately be necessary if the significant unmet burden of disease is to be addressed.

An Expanded Role for Specialist Sleep Nurses?

There has been increasing interest in the use of specialist nurses to manage chronic medical conditions in both the primary care and specialist settings. A review of RCTs of autonomous specialized nurse–led care versus physician-led care in primary health care settings for conditions such as diabetes, coronary artery disease, and heart failure found comparable outcomes in health resource use, disease-specific measures, quality of life, and patient satisfaction.[53] Nurses working in collaboration with PCPs versus physicians working alone resulted in disease-specific improvements, improved patient satisfaction, and lower hospitalization rates among patients with coronary artery disease. Another recent systematic review of RCTs of nurse-managed protocols for patients with diabetes, hyperlipidemia, and hypertension reported positive findings with respect to hemoglobin A1c levels and blood pressure and a trend to improved serum lipid levels.[54] A randomized controlled study in the Netherlands of a nurse-led clinic for the management of atrial fibrillation versus usual care showed a superior outcome for nurse-led management, with a significant reduction in the composite outcome of cardiovascular hospitalizations and mortality.[55] In the United States, the Department of Veterans Affairs is currently giving nurses and nurse practitioners a major role as care managers in the Patient Aligned Care Teams initiative in order to more effectively tackle the burden of chronic disease in the Veterans Affairs population.[56]

The authors previously evaluated a specialist nurse–led model of care for the management of OSA in 3 Australian tertiary sleep centers.[46] One-hundred and ninety-five patients found to have moderate to severe OSA (ie, >2% oxygen desaturation index >27/h by home oximetry, ESS ≥8, and history of snoring) were randomized to either a simplified, nurse-led model of care consisting of home APAP to determine a fixed CPAP pressure, or to traditional, physician-led management including laboratory-based PSG and CPAP titration. After 3 months, specialist nurse-led management was found to be noninferior to physician-led care with respect to the change in ESS score. There were no significant differences between the treatment arms in objective sleepiness, quality of life, executive neurocognitive function, or CPAP adherence. Several items in the Visit-specific Satisfaction Questionnaire favored the nurse-led model. Thus, selected patients with OSA can be managed by appropriately trained specialist nurses without compromising patient outcomes. The authors think that, in the future, sleep-trained nurses could also have an expanded role in helping address lifestyle-related OSA and cardiovascular disease risk factors (eg, obesity, excessive alcohol use, smoking), and in delivering cognitive behavior therapy and/or other psychosocial interventions to optimize CPAP adherence, or as part of the management of overlapping depression and insomnia.

In conclusion, OSA has increased markedly in prevalence in recent years and despite a rapid expansion in sleep medicine services there is evidence of a significant unmet burden of disease. This burden presents a serious challenge to specialists and requires, the authors believe, a reappraisal of how services are delivered, including a move toward lower-cost, simplified methods of diagnosis and treatment, an expansion of the sleep apnea workforce to include suitably trained and equipped PCPs and nurses, and the incorporation of chronic disease management principles that link patients to relevant community resources and empower them through new technologies to engage more fully in their own care.

REFERENCES

1. Marshall NS, Wilsmore BR, McEvoy RD, et al. Polysomnography in Australia–trends in provision. J Clin Sleep Med 2007;3(3):281–4.
2. Medicare Australia. Medicare benefits scheme item statistics reports. 2011. Available at: https://www.medicareaustralia.gov.au/statistics/mbs_item.shtml. Accessed July 5, 2011.
3. Adams R, Appleton S, Vakulin A, et al. High prevalence of undiagnosed OSA in a community sample of men aged 40 years and over. Sleep Biol Rhythms 2012;10(Suppl 1):42 (A117).
4. Epstein LJ, Kristo D, Strollo PJ Jr, et al. Clinical guideline for the evaluation, management and long-term care of obstructive sleep apnea in adults. J Clin Sleep Med 2009;5(3):263–76.
5. Fleetham J, Ayas N, Bradley D, et al. Canadian Thoracic Society 2011 guideline update: diagnosis and treatment of sleep disordered breathing. Can Respir J 2011;18(1):25–47.
6. Heinzer R, Vat S, Marques-Vidal P, et al. Prevalence of sleep-disordered breathing in the general population: the HypnoLaus study. Lancet Respir Med 2015;3(4):310–8.
7. Adams R, Appleton S, Taylor A, et al. Are the ICSD-3 criteria for sleep apnoea syndrome too inclusive? Lancet Respir Med 2016, in press.
8. Ahmadi N, Shapiro GK, Chung SA, et al. Clinical diagnosis of sleep apnea based on single night of polysomnography vs. two nights of polysomnography. Sleep Breath 2009;13(3):221–6.

9. Tregear S, Reston J, Schoelles K, et al. Obstructive sleep apnea and risk of motor vehicle crash: systematic review and meta-analysis. J Clin Sleep Med 2009;5(6):573–81.

10. Vakulin A, Catcheside PG, Baulk SD, et al. Individual variability and predictors of driving simulator impairment in patients with obstructive sleep apnea. J Clin Sleep Med 2014;10(6):647–55.

11. Shahar E, Whitney CW, Redline S, et al. Sleep-disordered breathing and cardiovascular disease: cross-sectional results of the Sleep Heart Health Study. Am J Respir Crit Care Med 2001;163(1): 19–25.

12. Redline S, Yenokyan G, Gottlieb DJ, et al. Obstructive sleep apnea-hypopnea and incident stroke: the Sleep Heart Health Study. Am J Respir Crit Care Med 2010;182(2):269–77.

13. Young T, Finn L, Peppard PE, et al. Sleep disordered breathing and mortality: eighteen-year follow-up of the Wisconsin sleep cohort. Sleep 2008;31(8): 1071–8.

14. Gottlieb DJ, Craig SE, Lorenzi-Filho G, et al. Sleep apnea cardiovascular clinical trials-current status and steps forward: the International Collaboration of Sleep Apnea Cardiovascular Trialists. Sleep 2013;36(7):975–80.

15. Iftikhar IH, Valentine CW, Bittencourt LR, et al. Effects of continuous positive airway pressure on blood pressure in patients with resistant hypertension and obstructive sleep apnea: a meta-analysis. J Hypertens 2014;32(12):2341–50 [discussion: 2350].

16. Montesi SB, Edwards BA, Malhotra A, et al. The effect of continuous positive airway pressure treatment on blood pressure: a systematic review and meta-analysis of randomized controlled trials. J Clin Sleep Med 2012;8(5):587–96.

17. Flemons WW, Whitelaw WA, Brant R, et al. Likelihood ratios for a sleep apnea clinical prediction rule. Am J Respir Crit Care Med 1994;150(5 Pt 1):1279–85.

18. Maislin G, Pack AI, Kribbs NB, et al. A survey screen for prediction of apnea. Sleep 1995;18(3): 158–66.

19. Rowley JA, Aboussouan LS, Badr MS. The use of clinical prediction formulas in the evaluation of obstructive sleep apnea. Sleep 2000;23(7):929–38.

20. Crocker BD, Olson LG, Saunders NA, et al. Estimation of the probability of disturbed breathing during sleep before a sleep study. Am Rev Respir Dis 1990;142(1):14–8.

21. Viner S, Szalai JP, Hoffstein V. Are history and physical examination a good screening test for sleep apnea? Ann Intern Med 1991;115(5):356–9.

22. Netzer NC, Stoohs RA, Netzer CM, et al. Using the Berlin Questionnaire to identify patients at risk for the sleep apnea syndrome. Ann Intern Med 1999; 131(7):485–91.

23. Chung F, Yegneswaran B, Liao P, et al. STOP questionnaire: a tool to screen patients for obstructive sleep apnea. Anesthesiology 2008;108(5):812–21.

24. Teculescu D, Guillemin F, Virion JM, et al. Reliability of the Wisconsin Sleep Questionnaire: a French contribution to international validation. J Clin Epidemiol 2003;56(5):436–40.

25. Takegami M, Hayashino Y, Chin K, et al. Simple four-variable screening tool for identification of patients with sleep-disordered breathing. Sleep 2009;32(7): 939–48.

26. Abrishami A, Khajehdehi A, Chung F. A systematic review of screening questionnaires for obstructive sleep apnea. Can J Anaesth 2010;57(5):423–38.

27. Kushida CA, Efron B, Guilleminault C. A predictive morphometric model for the obstructive sleep apnea syndrome. Ann Intern Med 1997;127(8 Pt 1): 581–7.

28. Tsai WH, Remmers JE, Brant R, et al. A decision rule for diagnostic testing in obstructive sleep apnea. Am J Respir Crit Care Med 2003;167(10):1427–32.

29. Chai-Coetzer CL, Antic NA, Rowland LS, et al. A simplified model of screening questionnaire and home monitoring for obstructive sleep apnoea in primary care. Thorax 2011;66(3):213–9.

30. Collop NA, Anderson WM, Boehlecke B, et al. Clinical guidelines for the use of unattended portable monitors in the diagnosis of obstructive sleep apnea in adult patients. Portable Monitoring Task Force of the American Academy of Sleep Medicine. J Clin Sleep Med 2007;3(7):737–47.

31. Chai-Coetzer CL, Douglas J, McEvoy D, et al. Guidelines for sleep studies in adults: prepared for the Australasian Sleep Association. 2014. Available at: http://www.sleep.org.au/professional-resources/sleep-documents/guidelines-for-sleep-studies-in-adults-2014.

32. Smith I, Lasserson TJ. Pressure modification for improving usage of continuous positive airway pressure machines in adults with obstructive sleep apnoea. Cochrane Database Syst Rev 2009;(4):CD003531.

33. McArdle N, Singh B, Murphy M, et al. Continuous positive airway pressure titration for obstructive sleep apnoea: automatic versus manual titration. Thorax 2010;65(7):606–11.

34. Morgenthaler TI, Aurora RN, Brown T, et al. Practice parameters for the use of autotitrating continuous positive airway pressure devices for titrating pressures and treating adult patients with obstructive sleep apnea syndrome: an update for 2007. An American Academy of Sleep Medicine report. Sleep 2008;31(1):141–7.

35. Dowrick C, Dixon-Woods M, Holman H, et al. What is chronic illness? Chronic Illn 2005;1(1):1–6.

36. Chai-Coetzer CL, Antic NA, McEvoy RD. Integrated care for obstructive sleep apnea. European Respiratory Society Monograph 2015;67:293–304.

37. Wagner EH, Austin BT, Von Korff M. Organizing care for patients with chronic illness. Milbank Q 1996; 74(4):511–44.

38. Kruis AL, Smidt N, Assendelft WJ, et al. Integrated disease management interventions for patients with chronic obstructive pulmonary disease. Cochrane Database Syst Rev 2013;(10):CD009437.

39. Seitz P, Rosemann T, Gensichen J, et al. Interventions in primary care to improve cardiovascular risk factors and glycated haemoglobin (HbA1c) levels in patients with diabetes: a systematic review. Diabetes Obes Metab 2011;13(6):479–89.

40. Gibson PG, McDonald VM, Marks GB. Asthma in older adults. Lancet 2010;376(9743):803–13.

41. Comin-Colet J, Verdu-Rotellar JM, Vela E, et al. Efficacy of an integrated hospital-primary care program for heart failure: a population-based analysis of 56,742 patients. Rev Esp Cardiol (Engl Ed) 2014; 67(4):283–93.

42. Fox N, Hirsch-Allen AJ, Goodfellow E, et al. The impact of a telemedicine monitoring system on positive airway pressure adherence in patients with obstructive sleep apnea: a randomized controlled trial. Sleep 2012;35(4):477–81.

43. Eland-de Kok P, van Os-Medendorp H, Vergouwe-Meijer A, et al. A systematic review of the effects of e-health on chronically ill patients. J Clin Nurs 2011;20(21–22):2997–3010.

44. Phillips B, Gozal D, Malhotra A. What is the future of sleep medicine in the United States? Am J Respir Crit Care Med 2015;192(8):915–7.

45. Chai-Coetzer CL, Antic NA, Rowland LS, et al. Primary care vs specialist sleep center management of obstructive sleep apnea and daytime sleepiness and quality of life: a randomized trial. JAMA 2013; 309(10):997–1004.

46. Antic NA, Buchan C, Esterman A, et al. A randomized controlled trial of nurse-led care for symptomatic moderate-severe obstructive sleep apnea. Am J Respir Crit Care Med 2009;179(6):501–8.

47. Sanchez-de-la-Torre M, Nadal N, Cortijo A, et al. Role of primary care in the follow-up of patients with obstructive sleep apnoea undergoing CPAP treatment: a randomised controlled trial. Thorax 2015;70(4):346–52.

48. Masa JF, Duran-Cantolla J, Capote F, et al. Efficacy of home single-channel nasal pressure for recommending continuous positive airway pressure treatment in sleep apnea. Sleep 2015;38(1):13–21.

49. Masa JF, Duran-Cantolla J, Capote F, et al. Effectiveness of home single-channel nasal pressure for sleep apnea diagnosis. Sleep 2014;37(12):1953–61.

50. Rofail LM, Wong KK, Unger G, et al. The utility of single-channel nasal airflow pressure transducer in the diagnosis of OSA at home. Sleep 2010;33(8): 1097–105.

51. Perraudin C, Fleury B, Pelletier-Fleury N. Effectiveness of intervention led by a community pharmacist for improving recognition of sleep apnea in primary care–a cohort study. J Sleep Res 2015;24(2): 167–73.

52. Perraudin C, Le Vaillant M, Pelletier-Fleury N. Cost-effectiveness of a community pharmacist-led sleep apnea screening program - a Markov model. PLoS One 2013;8(6):e63894.

53. Health Quality Ontario. Specialized nursing practice for chronic disease management in the primary care setting: an evidence-based analysis. Ont Health Technol Assess Ser 2013;13(10):1–66.

54. Shaw RJ, McDuffie JR, Hendrix CC, et al. Effects of nurse-managed protocols in the outpatient management of adults with chronic conditions: a systematic review and meta-analysis. Ann Intern Med 2014; 161(2):113–21.

55. Hendriks JM, de Wit R, Crijns HJ, et al. Nurse-led care vs. usual care for patients with atrial fibrillation: results of a randomized trial of integrated chronic care vs. routine clinical care in ambulatory patients with atrial fibrillation. Eur Heart J 2012;33(21): 2692–9.

56. Shaw RJ, McDuffie JR, Hendrix CC, et al. Effects of nurse-managed protocols in the outpatient management of adults with chronic conditions. Washington, DC: Department of Veterans Affairs; 2013.

Consequences of Obstructive Sleep Apnea

Cardiovascular Risk of Obstructive Sleep Apnea and Whether Continuous Positive Airway Pressure Reduces that Risk

Rami Khayat, MD[a], Adam Pleister, MD[b,c],*

KEYWORDS

- Obstructive sleep apnea • Sleep-disordered breathing • Cardiovascular disease
- Systemic hypertension • Intermittent hypoxia • Sympathetic activation • Coronary artery disease
- Heart failure

KEY POINTS

- Obstructive sleep apnea (OSA) is associated with unique perturbations that include intermittent hypoxia, sympathetic activation, and oxidative stress.
- OSA is a cause of hypertension, and can worsen the outcome of coronary artery disease, atrial fibrillation, and stroke.
- Treatment of OSA can improve the outcomes of all cardiovascular disorders.
- Expedited approaches to identification and treatment of OSA are important interventions in the management of cardiovascular disease.

INTRODUCTION

Obstructive sleep apnea (OSA) is increasingly recognized as an important modifiable risk factor for cardiovascular disease (CVD). The prevalence of OSA in the United States is estimated at 20% to 30% in adult men and 10% to 15% in adult women.[1,2] This prevalence is likely increasing because of increasing obesity and the aging population. With an incidence approaching 50%, CVD remains a leading cause of morbidity and mortality in Western societies.[3] Identification and treatment of modifiable CVD risk factors such as OSA is a critical part of the public health approach to CVD.

This article discusses the mechanistic link between OSA and CVD and presents an overview of the evidence for the causative relationship between OSA and CVD. It then addresses the relationship between OSA and the major manifestations of CVD, including systemic hypertension, coronary artery disease (CAD), cardiac arrhythmias, stoke,

Disclosure Statement: R. Khayat received research grant support from Philips Respironics; A. Pleister has no disclosures.
[a] Internal Medicine-Pulmonary, Allergy, Critical Care, and Sleep Medicine, Wexner Medical Center, The Ohio State University, Suite 200, 473 West 12th Avenue, Columbus, OH 43210-1267, USA; [b] Division of Cardiovascular Medicine (Advanced Heart Failure & Cardiac Transplant), Department of Internal Medicine, Wexner Medical Center, Davis Heart & Lung Research Institute, The Ohio State University, Suite 200, 473 West 12th Avenue, Columbus, OH 43210-1267, USA; [c] Division of Pulmonary, Allergy, Critical Care, and Sleep Medicine (Sleep Medicine), Department of Internal Medicine, Wexner Medical Center, Davis Heart & Lung Research Institute, The Ohio State University, Suite 200, 473 West 12th Avenue, Columbus, OH 43210-1267, USA
* Corresponding author.
E-mail address: adam.pleister@osumc.edu

Sleep Med Clin 11 (2016) 273–286
http://dx.doi.org/10.1016/j.jsmc.2016.05.002
1556-407X/16/$ – see front matter © 2016 Elsevier Inc. All rights reserved.

pulmonary hypertension, and heart failure (HF). It presents a focused discussion of the role and expected effects of OSA treatment on modifying the outcomes of these. In addition, it addresses practical approaches to OSA as a modifiable risk factor for CVD.

OVERVIEW OF SLEEP-DISORDERED BREATHING

The term sleep-disordered breathing (SDB) encompasses all respiratory disorders of sleep and includes both OSA and central sleep apnea (CSA). SDB is defined by the presence of 5 or more respiratory events (apneas or hypopneas) per 1 hour of sleep; that is, an apnea-hypopnea index (AHI) of 5 or more events per hour. The SDB is classified as OSA if more than half of the events are classified as obstructive and CSA if more than half of the events are central. Determination of the obstructive or central nature of a respiratory event relies mainly on the presence or absence of respiratory effort signal during the event. Regardless of type, sleep apnea is defined as mild if the AHI is 5 to 14, moderate if the AHI is 15 to 30, and severe if the AHI is more than 30. The presence or absence of reported sleep-related symptoms is sometimes used to further define the disorder as a syndrome. OSA syndrome is defined as an AHI of 5 to 15 events/h in the presence of significant sleep-related symptoms, or an AHI of 15 events/h or more regardless of symptoms. Likewise, CSA syndrome is defined as an AHI of 5 to 15 in the presence of significant sleep-related symptoms or an AHI of 15 or more regardless of symptoms. CSA is often found in patients with already established end-stage CVD, particularly HF and stroke. Note that a significant overlap between CSA and OSA can occur in the same patient. This overlap is most often seen in patients with HF.

MECHANISM OF CARDIOVASCULAR DISEASE IN OBSTRUCTIVE SLEEP APNEA

Extensive work in the past 3 decades has greatly expanded the understanding of the mechanism of CVD in patients with OSA. Several pathways have been identified as important for the development of CVD in OSA. These pathways may provide targets for therapeutic interventions in the near future.

Intermittent Hypoxia

Patients with OSA can experience recurrent episodes of apnea or hypopnea ranging in frequency from 5 to more than 100 events per hour. Each of

these obstructive respiratory events results in an episode of hypoxia followed by reoxygenation (after the termination of the respiratory episode and resumption of recovery breaths). Each episode of hypoxia stimulates the carotid chemoreceptors,[1] resulting in sympathetic nerve activation[2,4] and a secondary surge in blood pressure.[5] The recurrence of these respiratory events and their respective recovery phases produces a characteristic pattern of nocturnal intermittent hypoxia that is unique to OSA/SDB. As a result, patients with OSA spend their sleep periods in a state of intermittent hypoxia and a cycling pattern of recurrent surges of vasoconstriction.

The pattern of intermittent hypoxia is unique to OSA and results in a different profile of biological consequences from other types of hypoxia exposure.[6–9] The sympathetic activation seen in OSA, caused by intermittent hypoxia, during the sleep period persists through the daytime owing to a memory effect (plasticity) in the sympathetic activation.[10] This plasticity was recently shown to be mediated by a reactive oxygen species–dependent pathway unique to the intermittent hypoxia exposure.[6] Thus, the nocturnal intermittent hypoxia pattern of OSA mediates the vascular response to apnea.[2,5,11,12] Intermittent hypoxia is the critical abnormality in OSA leading to the immediate-term and long-term cardiovascular consequences of OSA, including systemic hypertension,[4,13] left ventricular hypertrophy,[14,15] and endothelial dysfunction.[16–18]

Sympathetic Activation, a Critical Mediator for Cardiovascular Disease in Obstructive Sleep Apnea

Hypoxia activates the sympathetic system, which induces vasoconstriction and increases in blood pressure. Sympathetic activation has several deleterious cardiovascular consequences in patients with SDB. Increased sympathetic tone exerts systemic changes that promote the persistence of increased blood pressure[19,20] and augment the response to subsequent sympathetic stimuli.[21] Sympathetic overactivity is the critical link between OSA and systemic hypertension.[22,23] Intermittent hypoxia not only increases basal sympathetic activity but also augments the sympathetic response to subsequent episodes of hypoxia.[24–26] The role of sympathetic activation is well established in the pathogenesis of systemic hypertension. Young patients with early essential hypertension have increased cardiac sympathetic tone compared with age-matched controls.[27] In a population-based study, increased heart rate (a manifestation of sympathetic activation) correlated with future development of systemic hypertension.[28]

The sympathetic interaction with the renin-angiotensin system may be another important element in the pathogenesis of systemic hypertension.[19,29,30] In animal models of OSA, intermittent hypoxia-induced systemic hypertension was mediated by renal sympathetic nerve activity[4,31] and the intact renin-angiotensin system was critical for this blood pressure response to intermittent hypoxia.[32]

Patients with OSA develop changes in their autonomic regulation of blood pressure (baroreflex) consistent with adaptation of the baroreceptors to higher blood pressure set point.[33,34] In normal individuals, blood pressure fluctuates in a circadian rhythm with pressures decreasing, or dipping, during sleep. However, in patients with systemic hypertension and in patients with SDB, this rhythm is altered, leading to a pattern of nondipping during the night.[35,36]

In addition, sympathetic activation–mediated vasoconstriction may induce long-lasting structural changes in resistance vessels that contribute to the persistence of hypertension.[37] Animal models of intermittent hypoxia show early structural and functional vascular changes,[17] along with impaired vasodilator response to hypoxia.[38]

Oxidative Stress

Accumulation of reactive oxygen species (ROS) in various organs and systems is more a recently recognized pathway of morbidity in SDB. Importantly, as mentioned earlier, intermittent hypoxia upregulates the carotid chemoreceptors via an ROS-dependent pathway resulting in ventilator and sympathetic overactivity.[10,39] Increased oxidative stress in the vascular milieu is involved in the pathogenesis of endothelial dysfunction[40–42] with likely contribution to vascular lesion formation and CAD. Furthermore, cognitive impairment,[43,44] inflammation,[45,46] atherosclerosis,[47] hypertension,[48] and myocardial injury[49] may all be direct consequences of the increased oxidative stress in OSA.

Metabolic Dysregulation in Obstructive Sleep Apnea

Sleep disturbance and restriction as found in OSA have been implicated as causes of metabolic dysregulation. Sleep restriction reduces glucose tolerance, increases evening cortisol concentrations, and decreases insulin release.[50] Likewise, short sleep duration has been associated with decreased leptin levels, increased ghrelin levels, and increased hunger and appetite.[51] Therefore, short sleep durations have been found to increase the risk of developing diabetes.[52] SDB decreases glucose tolerance and insulin release, and has been independently associated with the development of insulin resistance[53] and type 2 diabetes mellitus.[54]

CLINICAL LINK BETWEEN OBSTRUCTIVE SLEEP APNEA/SLEEP-DISORDERED BREATHING AND SPECIFIC CARDIOVASCULAR DISEASES

Systemic Hypertension and Obstructive Sleep Apnea: A Critical Causative Relationship

Systemic hypertension deserves special attention as the most common CVD leading to a significant portion of CVD-linked mortality in developed societies.[55] Systemic hypertension is the best-established cardiovascular consequence of OSA. Mounting evidence from experimental, observational, and clinical trials over the past 3 decades has established OSA as a modifiable risk factor for systemic hypertension.

The earliest compelling description of a dose-response relationship between OSA and systemic hypertension was provided by the Wisconsin Sleep Cohort.[56] In this landmark study, the investigators established a community-based cohort of otherwise healthy individuals who underwent research sleep studies and followed them for a period of 4 years. The investigators found a dose-response association between having OSA at baseline and the incidence of hypertension in this cohort. This association was independent of known risk factors of hypertension. This study provided the first compelling evidence for the causative relationship between SDB and systemic hypertension. A large cross-sectional study, the Sleep Heart Health Study, also found a strong independent association between OSA and systemic hypertension.[57] In this large multicenter study of cardiovascular risk factors, 6424 patients were evaluated with home sleep studies. The investigators also observed a linear relationship between the severity of OSA and the risk of having systemic hypertension.

Resistant hypertension is an important variant of this disease as it relates to coexisting SDB. Resistant hypertension is often defined as blood pressure that remains greater than a target level despite the use of 3 antihypertensive agents of different classes (one of which is in the diuretic class of medications). Patients whose blood pressure is controlled with 4 or more medications are also considered to have resistant hypertension. A case-control study of 126 patients with either controlled systemic hypertension or resistant hypertension (with both groups receiving medical therapy for increased blood pressure) revealed that OSA was found in 71% of patients with resistant hypertension versus 38% of patients with controlled systemic hypertension.[58]

A prospective cohort of 1889 patients referred to a sleep center for polysomnography testing was followed for a median of 12 years. An increased risk of systemic hypertension was noted in patients diagnosed with OSA who were noncompliant with continuous positive airway pressure (CPAP) therapy (because of refusal, nonadherence, or ineligibility) compared with controls.[59] Those patients with OSA who were appropriately treated with CPAP therapy had a lower risk of being diagnosed with incident hypertension compared with controls. Several randomized controlled trials have shown that treatment of OSA with CPAP therapy can improve blood pressure control in patients with systemic hypertension.

In attempt to quantify the contribution of CPAP to blood pressure decrease in patients with hypertension, 2 recent meta-analyses described modest but statistically significant decreases in blood pressure in patients with OSA treated with CPAP therapy.[9,10,60,61] Both studies showed a decrease in systolic blood pressure of 2.5 to 3.0 mm Hg. It is notable that previous data showed that even a decrease of 1.0 to 2.0 mm Hg in blood pressure is associated with a reduction in HF, stroke, and major cardiovascular events.[11,62] Furthermore, another recent meta-analysis suggested that patients with OSA with uncontrolled hypertension are likely to gain the largest benefit from CPAP in terms of a substantial reduction in blood pressure, even after controlling for disease severity.[12,63] Most studies analyzing the effect of CPAP therapy on patients with OSA with systemic hypertension included patients with daytime symptoms, such as excessive daytime sleepiness. However, some studies have suggested that the benefit of treatment may not occur in those patients without such symptoms. A recent multicenter, parallel-group, randomized controlled trial including 725 patients with moderate to severe SDB but no significant daytime symptoms (defined as an Epworth Sleepiness Scale score of 10 or less) revealed that the prescription of CPAP compared with usual care did not result in a statistically significant reduction in the incidence of hypertension or cardiovascular events.[13,64] In addition, CPAP seems to improve blood pressure control more than nocturnal supplemental oxygen via nasal cannula: a multicenter randomized controlled trial of 318 patients revealed that, in patients with CVD or multiple cardiovascular risk factors, the treatment of OSA with CPAP compared with nocturnal supplemental oxygen resulted in a significant reduction in blood pressure (-2.8 mm

Hg; 95% confidence interval [CI], -5.1 to -0.5; $P = .02$).[14,65] Similar findings were noted when comparing the CPAP arm with controls (-2.4 mm Hg; 95% CI, -4.7 to -0.1; $P = .04$). There was no significant difference in the 24-hour mean arterial pressure between the control group and the group receiving oxygen. Therefore, emerging evidence has shown strong association between OSA/SDB and systemic hypertension, as well as potential benefits of treatment of OSA on blood pressure control in select populations.

Coronary Artery Disease and Obstructive Sleep Apnea

Similar to hypertension, CAD shares several pathophysiologic pathways with OSA, making a causative relationship very likely. Vascular endothelial dysfunction (VED) is an important vascular abnormality that precedes the clinical manifestations of CVD, including CAD and systemic hypertension.[66,67] Impairment in endothelial function facilitates the development of atherosclerotic changes and can contribute to arterial lesion development and subsequent clinical complications, including myocardial infarction and chronic ischemic heart disease.[68] VED is found in patients with OSA who have no manifested CVD.[40,69] The severity of OSA correlates with the severity of endothelial dysfunction in these patients. Treatment of OSA reverses the VED, further supporting the causative relationship between OSA and endothelial dysfunction.

In addition to VED, OSA is associated with several perturbations that trigger accelerated atherosclerosis and vascular lesion formation. Therefore, OSA is likely causative in the pathogenesis of CAD. Clinical studies have provided significant evidence to support the association between OSA and an increased incidence of CAD, as well as increased CAD related events. A large, prospective, cohort study followed more than 1650 men for a mean of 10 years after initial sleep studies.[70] Compared with mild to moderate OSA (AHI<30), simple snorers, and healthy patients, those patients with more severe OSA were noted to have a significantly higher independent risk of fatal and nonfatal cardiovascular events. In this study, cardiovascular events included acute coronary syndrome, myocardial infarction, and stroke. Other studies have confirmed that patients with diagnosed but poorly treated severe OSA have an increased risk of cardiovascular events and mortality compared with patients without OSA.[71,72]

Treatment of OSA with CPAP therapy can reduce the incidence of fatal and nonfatal events related to CAD. The previously described large, prospective, cohort study analyzed patients with severe OSA who were successfully treated with CPAP and those patients whose severe OSA remained untreated.[70] Patients on CPAP therapy had a lower incidence of fatal and nonfatal cardiovascular events. In addition, the incidence of these events did not differ significantly between patients with severe OSA successfully treated with CPAP therapy and those patients without OSA. Another prospective study analyzed 54 patients with both CAD and OSA; approximately half were treated with CPAP therapy and the remaining patients declined treatment.[73] OSA treatment significantly reduced the risk of occurrence of the study end point (a composite of cardiovascular death, acute coronary syndrome, hospitalization for HF, or need for coronary revascularization), indicating that the treatment of OSA in patients with CAD is associated with a decrease in the occurrence of new cardiovascular events, as well as an increase in the time to such events. Therefore, existing evidence for the association between OSA and CAD lies primarily in those patients with severe OSA, and it seems that treating these patients with CPAP therapy may improve cardiovascular outcomes.

Cardiac Arrhythmia (with a Focus on Atrial Fibrillation) and Obstructive Sleep Apnea

Over the past 2 decades, a strong relationship between OSA and cardiac dysrhythmia has emerged. Atrial fibrillation (AF), the most common cardiac arrhythmia, seems to have the strongest association with OSA. However, in patients with HF, most tachyarrhythmias (particularly ventricular tachycardia) seem to be strongly associated with SDB as well.[74]

The relationship between OSA and AF has received increasing attention in recent years. AF is an important cause of stroke and cardiovascular morbidity. Studies have supported a high prevalence of previously undiagnosed OSA in patients with AF. Independent of cofounders such as systemic hypertension, HF, and obesity, the prevalence of OSA in patients with AF has been shown to be significant.[75,76] In addition, several case-control and cross-sectional studies have revealed an increased prevalence of AF in patients with OSA. One large cross-sectional study assessed the prevalence of AF with and without SDB as diagnosed by polysomnography: 5% in patients with SBD and 1% in patients without SBD. Again, this was independent of CVD, including HF, body mass index, age, and gender.[77] Another study showed that type of SDB (CSA or OSA) and the severity of SDB increased the prevalence of AF[78]: in a cohort of almost 3000 men, both more severe SDB and the presence of CSA compared with OSA correlated with a higher chance of a coexisting diagnosis of AF.

A meta-analysis of 6 observational studies suggested that the risk of recurrent AF after radiofrequency catheter-guided ablation increased with a preexisting diagnosis of OSA by 25%.[79] Importantly, emerging data (although primarily observational studies) have shown that OSA may be a modifiable risk factor for recurrent AF after ablation or cardioversion. Treatment of OSA may reduce the risk of recurrent AF after treatment of AF by radiofrequency catheter ablation. A prospective study followed 153 patients who underwent extensive encircling pulmonary vein isolation for AF.[80] Those patients with OSA who were appropriately treated with CPAP therapy had a lower risk of AF recurrence compared with untreated patients (hazard ratio [HR] 0.41; 95% CI, 0.22–0.76; $P<.01$). An observational study of 62 patients undergoing pulmonary vein isolation revealed that CPAP therapy resulted in a lower rate of AF recurrence compared with those patients not compliant with CPAP (28% vs 63%, respectively; $P = .01$) as well as a lower rate of AF recurrence when off antiarrhythmic medications (66% vs 33%, respectively; $P = .02$).[81] Taken as a whole, these data support a strong etiologic and pathophysiologic relationship between OSA and AF and potential treatment benefits of OSA in patients with AF in certain populations.

Cerebrovascular Accidents and Obstructive Sleep Apnea

Independent of cardiovascular risk factors, OSA has been associated with an increased risk for strokes or cerebral vascular accidents (CVAs) of ischemic origin. Several prospective cohort studies have shown this association, as well as a dose-dependent effect: the more severe the OSA, the higher the risk of stroke.[82–85] A prospective cohort study followed more than 5400 individuals with no prior CVA for almost 9 years.[84] After adjustment for confounding agents, a higher AHI was associated with a higher risk of ischemic CVA (adjusted HR, 2.86; 95% CI, 1.10–7.39). A gender effect was noted: although this association was clearly shown in men, it was not statistically significant in women.

With regard to potential treatment benefits of CPAP therapy on OSA in patients with stroke, limited data exist currently. Several investigators have suggested that, because systemic hypertension is an established risk factor for stroke and treatment of OSA with CPAP therapy has been shown to significantly reduce blood pressure, such treatment therefore decreases stroke risk. One randomized controlled trial that analyzed the effect of OSA treatment on stroke risk did not show a benefit to treatment,[64] although the investigators concluded that the study may have had limited power to detect a significant difference.

Small randomized trials have shown a decrease in stroke severity in those acute post-CVA patients who received CPAP therapy for OSA; however, the level of compliance was a confounding issue in this patient population.[86,87] Other studies have shown no benefit to treatment in this patient population, but again adherence remained a significant issue because of cognitive dysfunction, age, and poor tolerance to CPAP therapy.[87,88] However, an observational study of almost 100 patients with ischemic stroke showed decreased mortality at 5 years[89] as well as decreased nonfatal cardiovascular events at 7 years.[90]

Overall, these limited data suggest that OSA may be associated with a higher risk of CVA, especially in more severe OSA cases, but the impact of treatment of OSA on CVA risk is not yet well defined. Emerging evidence indicates potential benefits of treatment of OSA in patients after CVA.

Pulmonary Hypertension and Obstructive Sleep Apnea

An association between OSA and pulmonary hypertension has been shown in several studies. Patients with moderate to severe OSA have a prevalence of coexisting pulmonary hypertension of approximately 20%.[91,92] Risk factors for pulmonary hypertension in patients with OSA included coexisting lung disease or obesity-hypoventilation syndrome, higher AHI, and daytime hypoxemia. In addition, the presence of pulmonary hypertension may have prognostic implications for patients who are diagnosed with OSA. A group of 83 patients diagnosed with OSA were included in an observational study; all patients underwent pulmonary artery catheterization and were followed up at 1, 4, and 8 years. Survival rates were lower in those patients with OSA with pulmonary hypertension versus those without pulmonary hypertension: 93%, 74%, and 43% in patients with pulmonary hypertension versus 100%, 90%, and 76% in patients without pulmonary hypertension at 1, 4, and 8 years, respectively.[93] The results also showed that, although generally mild to moderate, severe pulmonary hypertension can occur in patients with OSA. Female gender, younger age, obesity, and nocturnal desaturation were associated with pulmonary hypertension, and pulmonary hypertension caused functional limitations and increased mortality in patients with OSA.

Changes in right ventricle structure and function have been reported in association with OSA, although the clinical significance of these changes is uncertain.[94] Failure of the right ventricle in patients with OSA is uncommon, but is more likely to occur in the setting of left-sided heart disease or chronic hypoxic respiratory disease.[94]

Several recent studies have shown not only that pulmonary hypertension occurs in at least 20% of patients with OSA without other known cardiopulmonary disorders but also that CPAP therapy can reduce pulmonary artery pressures.[94,95] A randomized crossover trial followed 33 patients either with or without OSA to examine the effect of CPAP therapy on pulmonary artery pressures.[95] At baseline, patients with OSA had higher pulmonary artery systolic pressures than controls (29.8 ± 8.8 mm Hg vs 23.4 ± 4.1 mm Hg, respectively; $P = .036$). None of the control patients had pulmonary hypertension at baseline. Patients with OSA were given either therapeutic CPAP or a sham device; effective CPAP therapy significantly reduced pulmonary artery systolic pressures (from 28.9 ± 8.6 mm Hg to 24.0 ± 5.8 mm Hg; $P<.0001$). The reduction was greatest in patients with either pulmonary or left ventricular diastolic dysfunction at baseline. In addition to these therapeutic benefits, the study showed that severe OSA is independently associated with pulmonary hypertension in a direct relationship with disease severity and presence of diastolic dysfunction. Although not as robust as the data regarding systemic hypertension, existing data suggest an association between OSA and pulmonary hypertension as well as some evidence for a treatment benefit of OSA in patients with pulmonary hypertension.

Cardiomyopathy, Heart Failure, and Sleep-disordered Breathing

An increase in the incidence of HF in recent decades is attributed to improved survival of initial CVD (eg, systemic hypertension and CAD), increased prevalence of diabetes,[96] and aging of the population.[97] The lifelong risk of developing HF at age 40 years is estimated at 20%.[98] The mortality of HF is estimated as 20% in 1 year and remains largely unchanged despite advances in the management of CVD.[98] SDB is likely the most common comorbidity in patients with HF. Several studies have shown a prevalence of SDB in patients with HF approaching 50% to 70%.[99,100] The prevalence of OSA in patients with systolic HF approaches 40% and provides an important target for treatment and improvement of HF outcomes.[101] Clinicians caring for cardiovascular patients should view SDB as both a

CVD that interacts with other CVDs leading to the development of HF and also as an important co-morbidity in patients with HF that can lead to decompensation, hospitalization, and death. It is well established that OSA exacerbates hypertension,[102] CAD,[103] and arrhythmia,[104,105] leading to both acute and chronic HF.[106] As discussed earlier, respiratory events including apneas and hypopneas result in recurrent episodes of intermittent hypoxia, sympathetic activation, and surges in blood pressure. In addition to these perturbations, the increased respiratory effort against closed airways during apneas is associated with further detrimental effects on the heart. These futile inspiratory incursions against occluded pharynx increase the negative intrathoracic pressure. Subsequently, this leads to an increase in left ventricular transmural gradient causing increased cardiac afterload and decreased cardiac output.[107] Augmentation of this negative intrathoracic pressure enhances right ventricular venous return. Overfilling of the right ventricle can push the interventricular septum toward the left ventricular cavity, thereby compromising left-sided filling mechanics and decreasing left ventricular filling.[108] In addition, this negative intrathoracic pressure may affect the balance of forces governing the transudation of fluid into the interstitial space, resulting in pulmonary edema.[109] Therefore, the effect of this respiratory effort may be more important in patients with existing cardiac dysfunction[110,111] than in otherwise healthy individuals with OSA. It is established that patients with HF and OSA experience immediate improvement in their cardiac work index with elimination of OSA events.[112,113]

Evidence of the benefit of treatment of SDB in patients with HF has shown that optimal management of the primary HF syndrome may improve SDB. Such treatment includes standard medical therapy for HF, including diuretics and angiotensin-converting enzyme inhibitors[114,115] and device therapy including biventricular pacemaker implantation cardiac resynchronization therapy.[116,117] Treatment of HF with either cardiac transplant or mechanical circulatory support with left ventricular assist device implantation (and the known optimization of hemodynamics and end-organ function that these therapies provide) does not seem to reverse existing SDB, although data are limited.[118,119]

The mainstay of OSA treatment in HF as well as in the general population is CPAP. These devices function as a pneumatic splint, and are highly effective in eliminating the upper airway collapse that is pathognomonic to OSA. In addition to elimination of the upper airway obstruction, these devices provide positive end-expiratory pressure, which has multiple physiologic effects relevant to the patients with HF. Positive end-expiratory pressure can reduce preload, decrease left ventricular afterload because of reduced wall stress, increase lung compliance because of reduced extravascular lung fluid levels, decrease negative pleural pressure with inspiration, and suppress catecholamine levels because of improved cardiac output and oxygenation and reduced mitral regurgitation.[120] In patients with chronic HF, nocturnal CPAP increases the left ventricular ejection fraction (LVEF) and improves the quality of life. In one trial of patients with HF with OSA, the treatment group experienced a 9% improvement in LVEF as well as improvement in left ventricular size, heart rate, and systolic blood pressure after 1 month of CPAP treatment.[121] Another small randomized controlled trial in patients with chronic systolic HF with OSA showed a significant improvement in LVEF, sympathetic activity, and quality of life with CPAP treatment.[122]

Earlier studies in patients with HF and predominantly CSA (as opposed to OSA) suggested that CPAP can improve HF outcomes. Two randomized trials and 1 meta-analysis have shown an improvement in LVEF in patients with HF with SDB who were treated with CPAP.[122–124] More recently, a treatment modality that can deliver breaths during central apneas in addition to continuous pressure, adaptive servoventilation (ASV), emerged as treatment of CSA. A recent randomized controlled trial (SERVE-HF) examined the effect of ASV in patients who had HF with reduced ejection fraction and predominantly CSA. The study showed no significant effect on the primary end point; the primary end point in the time-to-event analysis was the first event of death from any cause, lifesaving cardiovascular intervention (cardiac transplant, implantation of a ventricular assist device, resuscitation after sudden cardiac arrest, or appropriate lifesaving shock), or unplanned hospitalization for worsening HF. Several questions remain regarding the population studied, device use, and cause of death.[125–127] Therefore, although appropriate therapy for CSA in patients with HF remains controversial, CPAP remains widely accepted for OSA in patients with HF.

Treatment of Sleep-disordered Breathing as a Therapeutic Intervention to Modify Cardiovascular Disease Risk

As detailed earlier, several observational studies, single-center or smaller randomized trials, and meta-analyses have addressed both the association and potential treatment benefits of SDB on

CVD. Clear demonstration of a direct causal pathway from SDB to CVD is lacking in most areas and large, multicenter, double-blinded, randomized controlled trials are needed in order to make definite recommendations for the diagnosis and treatment of SDB in the CVD disease population. Given current available evidence as well as our clinical experience at The Ohio State University Sleep-Heart Program, this article provides treatment recommendations regarding appropriate therapy for SDB in patients with CVD.

First, note that although most of the clinical literature regarding the therapy for SDB in both the CVD population and general population is based on CPAP therapy, other therapies have been studied and may be beneficial to select patients. For patients with mild OSA with no symptoms, the addition of simple behavioral or lifestyle modifications may be all that is needed to reduce or abolish OSA.[128] Weight loss and maintenance of a normal body mass index, avoidance of alcohol and sedative medications before bedtime, and positional therapy can be recommended.

Other therapies have been developed to treat OSA, including custom-made mandibular advancement devices to prevent tongue-related pharyngeal obstruction during sleep, nasal devices worn inside each nostril that create increased expiratory nasal resistance to maintain a patent upper airway, and various surgical procedures used to enlarge the pharyngeal airway.[128,129] None of these therapies have been to be shown to be as effective as CPAP at treating OSA, nor have they been specifically tested on patients with HF. In addition, none of these devices have been shown to benefit patients with CSA. We only recommend the mandibular advancement devices to patients with CVD with mild OSA and not CSA, only if they could not tolerate CPAP therapy.

The strongest evidence for a benefit of SDB treatment in CVD is for systemic hypertension. The authors recommend treatment of all patients with systemic hypertension with sleep-related symptoms, resistant hypertension, controlled hypertension on 2 or more antihypertensive medications, and moderate to severe OSA in patients without significant sleep-related symptoms. The evidence for treatment of patients with mild OSA without significant symptoms is not well defined.

The data supporting the treatment of SDB in patients with CAD are less robust than the systemic hypertension or AF evidence. The authors recommend treatment of severe OSA in patients with CAD regardless of symptoms as well as mild to moderate OSA in patients with significant sleep-related symptoms. Patients with complex or progressive CAD should also be considered for treatment, regardless of symptoms or severity of OSA. The subgroup of patients with AF that seem to benefit most from SDB treatment is those with recurrent AF after cardioversion or ablation therapy. Given the high prevalence of SDB in patients with AF, the authors recommend treatment in all patients with significant sleep-related symptoms, recurrent AF, AF requiring antiarrhythmia medications, and moderate to severe OSA in patients without significant sleep-related symptoms. Consideration for treatment of patients with mild OSA without significant sleep-related symptoms should be considered in the setting of recurrent AF or AF requiring antiarrhythmia medications.

Patients with pulmonary hypertension should be considered for SDB treatment in the setting of coexisting lung disease, such as chronic obstructive pulmonary disease or interstitial lung disease, obesity-hypoventilation syndrome, daytime hypoxemia, significant sleep-related symptoms, moderate to severe OSA in the absence of significant sleep-related symptoms, or moderate to severe pulmonary hypertension. Reevaluation of pulmonary artery pressures by either pulmonary artery catheterization or echocardiography should be done both before and after treatment of SDB may be useful in evaluating the effectiveness of CPAP therapy. A noninvasive evaluation with transthoracic echocardiography may be the best first option for the evaluation of changes in pulmonary artery pressures in the setting of CPAP therapy.

The American College of Cardiology/American Heart Association guidelines on the diagnosis and treatment of chronic HF indicate that screening for SDB is reasonable in selected patients; namely those with risk factors.[130] However, similar to patients with stroke, the typical symptoms of SDB are not always present in patients with HF and questionnaire data have low sensitivity and specificity for the diagnosis of SDB.[131] In our practice, we collaborate with our cardiovascular medicine and advanced HF physicians to ensure that patients are optimally treated in terms of evidence-based medical therapy and device therapy for HF. We also recommend treatment of any patient with significant sleep-related symptoms and also those with moderate to severe OSA, regardless of symptoms. In addition, we recommend treatment in any patient with progressive or end-stage HF, as tolerated.

With the recent US Food and Drug Administration approval of wireless hemodynamic pulmonary artery pressure monitors for the management of HF,[132] the effect of treatment of SDB in patients with HF may be better evaluated and managed in the outpatient setting and CPAP therapy may help to reduce hospitalizations in patients with HF implanted with such a device. The CardioMEMs HF system may also provide guidance as to the optimal timing of CPAP therapy (while hospitalized, immediately after hospital discharge, or within 2 to 3 months of hospital discharge).

In addition, treatment decisions should be considered dynamic and not static. The authors recommend that patients with CVD be reevaluated for sleep-related symptoms and, in the context of SDB risk, progression of their CVD on at least a yearly basis. This recommendation does not imply yearly in-laboratory polysomnography but instead evaluation in a sleep medicine clinic or by a well-educated primary care physician or cardiovascular medicine specialist. Because sleep-related symptoms and severity of potential SDB may progress with age and CVD burden, the likelihood of the development of significant SDB and indications for treatment may change over time.

SUMMARY

As discussed in this article, significant evidence has shown a pathophysiologic link between OSA/SDB and CVD/VED. In addition, emerging clinical trial data have shown a relationship between OSA/SDB and a variety of CVD states. Potential treatment benefits of SDB on CVD risk in certain patient populations have also been shown. However, a clear demonstration of a direct causal pathway from SDB to CVD is lacking with most CVDs and large, multicenter, double-blinded, randomized controlled trials are needed in order to make definitive recommendations for the diagnosis and treatment of SDB in the CVD disease population. Further basic and translational research is also needed. Well-defined evidence-based guidelines are not possible at the current time but general recommendations can be made for clinical decision making based on available evidence, as provided here. Ongoing and future basic, translational, and clinical studies will better define the relationship between SDB and CVD, with the goal of lessening the overall burden of CVD mortality and morbidity.

REFERENCES

1. Fletcher EC, Lesske J, Behm R, et al. Carotid chemoreceptors, systemic blood pressure, and chronic episodic hypoxia mimicking sleep apnea. J Appl Physiol (1985) 1992;72(5):1978–84.
2. Morgan BJ, Denahan T, Ebert TJ. Neurocirculatory consequences of negative intrathoracic pressure vs. asphyxia during voluntary apnea. J Appl Physiol (1985) 1993;74(6):2969–75.
3. Rapsomaniki E, Timmis A, George J, et al. Blood pressure and incidence of twelve cardiovascular diseases: lifetime risks, healthy life-years lost, and age-specific associations in 1.25 million people. Lancet 2014;383(9932):1899–911.
4. Lesske J, Fletcher EC, Bao G, et al. Hypertension caused by chronic intermittent hypoxia–influence of chemoreceptors and sympathetic nervous system. J Hypertens 1997;15(12 Pt 2):1593–603.
5. Katragadda S, Xie A, Puleo D, et al. Neural mechanism of the pressor response to obstructive and nonobstructive apnea. J Appl Physiol (1985) 1997;83(6):2048–54.
6. Peng YJ, Prabhakar NR. Reactive oxygen species in the plasticity of respiratory behavior elicited by chronic intermittent hypoxia. J Appl Physiol (1985) 2003;94(6):2342–9.
7. Prabhakar NR, Fields RD, Baker T, et al. Intermittent hypoxia: cell to system. Am J Physiol Lung Cell Mol Physiol 2001;281(3):L524–8.
8. Prabhakar NR, Kline DD. Ventilatory changes during intermittent hypoxia: importance of pattern and duration. High Alt Med Biol 2002;3(2):195–204.
9. Cutler MJ, Swift NM, Keller DM, et al. Periods of intermittent hypoxic apnea can alter chemoreflex control of sympathetic nerve activity in humans. Am J Physiol Heart Circ Physiol 2004;287(5): H2054–60.
10. Narkiewicz K, van de Borne PJ, Montano N, et al. Contribution of tonic chemoreflex activation to sympathetic activity and blood pressure in patients with obstructive sleep apnea. Circulation 1998;97(10): 943–5.
11. Bao G, Metreveli N, Li R, et al. Blood pressure response to chronic episodic hypoxia: role of the sympathetic nervous system. J Appl Physiol (1985) 1997;83(1):95–101.
12. Xie A, Skatrud JB, Crabtree DC, et al. Neurocirculatory consequences of intermittent asphyxia in humans. J Appl Physiol (1985) 2000;89(4):1333–9.
13. Brooks D, Horner RL, Kozar LF, et al. Obstructive sleep apnea as a cause of systemic hypertension. Evidence from a canine model. J Clin Invest 1997; 99(1):106–9.
14. Alchanatis M, Tourkohoriti G, Kosmas EN, et al. Evidence for left ventricular dysfunction in patients with obstructive sleep apnoea syndrome. Eur Respir J 2002;20(5):1239–45.
15. Amin RS, Kimball TR, Bean JA, et al. Left ventricular hypertrophy and abnormal ventricular geometry in children and adolescents with obstructive sleep apnea. Am J Respir Crit Care Med 2002;165(10): 1395–9.
16. Dopp JM, Philippi NR, Marcus NJ, et al. Xanthine oxidase inhibition attenuates endothelial dysfunction caused by chronic intermittent hypoxia in rats. Respiration 2011;82(5):458–67.

17. Phillips SA, Olson EB, Lombard JH, et al. Chronic intermittent hypoxia alters NE reactivity and mechanics of skeletal muscle resistance arteries. J Appl Physiol (1985) 2006;100(4):1117–23.

18. Varadharaj S, Porter K, Pleister A, et al. Endothelial nitric oxide synthase uncoupling: a novel pathway in OSA induced vascular endothelial dysfunction. Respir Physiol Neurobiol 2015;207:40–7.

19. Esler M, Julius S, Randall O, et al. High-renin essential hypertension: adrenergic cardiovascular correlates. Clin Sci Mol Med Suppl 1976;3:181s–4s.

20. Oparil S, Zaman MA, Calhoun DA. Pathogenesis of hypertension. Ann Intern Med 2003;139(9):761–76.

21. Guo GB, Abboud FM. Angiotensin II attenuates baroreflex control of heart rate and sympathetic activity. Am J Physiol 1984;246(1 Pt 2):H80–9.

22. Somers VK, Dyken ME, Clary MP, et al. Sympathetic neural mechanisms in obstructive sleep apnea. J Clin Invest 1995;96(4):1897–904.

23. Fletcher EC. Sympathetic over activity in the etiology of hypertension of obstructive sleep apnea. Sleep 2003;26(1):15–9.

24. Dick TE, Hsieh YH, Wang N, et al. Acute intermittent hypoxia increases both phrenic and sympathetic nerve activities in the rat. Exp Physiol 2007; 92(1):87–97.

25. Sica AL, Greenberg HE, Ruggiero DA, et al. Chronic-intermittent hypoxia: a model of sympathetic activation in the rat. Respir Physiol 2000; 121(2–3):173–84.

26. Greenberg HE, Sica A, Batson D, et al. Chronic intermittent hypoxia increases sympathetic responsiveness to hypoxia and hypercapnia. J Appl Physiol (1985) 1999;86(1):298–305.

27. Rumantir MS, Jennings GL, Lambert GW, et al. The 'adrenaline hypothesis' of hypertension revisited: evidence for adrenaline release from the heart of patients with essential hypertension. J Hypertens 2000;18(6):717–23.

28. Kim JR, Kiefe CI, Liu K, et al. Heart rate and subsequent blood pressure in young adults: the CARDIA study. Hypertension 1999;33(2):640–6.

29. Farsang C, Juhász I, Kapocsi J, et al. Effect of prazosin and oxprenolol on plasma renin activity and blood pressure in patients with essential hypertension. Cardiology 1981;67(3):164–71.

30. Winternitz SR, Katholi RE, Oparil S. Role of the renal sympathetic nerves in the development and maintenance of hypertension in the spontaneously hypertensive rat. J Clin Invest 1980;66(5):971–8.

31. Fletcher EC, Bao G, Li R. Renin activity and blood pressure in response to chronic episodic hypoxia. Hypertension 1999;34(2):309–14.

32. Fletcher EC, Orolinova N, Bader M. Blood pressure response to chronic episodic hypoxia: the renin-angiotensin system. J Appl Physiol (1985) 2002; 92(2):627–33.

33. Somers VK, Mark AL, Abboud FM. Interaction of baroreceptor and chemoreceptor reflex control of sympathetic nerve activity in normal humans. J Clin Invest 1991;87(6):1953–7.

34. Chapleau MW, Hajduczok G, Abboud FM. Mechanisms of resetting of arterial baroreceptors: an overview. Am J Med Sci 1988;295(4):327–34.

35. Davies CW, Crosby JH, Mullins RL, et al. Case-control study of 24 hour ambulatory blood pressure in patients with obstructive sleep apnoea and normal matched control subjects. Thorax 2000; 55(9):736–40.

36. Suzuki M, Guilleminault C, Otsuka K, et al. Blood pressure "dipping" and "non-dipping" in obstructive sleep apnea syndrome patients. Sleep 1996; 19(5):382–7.

37. Rouwet EV, Tintu AN, Schellings MW, et al. Hypoxia induces aortic hypertrophic growth, left ventricular dysfunction, and sympathetic hyperinnervation of peripheral arteries in the chick embryo. Circulation 2002;105(23):2791–6.

38. Phillips SA, Olson EB, Morgan BJ, et al. Chronic intermittent hypoxia impairs endothelium-dependent dilation in rat cerebral and skeletal muscle resistance arteries. Am J Physiol Heart Circ Physiol 2004; 286(1):H388–93.

39. Peng YJ, Overholt JL, Kline D, et al. Induction of sensory long-term facilitation in the carotid body by intermittent hypoxia: implications for recurrent apneas. Proc Natl Acad Sci U S A 2003;100(17):10073–8.

40. Patt BT, Jarjoura D, Haddad DN, et al. Endothelial dysfunction in the microcirculation of patients with obstructive sleep apnea. Am J Respir Crit Care Med 2010;182(12):1540–5.

41. Grebe M, Eisele HJ, Weissmann N, et al. Antioxidant vitamin C improves endothelial function in obstructive sleep apnea. Am J Respir Crit Care Med 2006;173(8):897–901.

42. Teramoto S, Kume H, Yamaguchi Y, et al. Improvement of endothelial function with allopurinol may occur in selected patients with OSA: effect of age and sex. Eur Respir J 2007;29(1):216–7 [author reply: 217–8].

43. Veasey SC, Davis CW, Fenik P, et al. Long-term intermittent hypoxia in mice: protracted hypersomnolence with oxidative injury to sleep-wake brain regions. Sleep 2004;27(2):194–201.

44. Xu W, Chi L, Row BW, et al. Increased oxidative stress is associated with chronic intermittent hypoxia-mediated brain cortical neuronal cell apoptosis in a mouse model of sleep apnea. Neuroscience 2004;126(2):313–23.

45. Schulz R, Mahmoudi S, Hattar K, et al. Enhanced release of superoxide from polymorphonuclear neutrophils in obstructive sleep apnea. Impact of continuous positive airway pressure therapy. Am J Respir Crit Care Med 2000;162(2 Pt 1):566–70.

46. Row BW, Kheirandish L, Li RC, et al. Platelet-activating factor receptor-deficient mice are protected from experimental sleep apnea-induced learning deficits. J Neurochem 2004;89(1):189–96.

47. Tan KC, Chow WS, Lam JC, et al. HDL dysfunction in obstructive sleep apnea. Atherosclerosis 2006; 184(2):377–82.

48. Troncoso Brindeiro CM, da Silva AQ, Allahdadi KJ, et al. Reactive oxygen species contribute to sleep apnea-induced hypertension in rats. Am J Physiol Heart Circ Physiol 2007;293(5):H2971–6.

49. Park AM, Suzuki YJ. Effects of intermittent hypoxia on oxidative stress-induced myocardial damage in mice. J Appl Physiol (1985) 2007;102(5):1806–14.

50. Spiegel K, Leproult R, Van Cauter E. Impact of sleep debt on metabolic and endocrine function. Lancet 1999;354(9188):1435–9.

51. Spiegel K, Tasali E, Penev P, et al. Brief communication: sleep curtailment in healthy young men is associated with decreased leptin levels, elevated ghrelin levels, and increased hunger and appetite. Ann Intern Med 2004;141(11):846–50.

52. Yaggi HK, Araujo AB, McKinlay JB. Sleep duration as a risk factor for the development of type 2 diabetes. Diabetes Care 2006;29(3):657–61.

53. Ip MS, Lam B, Ng MM, et al. Obstructive sleep apnea is independently associated with insulin resistance. Am J Respir Crit Care Med 2002;165(5): 670–6.

54. Botros N, Concato J, Mohsenin V, et al. Obstructive sleep apnea as a risk factor for type 2 diabetes. Am J Med 2009;122(12):1122–7.

55. Go AS, Mozaffarian D, Roger VL, et al. Heart disease and stroke statistics–2014 update: a report from the American Heart Association. Circulation 2014;129(3):e28–292.

56. Peppard PE, Young T, Palta M, et al. Prospective study of the association between sleep-disordered breathing and hypertension. N Engl J Med 2000; 342(19):1378–84.

57. Nieto FJ, Young TB, Lind BK, et al. Association of sleep-disordered breathing, sleep apnea, and hypertension in a large community-based study. Sleep Heart Health Study. JAMA 2000;283(14): 1829–36.

58. Goncalves SC, Martinez D, Gus M, et al. Obstructive sleep apnea and resistant hypertension: a case-control study. Chest 2007;132(6):1858–62.

59. Marin JM, Agusti A, Villar I, et al. Association between treated and untreated obstructive sleep apnea and risk of hypertension. JAMA 2012;307(20): 2169–76.

60. Montesi SB, Edwards BA, Malhotra A, et al. The effect of continuous positive airway pressure treatment on blood pressure: a systematic review and meta-analysis of randomized controlled trials. J Clin Sleep Med 2012;8(5):587–96.

61. Fava C, Dorigoni S, Dalle Vedove F, et al. Effect of CPAP on blood pressure in patients with OSA/hypopnea a systematic review and meta-analysis. Chest 2014;145(4):762–71.

62. Turnbull F, Blood Pressure Lowering Treatment Trialists Collaboration. Effects of different blood-pressure-lowering regimens on major cardiovascular events: results of prospectively-designed overviews of randomised trials. Lancet 2003; 362(9395):1527–35.

63. Bakker JP, Edwards BA, Gautam SP, et al. Blood pressure improvement with continuous positive airway pressure is independent of obstructive sleep apnea severity. J Clin Sleep Med 2014; 10(4):365–9.

64. Barbe F, Durán-Cantolla J, Sánchez-de-la-Torre M, et al. Effect of continuous positive airway pressure on the incidence of hypertension and cardiovascular events in nonsleepy patients with obstructive sleep apnea: a randomized controlled trial. JAMA 2012;307(20):2161–8.

65. Gottlieb DJ, Punjabi NM, Mehra R, et al. CPAP versus oxygen in obstructive sleep apnea. N Engl J Med 2014;370(24):2276–85.

66. Koller A, Huang A. Impaired nitric oxide-mediated flow-induced dilation in arterioles of spontaneously hypertensive rats. Circ Res 1994;74(3):416–21.

67. Brevetti G, Silvestro A, Schiano V, et al. Endothelial dysfunction and cardiovascular risk prediction in peripheral arterial disease: additive value of flow-mediated dilation to ankle-brachial pressure index. Circulation 2003;108(17):2093–8.

68. Ross R. The pathogenesis of atherosclerosis: a perspective for the 1990s. Nature 1993;362(6423): 801–9.

69. Ip MS, Tse HF, Lam B, et al. Endothelial function in obstructive sleep apnea and response to treatment. Am J Respir Crit Care Med 2004;169(3): 348–53.

70. Marin JM, Carrizo SJ, Vicente E, et al. Long-term cardiovascular outcomes in men with obstructive sleep apnoea-hypopnoea with or without treatment with continuous positive airway pressure: an observational study. Lancet 2005;365(9464):1046–53.

71. Gottlieb DJ, Yenokyan G, Newman AB, et al. Prospective study of obstructive sleep apnea and incident coronary heart disease and heart failure: the sleep heart health study. Circulation 2010;122(4): 352–60.

72. Martinez-Garcia MA, Campos-Rodríguez F, Catalán-Serra P, et al. Cardiovascular mortality in obstructive sleep apnea in the elderly: role of long-term continuous positive airway pressure treatment: a prospective observational study. Am J Respir Crit Care Med 2012;186(9):909–16.

73. Milleron O, Pillière R, Foucher A, et al. Benefits of obstructive sleep apnoea treatment in coronary

artery disease: a long-term follow-up study. Eur Heart J 2004;25(9):728–34.

74. Javaheri S. Effects of continuous positive airway pressure on sleep apnea and ventricular irritability in patients with heart failure. Circulation 2000; 101(4):392–7.

75. Porthan KM, Melin JH, Kupila JT, et al. Prevalence of sleep apnea syndrome in lone atrial fibrillation: a case-control study. Chest 2004;125(3):879–85.

76. Gami AS, Pressman G, Caples SM, et al. Association of atrial fibrillation and obstructive sleep apnea. Circulation 2004;110(4):364–7.

77. Mehra R, Benjamin EJ, Shahar E, et al. Association of nocturnal arrhythmias with sleep-disordered breathing: the Sleep Heart Health Study. Am J Respir Crit Care Med 2006;173(8):910–6.

78. Mehra R, Stone KL, Varosy PD, et al. Nocturnal arrhythmias across a spectrum of obstructive and central sleep-disordered breathing in older men: outcomes of sleep disorders in older men (MrOS sleep) study. Arch Intern Med 2009;169(12):1147–55.

79. Ng CY, Liu T, Shehata M, et al. Meta-analysis of obstructive sleep apnea as predictor of atrial fibrillation recurrence after catheter ablation. Am J Cardiol 2011;108(1):47–51.

80. Naruse Y, Tada H, Satoh M, et al. Concomitant obstructive sleep apnea increases the recurrence of atrial fibrillation following radiofrequency catheter ablation of atrial fibrillation: clinical impact of continuous positive airway pressure therapy. Heart Rhythm 2013;10(3):331–7.

81. Fein AS, Shvilkin A, Shah D, et al. Treatment of obstructive sleep apnea reduces the risk of atrial fibrillation recurrence after catheter ablation. J Am Coll Cardiol 2013;62(4):300–5.

82. Yaggi HK, Concato J, Kernan WN, et al. Obstructive sleep apnea as a risk factor for stroke and death. N Engl J Med 2005;353(19):2034–41.

83. Valham F, Mooe T, Rabben T, et al. Increased risk of stroke in patients with coronary artery disease and sleep apnea: a 10-year follow-up. Circulation 2008; 118(9):955–60.

84. Redline S, Yenokyan G, Gottlieb DJ, et al. Obstructive sleep apnea-hypopnea and incident stroke: the Sleep Heart Health Study. Am J Respir Crit Care Med 2010;182(2):269–77.

85. Loke YK, Brown JW, Kwok CS, et al. Association of obstructive sleep apnea with risk of serious cardiovascular events: a systematic review and meta-analysis. Circ Cardiovasc Qual Outcomes 2012; 5(5):720–8.

86. Bravata DM, Concato J, Fried T, et al. Continuous positive airway pressure: evaluation of a novel therapy for patients with acute ischemic stroke. Sleep 2011;34(9):1271–7.

87. Minnerup J, Ritter MA, Wersching H, et al. Continuous positive airway pressure ventilation for acute ischemic stroke: a randomized feasibility study. Stroke 2012;43(4):1137–9.

88. Hsu CY, Vennelle M, Li HY, et al. Sleep-disordered breathing after stroke: a randomised controlled trial of continuous positive airway pressure. J Neurol Neurosurg Psychiatry 2006;77(10):1143–9.

89. Martinez-Garcia MA, Soler-Cataluña JJ, Ejarque-Martínez L, et al. Continuous positive airway pressure treatment reduces mortality in patients with ischemic stroke and obstructive sleep apnea: a 5-year follow-up study. Am J Respir Crit Care Med 2009;180(1):36–41.

90. Martinez-Garcia MA, Campos-Rodríguez F, Soler-Cataluña JJ, et al. Increased incidence of nonfatal cardiovascular events in stroke patients with sleep apnoea: effect of CPAP treatment. Eur Respir J 2012;39(4):906–12.

91. Yamakawa H, Shiomi T, Sasanabe R, et al. Pulmonary hypertension in patients with severe obstructive sleep apnea. Psychiatry Clin Neurosci 2002; 56(3):311–2.

92. Chaouat A, Weitzenblum E, Krieger J, et al. Pulmonary hemodynamics in the obstructive sleep apnea syndrome. Results in 220 consecutive patients. Chest 1996;109(2):380–6.

93. Minai OA, Ricaurte B, Kaw R, et al. Frequency and impact of pulmonary hypertension in patients with obstructive sleep apnea syndrome. Am J Cardiol 2009;104(9):1300–6.

94. Sajkov D, McEvoy RD. Obstructive sleep apnea and pulmonary hypertension. Prog Cardiovasc Dis 2009;51(5):363–70.

95. Arias MA, García-Río F, Alonso-Fernández A, et al. Pulmonary hypertension in obstructive sleep apnoea: effects of continuous positive airway pressure: a randomized, controlled cross-over study. Eur Heart J 2006;27(9):1106–13.

96. From AM, Leibson CL, Bursi F, et al. Diabetes in heart failure: prevalence and impact on outcome in the population. Am J Med 2006;119(7): 591–9.

97. Barker WH, Mullooly JP, Getchell W. Changing incidence and survival for heart failure in a well-defined older population, 1970-1974 and 1990-1994. Circulation 2006;113(6):799–805.

98. Lloyd-Jones D, Adams RJ, Brown TM, et al. Heart disease and stroke statistics–2010 update: a report from the American Heart Association. Circulation 2010;121(7):e46–215.

99. Khayat R, Jarjoura D, Patt B, et al. In-hospital testing for sleep-disordered breathing in hospitalized patients with decompensated heart failure: report of prevalence and patient characteristics. J Card Fail 2009;15(9):739–46.

100. Oldenburg O, Lamp B, Faber L, et al. Sleep-disordered breathing in patients with symptomatic heart failure: a contemporary study of prevalence in and

characteristics of 700 patients. Eur J Heart Fail 2007;9(3):251–7.

101. Khayat R, Jarjoura D, Porter K, et al. Sleep disordered breathing and post-discharge mortality in patients with acute heart failure. Eur Heart J 2015;36(23):1463–9.

102. Logan AG, Tkacova R, Perlikowski SM, et al. Refractory hypertension and sleep apnoea: effect of CPAP on blood pressure and baroreflex. Eur Respir J 2003;21(2):241–7.

103. Peker Y, Carlson J, Hedner J. Increased incidence of coronary artery disease in sleep apnoea: a longterm follow-up. Eur Respir J 2006;28(3):596–602.

104. Yang A, Schäfer H, Manka R, et al. Influence of obstructive sleep apnea on heart rate turbulence. Basic Res Cardiol 2005;100(5):439–45.

105. Roche F, Court-Fortune I, Pichot V, et al. Reduced cardiac sympathetic autonomic tone after longterm nasal continuous positive airway pressure in obstructive sleep apnoea syndrome. Clin Physiol 1999;19(2):127–34.

106. Nieminen MS, Brutsaert D, Dickstein K, et al. EuroHeart Failure Survey II (EHFS II): a survey on hospitalized acute heart failure patients: description of population. Eur Heart J 2006;27(22):2725–36.

107. Bradley TD, Hall MJ, Ando S, et al. Hemodynamic effects of simulated obstructive apneas in humans with and without heart failure. Chest 2001;119(6):1827–35.

108. Brinker JA, Weiss JL, Lappé DL, et al. Leftward septal displacement during right ventricular loading in man. Circulation 1980;61(3):626–33.

109. Fletcher EC, Proctor M, Yu J, et al. Pulmonary edema develops after recurrent obstructive apneas. Am J Respir Crit Care Med 1999;160(5 Pt 1):1688–96.

110. Chen L, Shi Q, Scharf SM. Hemodynamic effects of periodic obstructive apneas in sedated pigs with congestive heart failure. J Appl Physiol (1985) 2000;88(3):1051–60.

111. Hall MJ, Ando S, Floras JS, et al. Magnitude and time course of hemodynamic responses to Mueller maneuvers in patients with congestive heart failure. J Appl Physiol (1985) 1998;85(4):1476–84.

112. Naughton MT. Impact of treatment of sleep apnoea on left ventricular function in congestive heart failure. Thorax 1998;53(Suppl 3):S37–40.

113. Tkacova R, Rankin F, Fitzgerald FS, et al. Effects of continuous positive airway pressure on obstructive sleep apnea and left ventricular afterload in patients with heart failure. Circulation 1998;98(21):2269–75.

114. Brack T, Thüer I, Clarenbach CF, et al. Daytime Cheyne-Stokes respiration in ambulatory patients with severe congestive heart failure is associated with increased mortality. Chest 2007;132(5):1463–71.

115. Walsh JT, Andrews R, Starling R, et al. Effects of captopril and oxygen on sleep apnoea in patients with mild to moderate congestive cardiac failure. Br Heart J 1995;73(3):237–41.

116. Sinha AM, Skobel EC, Breithardt OA, et al. Cardiac resynchronization therapy improves central sleep apnea and Cheyne-Stokes respiration in patients with chronic heart failure. J Am Coll Cardiol 2004;44(1):68–71.

117. Stanchina ML, Ellison K, Malhotra A, et al. The impact of cardiac resynchronization therapy on obstructive sleep apnea in heart failure patients: a pilot study. Chest 2007;132(2):433–9.

118. Mansfield DR, Solin P, Roebuck T, et al. The effect of successful heart transplant treatment of heart failure on central sleep apnea. Chest 2003;124(5):1675–81.

119. Padeletti M, Henriquez A, Mancini DM, et al. Persistence of Cheyne-Stokes breathing after left ventricular assist device implantation in patients with acutely decompensated end-stage heart failure. J Heart Lung Transplant 2007;26(7):742–4.

120. Malhotra A, Muse VV, Mark EJ. Case records of the Massachusetts General Hospital. Weekly clinicopathological exercises. Case 12-2003. An 82-year-old man with dyspnea and pulmonary abnormalities. N Engl J Med 2003;348(16):1574–85.

121. Kaneko Y, Floras JS, Usui K, et al. Cardiovascular effects of continuous positive airway pressure in patients with heart failure and obstructive sleep apnea. N Engl J Med 2003;348(13):1233–41.

122. Mansfield DR, Gollogly NC, Kaye DM, et al. Controlled trial of continuous positive airway pressure in obstructive sleep apnea and heart failure. Am J Respir Crit Care Med 2004;169(3):361–6.

123. Bradley TD, Logan AG, Kimoff RJ, et al. Continuous positive airway pressure for central sleep apnea and heart failure. N Engl J Med 2005;353(19):2025–33.

124. Sun H, Shi J, Li M, et al. Impact of continuous positive airway pressure treatment on left ventricular ejection fraction in patients with obstructive sleep apnea: a meta-analysis of randomized controlled trials. PLoS One 2013;8(5):e62298.

125. Cowie MR, Woehrle H, Wegscheider K, et al. Adaptive servo-ventilation for central sleep apnea in systolic heart failure. N Engl J Med 2015;373(12):1095–105.

126. Randerath W, Khayat R, Arzt M, et al. Missing links. Sleep Med 2015;16(12):1495–6.

127. Javaheri S, Brown LK, Randerath W, et al. SERVE-HF: more questions than answers. Chest 2016;149(4):900–4.

128. Khayat R, Small R, Rathman L, et al. Sleep-disordered breathing in heart failure: identifying and treating an important but often unrecognized

comorbidity in heart failure patients. J Card Fail 2013;19(6):431–44.

129. Augostini R. A novel approach to the treatment of central sleep apnea in patients with heart failure. Herzschrittmacherther Elektrophysiol 2012;23(1): 9–13.

130. Yancy CW, Jessup M, Bozkurt B, et al. 2013 ACCF/ AHA guideline for the management of heart failure: executive summary: a report of the American College of Cardiology Foundation/American Heart Association Task Force on Practice Guidelines. Circulation 2013;128(16):1810–52.

131. Bitter T, Westerheide N, Hossain SM, et al. Symptoms of sleep apnoea in chronic heart failure–results from a prospective cohort study in 1,500 patients. Sleep Breath 2012;16(3):781–91.

132. Abraham WT, Adamson PB, Bourge RC, et al. Wireless pulmonary artery haemodynamic monitoring in chronic heart failure: a randomised controlled trial. Lancet 2011;377(9766):658–66.

Impact of Obstructive Sleep Apnea on Neurocognitive Function and Impact of Continuous Positive Air Pressure

Charles R. Davies, MD, PhD[a],*, John J. Harrington, MD, MPH[b]

KEYWORDS

- Obstructive sleep apnea • Neurocognitive function • Cognition
- Continuous positive airway pressure (CPAP)

KEY POINTS

- Obstructive sleep apnea is associated with impairment of multiple aspects of cognition, including attention, delayed visual and verbal memory, visuospatial skills, and some aspects of executive function.
- The mechanism of this impairment includes neuro-inflammation, oxidative stress, and sympathetic overactivity.
- Treatment with continuous positive air pressure (CPAP) is shown to improve executive function and verbal memory at 2 to 3 months.
- CPAP use of at least 6 hours per night may lead to further improvements in neurocognitive function.

INTRODUCTION

Obstructive sleep apnea (OSA) is a relatively common breathing disorder known to increase in prevalence with obesity and age.[1,2] The repetitive interruptions in breathing typically cause fragmented, poor quality sleep as well as oxygen desaturations. Other sleep disorders, including insomnia, restless legs syndrome, and parasomnias, such as sleepwalking, can be exacerbated by sleep-disordered breathing. OSA has been associated with excessive daytime sleepiness,[3] hypertension,[4] cardiovascular disease,[5] stroke,[6] depression,[7] impaired glucose tolerance,[8] endocrine dysfunction,[9] and increased risk of motor vehicle accidents (MVAs).[10] Hospitalization days and medical costs are increased per annum for persons with OSA.[11] In addition, multiple aspects of cognition can be affected; this is not only due to the sleepiness that often accompanies OSA but also because of direct pathologic effects on the brain. Although continuous positive air pressure (CPAP) has been shown to improve many of the conditions mentioned, opinions vary regarding improvement of neurocognitive impairments with CPAP. In this article, literature from the last 5 years on the neurocognitive impact of OSA, proposed mechanisms of these sequelae, and effect of CPAP, are reviewed.

Disclosure Statement: The authors have no relationship to disclose.
[a] Carle Neuroscience Institute, Carle Foundation Hospital, College of Medicine, University of Illinois at Urbana-Champaign, 602 West University Avenue, Urbana, IL 61801, USA; [b] Division of Pulmonary, Critical Care, Sleep and Allergy, Department of Medicine, 985990 Nebraska Medical Center, Omaha, NE 68159-5990, USA
* Corresponding author.
E-mail address: charles.davies@carle.com

Sleep Med Clin 11 (2016) 287–298
http://dx.doi.org/10.1016/j.jsmc.2016.04.006
1556-407X/16/$ – see front matter © 2016 Elsevier Inc. All rights reserved.

OBSTRUCTIVE SLEEP APNEA EFFECTS ON ATTENTION AND VIGILANCE

Attention is the ability to maintain focus on certain sensory stimuli while de-emphasizing other stimuli. Vigilance is the ability to sustain focus over an extended period of time. These neurocognitive domains are among the most consistently affected by OSA.[12–14] Although differences are seen when treating OSA as a dichotomous variable, a dose-response relationship between OSA severity and level of inattention has not been shown.[15] Batool-Anwar and coworkers[15] found significant worsening of attention as measured by the psychomotor vigilance test (PVT) associated with the Epworth Sleepiness Scale (ESS) and Pittsburgh Sleep Quality Index. Results were adjusted for age but not IQ. Olaithe and colleagues[16] also failed to find a correlation between measures of attention and apnea hypopnea index (AHI), even when controlling for age and premorbid intelligence. The investigators hypothesized that hypercapnia is inversely proportional to cognition given evidence that hypercapnia severity correlates with overall neurocognitive impairment.[17] Given the clear association between vigilance and driving ability, with implications for public safety, efforts have been underway to predict risk for MVAs in persons with OSA. Wong and colleagues[18] investigated the effects of 40 hours of sleep deprivation on cognition and simulated driving performance in OSA patients as compared with healthy controls. Vigilance was measured with the PVT. They found no association between OSA and attention, driving performance, or subjective sleepiness. Vakulin and colleagues[19] used the Stroop test to measure focused and selective attention in OSA patients undergoing driving simulator testing after normal sleep with or without alcohol, or sleep restriction. There was no association between poor driving performance and Stroop test outcomes. Recently, Karimi and colleagues[20] used the Gothenburg Sleep Resistance Test (GOSLING) to assess sustained attention in OSA patients with and without a MVA. Both reaction time and the proportion of lapses were significantly higher in OSA patients with a MVA. This study failed to show a dose-response relationship between OSA severity and MVA risk. Gozal and colleagues[21] proposed genetic differences to explain susceptible versus resilient OSA patients.

OBSTRUCTIVE SLEEP APNEA EFFECTS ON VERBAL MEMORY

Verbal memory can be divided into immediate recall, verbal learning, verbal delayed recall, and verbal recognition. A meta-analysis compiled by Wallace and Bucks[22] included studies using tests designed to provide delineation of these memory domains such as the Buschke Selective Reminding Test and the California Verbal Learning Test. OSA was found to have a medium adverse effect on verbal immediate recall compared with norm and control referenced data. OSA had a medium effect on verbal learning compared with controls and no significant effect compared with norms. There was a more consistent medium effect on verbal delayed recall using these reference sets. Verbal recognition, however, was not affected when comparing OSA to norm subjects and significantly affected compared with patients without OSA. The variability for verbal data could not be explained by age, publication status, study design, sample source, or disease severity. In addition, screening by polysomnogram or questionnaire did not affect the significance of results. A recent study by Hoth and colleagues[23] examined the differential effects of hypoxemia on memory. Forty subjects with an average AHI of 37.8/h of sleep were divided into relatively mild and severe hypoxemia groups based on minimum oxygen saturation and time less than 90% blood oxygenation. The mild group spent no more than 6% of sleep time less than 90%, whereas this was at least 20% for the severe group. Surprisingly, the severe hypoxemia group performed better on tests of immediate and delayed verbal recall. Compared with normative data, the severe hypoxemia group was average, but the low hypoxemia group was borderline low. This counterintuitive result is supported by studies in humans and animals demonstrating protective effects of intermittent hypoxemia for the brain and cardiovascular system.[24] Another study suggested that intermittent hypoxemia in rat brains can decrease nitric oxide related toxicity.[25]

Ramos and coworkers[26] evaluated the effects of OSA in a Hispanic/Latino population. Neurocognitive tests included the Brief-Spanish English Verbal Learning Test. The mean AHI was 9.0 with a range of 0 to 142. One of the important findings was that women were more likely to have verbal memory and learning deficits associated with OSA compared with men. Although the prevalence of OSA is higher in men,[1] there has been some suggestion that women are more susceptible to the effects of OSA at lower AHI levels.[27]

Edwards and colleagues[28] examined the effect of moderate to severe OSA on several neurocognitive domains, including learning and memory (L/M). OSA severity was based on AHI and oxygen desaturation index (ODI). Verbal and visual test results were grouped. In addition, blood cortisol levels were measured over a 24-hour period. ODI, but not AHI, severity was associated with 24-hour cortisol levels. AHI, ODI, and cortisol levels were all associated with L/M deficits. The investigators hypothesized that sympathetic overactivity manifest through the hypothalamic-pituitary-adrenal axis, as opposed to the apneas themselves, was responsible for neurocognitive impairment.

A review by Vaessen and colleagues[29] focused on subjective neurocognitive complaints comparing OSA patients to controls. They did not find a consistent memory complaint for OSA patients and attributed this in part to small sample sizes. It should also be noted that due to the gradual progression of OSA, these persons are not always aware of their deficits, which has significant implications for identification and treatment of OSA and undoubtedly contributes to the estimated large percentage of untreated individuals.[30]

OBSTRUCTIVE SLEEP APNEA EFFECTS ON VISUAL AND VISUOSPATIAL MEMORY

Analogous to verbal memory, visual memory consists of immediate recall, delayed recall, and recognition. There is a paucity of data examining the effect of OSA on this neurocognitive domain. The meta-analysis of Wallace and Bucks[22] showed visual immediate recall to be unimpaired for OSA patients compared with norms and controls. This unexpected finding was thought to be due to limitations in matching OSA to non-OSA data. They did not identify enough studies to qualify for meta-analysis of visual delayed recall or recognition.

Visuospatial memory involves recall of how image components relate to each other and is typically tested using a drawing task or recalling a specific image location. Effects of OSA vary depending on the comparison data.[22] Using control references, medium deficits were found in immediate and delayed visuospatial recall. No significant deficit was found compared with norms. The 2 studies identified testing visuospatial learning had conflicting results rendering the overall analysis insignificant. There were insufficient data to draw any conclusions regarding visuospatial recognition.

Lau and colleagues[31] recently reported effects of OSA on cognition including immediate and delayed visual memory in a Chinese cohort. Subjects with moderate to severe OSA (AHI >15) were compared with controls. They found a significant medium negative effect on delayed visual recall but no significant effect on visual learning. Further studies are needed to explore the effects of OSA on visual memory.

OBSTRUCTIVE SLEEP APNEA EFFECTS ON PSYCHOMOTOR FUNCTION AND PROCEDURAL MEMORY

Psychomotor function represents neurocognitive processing speed and is often measured by 2-hand coordination or reaction times. The meta-review by Bucks and colleagues[12] found an effect of OSA on psychomotor function in only 2 of 5 studies. No clear relationship with disease severity was identified. Only 2 of the 5 reviews considered age as a potential influence but found no relationship with cognition. None of the studies considered premorbid IQ as confounding factor. Kilpinen and colleagues[32] reviewed the effects of OSA on information processing, including psychomotor performance. Six of the studies reviewed used tests assessing pure psychomotor speed. Four of the 6 studies showed deficits associated with OSA. The review by Lal and colleagues[33] indicated fine-motor coordination to be diminished by OSA but motor speed was unimpaired.

The study by Ramos and colleagues[26] examined the effects of mild to moderate OSA on processing speed using the digit symbol substitution test (DSST). A deficit was seen for older women but not men in the unadjusted model. Accounting for age, education, sex, and other comorbidities eliminated a significant relationship. Although a large cohort of 8000 was included, the relatively lower mean AHI of 9.0 per hour may explain the lack of effect. Bawden and colleagues[34] also used the DSST to study the effects of OSA on psychomotor performance. Roughly 75% of the OSA subjects had moderate to severe disease. Control subjects were matched for age and education. OSA subjects were slower than controls but had fewer errors.

There is evidence that motor skill learning is also affected by OSA. Landry and colleagues[35] compared subjects with moderate OSA (mean AHI: 25.0) to controls matched for age and education. Performance on the sequential finger tapping task showed similar rates of improvement for OSA and control subjects in the evening. There was however a trend toward worse performance by OSA subjects with fewer typed sequences. The following morning, control subjects showed a significantly greater rate of improvement (15.4%) over baseline compared with OSA sufferers (1.8%). This greater rate of improvement was thought to reflect impaired memory consolidation and learning due to worse sleep quality for the OSA group. In a similar study, Djonlagic and colleagues[36] compared performance on a motor sequence learning task (MST) for moderate OSA subjects (mean AHI: 17.1) with age and subjective sleepiness-matched controls. There was no difference in rate of improvement with practice in the evening. Significantly greater improvement was noted the following morning for the control group. Subjects without OSA showed 14.7% improvement after a night of sleep compared with just 1.1% improvement for the OSA group. These results were not explained by diminished attention in the OSA subjects as PVT results were similar for both groups. This difference remained despite multiple learning trials in the morning. By matching sleep architecture for the 2 groups, the investigators were able to demonstrate a significant inverse correlation between arousal index and MST improvement. The same relationship was noted but less robust for AHI and MST scores. There was no such finding for oxygen saturation measures. Therefore, consolidation of procedure memory appears to be affected by sleep fragmentation but not oxygen desaturations.

OBSTRUCTIVE SLEEP APNEA EFFECTS ON EXECUTIVE FUNCTION

Olaithe and Bucks[37] examined the effects of OSA on various aspects of executive function, including shifting or mental flexibility, updating or changing working memory, inhibition, generativity or ability to access long term memory, and fluid reasoning, in a recent meta-analysis. Studies included patients with AHI greater than 5.0 compared with controls. Medium effect sizes were seen for shifting and generativity. Large effects were seen for updating and fluid reasoning. A very large effect was seen for inhibition. Because there were relatively few subjects with mild or moderate OSA, a dose-response over the full range of AHI severity could not be determined. Nonetheless, comparison of severe to very severe OSA did not reveal a graded effect on cognition. This review was not able to distinguish whether the deficits in executive function were directly due to OSA or to excessive daytime sleepiness from OSA.

Executive function can be divided into several subdomains. In addition to more traditional aspects of executive function including planning, cognitive shifting, and inhibition, Borges and colleagues[38] chose updating or the ability to change the content of working memory as well as dual task performance, and efficient access to long-term memory to analyze effects of OSA. Moderate to severe OSA subjects were compared with controls matched for age, IQ, and education. All subjects were free of diabetes, hypertension, or depression and had body mass indexes less than 26 kg/m^2. No significant differences were found for any aspects of executive function

between the OSA and control groups. The investigators suggested that comorbidities, including obesity, hypertension, diabetes, and depression, alone or in combination with OSA, may play a greater role in executive dysfunction than OSA alone.

Several studies have looked at effects of OSA on certain aspects of executive function as part of a larger examination of neurocognitive domains in the setting of sleep-disordered breathing.[16,39–44] Four of the studies showed executive function deficits associated with OSA.[39,41,43,44] Two of the studies did not show any effect of OSA on executive function.[16,40] One study had mixed results.[42] Although all studies except one[42] used the trail making test B, results were not consistently itemized for each test. Therefore, it was difficult to make direct comparisons as to the relative significance of individual findings.

OBSTRUCTIVE SLEEP APNEA EFFECTS ON OVERALL IQ

Several reviews have reported on the effects of OSA on global cognitive function.[14,33,45] The meta-review by Bucks and colleagues[12] found deficits in 2 of 4 reviews. It was suggested that hypoxemia may have more of an impact on overall IQ than sleep fragmentation. More recently, Canessa and colleagues[41] used the Mini-Mental State Evaluation (MMSE) to assess global cognition in controls and subjects with severe OSA. They found no significant difference in MMSE scores. The MrOS study[40] also examined cognition in a large cohort (n = 2636) of community-dwelling older men with mild versus moderate OSA followed an average of 3.4 years. The Modified MMSE (3MS), a more sensitive instrument than the MMSE, was used to measure overall cognition. They found that men with 1% or more of sleep time with oxygen saturation less than 90% had a greater decline on the 3MS compared with men with less than 1% of their sleep time less than 90%. No significant association between AHI and 3MS was found. A previous cross-sectional study of the same cohort did not reveal any association between sleep-related hypoxemia and the 3MS. It was hypothesized that oxidative stress, impaired glucose tolerance, and inflammation represented the pathologic response to sleep-related hypoxemia resulting in neurocognitive decline.

The effect of OSA on cognition has also been evaluated in older women. A prospective study by Yaffe and colleagues[46] evaluated 298 women (average age 82.3 years) without dementia and found that those with at least moderate OSA (defined as an AHI $\geq$ 15 per hour of sleep) at mean follow-up of 4.7 years were more likely to have mild cognitive impairment or dementia compared with women with AHI less than 15 per hour of sleep, even after adjusting for potential confounders (odds ratio 1.85; 95% confidence interval, 1.11–3.08). ODI and increased sleep time in apnea or hypopnea were also associated with cognitive decline; however, measures of sleep fragmentation were not.

NEUROCOGNITIVE EFFECTS OF OBSTRUCTIVE SLEEP APNEA FOR CHILDREN

The prevalence of OSA has been estimated at 13% to 66% in obese children[47–50] and 1.2% to 5.7% in nonobese children.[51] Neurocognitive development is a particularly critical aspect of maturation during childhood. These findings may have implications for overall IQ in later years. A recent review[52] noted any severity of OSA and even snoring increases the risk for problems with attention, executive function, behavior, and scholastic performance in children.

Bourke and colleagues[53] looked at children aged 7 to 12 classified as controls, snorers, mild OSA, and moderate/severe OSA. Overall cognition and executive function were measured. In addition, reading, spelling, and arithmetical skills were assessed. They found significantly lower full-scale and verbal IQ scores for all other groups compared with controls. Although nonverbal and performance IQ scores were lower than controls, these findings did not reach statistical significance. Executive function was not significantly different for snorers or OSA subjects as compared with controls. Similarly, reading, spelling, and arithmetical skills did not differ between snorers, OSA subjects, and controls. These results support the importance of treating snoring as well as mild and severe sleep-disordered breathing in children.

Another study by Jackman and colleagues[54] evaluated behavior as well as cognition in preschool children (age 3–5) also divided into controls, snorers, mild, and moderate/severe OSA. Behavior in the home was assessed by standardized parental rating. Snorers and mild OSA subjects were found to have poorer behavior compared with controls. For some behaviors, these 2 groups were even worse than the moderate/severe OSA group. No differences were seen for measures of global intelligence, attention, language, visuospatial ability, fine-motor skills, memory, or executive function. The investigators speculated that behavioral dysfunction was due to a higher degree of sleep fragmentation not captured by current measurement techniques in this pediatric population. They furthermore

reasoned that a greater drive to protect the brain from hypoxia at the expense of sleep consolidation produced these findings.

Landau and coworkers[55] studied children with of mean age 45 months (±9 months) with OSA (mean AHI 13.2 ± 10.7) compared with age-matched controls. They assessed cognition, behavior, and quality of life. Impairment of executive function (planning and fluency), attention, and receptive vocabulary were noted for OSA subjects compared with controls using the Kaufman assessment battery for children but not for the Behavior Rating Inventory of Executive Function-Preschool version (BRIEF-P). This correlates with the Jackman study that also used the BRIEF-P to assess executive function. Landau, like Jackman, also found more behavior problems in the OSA group. In addition, Landau documented worse quality of life in OSA children compared with controls. This study underscores the impact of OSA in early childhood and the importance of identifying and treating OSA in this population.

Other reports in children age 7 to 15 with OSA have shown deficits in working memory,[56,57] psychomotor efficiency,[57] executive function,[58] and IQ.[59] Variability of results can in part be seen due to varying tests to assess particular neurocognitive domains.

IMAGING: MAGNETIC RESONANCE SPECTROSCOPY, DIFFUSION TENSOR IMAGING, FUNCTIONAL MRI STUDIES

In the last few years, imaging modalities, including MRI, magnetic resonance spectroscopy (MRS), functional MRI (fMRI), and diffusion tensor imaging (DTI), have provided insights into structural, functional, and metabolic correlates of the neurocognitive effects of OSA. Recent reviews[60–62] have highlighted volume loss in the anterior cingulate, hippocampus, frontal, parietal, and temporal lobes associated with OSA severity. The study by Canessa and colleagues[41] used voxel-based morphometry (VBM) analysis of MRI-T1 images to assess gray-matter (GM) volumes and cognition in subjects with severe OSA compared with age- and education-matched controls. Reduced GM volume in left hippocampus, left posterior parietal cortex, and right superior frontal gyrus correlated with significant impairment in short- and long-term verbal memory, constructional ability, attention, and especially executive function.

Castronovo and coworkers[43] examined white matter (WM) tracts with DTI along with assessments of similar neurocognitive domains in severe OSA subjects compared with age- and education-matched controls. As opposed to correlating with gross numbers of neurons such as with VBM techniques, the fractional anisotropy evaluation of DTI attempts to determine the integrity of groups of neurons working together as functional units. Neurocognitive deficits involving attention, executive function, and memory were associated with diffuse reduction of WM tract integrity involving the bilateral parietal and frontal lobes. These changes are thought to contribute to slowed information processing.

O'Donoghue and colleagues[44] applied MRS to elucidate effects of severe OSA on neuronal viability. Vigilance, memory, and executive function were quantified as well and compared with age-matched controls. Although changes suggestive of decreased frontal lobe neuronal viability were seen, there were no correlations with neurocognitive function. Cerebral metabolite concentrations did, however, correlate with OSA severity.

Zhang and colleagues[63] used a visual mismatch task to show changes in fMRI activation for severe OSA subjects compared with age- and education-matched controls. They found reduced frontal activation in the anterior cingulate cortices (ACC), middle frontal gyri, and inferior frontal gyri, but increased activity in the right anterior prefrontal gyri (aPFG). Reaction times were significantly slower for OSA subjects. These results along with lower frontal activation were associated with duration of time below oxygen saturation less than 80% and arousal index. Other measures of sleep-disordered breathing, such as the apnea, hypopnea, and desaturation indices, showed no such relationship. These data indicate that oxygen desaturation and sleep fragmentation play a role in executive dysfunction for tasks such as this. Effects on reaction time implicate circuits responsible for the transfer of information as opposed to a primary failure of neuronal units per se. Furthermore, the increased right aPFG activity suggests a compensatory response needed for OSA subjects to complete the mismatch task.

MECHANISMS OF OBSTRUCTIVE SLEEP APNEA EFFECTS ON COGNITION

The intermittent hypoxia (IH) and sleep fragmentation seen in OSA provide a link between sleep-disordered breathing and impairment over a range of neurocognitive domains as asserted by Gozal.[64] To further elucidate the mechanisms of neuronal damage due to IH, Sapin and colleagues[65] exposed mice to 1 day (acute) versus 6 or 24 weeks (chronic) of IH. They found that chronic but not acute IH was associated with significant microglial changes in the dorsal hippocampus. Acute but not chronic IH increased cytokines associated with neuro-inflammation. These findings complement the data showing impaired memory and learning in human OSA subjects. Smith and colleagues[66] showed increases in inflammatory gene expression of cortical microglia for rats exposed to IH.

Sales and colleagues[67] measured cognition and biomarkers of oxidative stress in subjects with severe OSA and age-matched controls. Vitamin E, superoxide dismutase (SOD), and vitamin B11 were lower, while homocysteine was higher in OSA subjects. These subjects also performed worse on measures of attention, executive function, working, verbal, and delayed visual memory. An association was found between executive function measures and vitamin E levels as well as SOD. Nair and colleagues[68] identified NADPH oxidase as the driving force of oxidative stress induced spatial learning impairments in mice exposed to IH.

Sleep fragmentation has also been implicated in neurocognitive dysfunction mediated by neuro-inflammation. Ramesh and colleagues[69] used a mouse model to examine the effects of disrupted sleep without reduced total sleep on cognition in mice. They found an association between poor spatial learning, memory, sleepiness, and increased cortical expression of tumor necrosis factor-α (TNF-α). They further demonstrated the absence of sleepiness or neurocognitive dysfunction in TNF-α double receptor knockout mice. Last, mice treated with a TNF-α neutralizing antibody did not develop sleepiness or neurocognitive dysfunction despite sleep fragmentation.

Sympathetic overdrive is another potential mechanism by which OSA affects cognition. Goya and colleagues[70] measured muscle sympathetic nerve activity (MSNA) in subjects with severe OSA and persons with mild OSA matched for age and education. Baseline MSNA was higher in severe OSA subjects. Further MSNA increases and worse executive function were seen in severe versus mild OSA subjects. The study by Fatouleh and colleagues[71] showed increased activation in the bilateral dorsolateral PFC, medial PFC, dorsal precuneus, ACC, retrosplenial cortex, and caudate nucleus associated with increased MSNA in OSA subjects. These cerebral areas are known to be involved in modulation of sympathetic outflow.

IMPACT OF CONTINUOUS POSITIVE AIR PRESSURE

CPAP is the most commonly prescribed treatment of OSA. This therapy has been shown to eliminate respiratory disturbances and improve daytime alertness.[72] Its effect on domains of neuro-cognitive function has been less consistently demonstrated.

The previously described meta-analysis by Olaithe and Bucks described reductions in OSA-related impairment across 5 subcomponents of executive function (ie, shifting, updating, inhibiting, generating, and fluid reasoning) with CPAP therapy.[37] Although age and disease severity did not moderate these outcomes, this review was unable to exclude the effects of premorbid intelligence because not all included studies provided this information.

In a multicenter study of 174 subjects with moderate to severe OSA, measures of subjective and objective sleepiness and neurocognitive function were assessed before and after 3 months of CPAP therapy.[73] In regard to daytime sleepiness, CPAP treatment resulted in a marked and dose-dependent reduction in subjective daytime sleepiness (ESS) but did not affect Maintenance of Wakefulness Test–derived mean sleep latencies. Nearly 20% of subjects who used CPAP for more than 7 hours per night had abnormal sleepiness scores despite seemingly adequate use. There were significant improvements in verbal memory and executive function but not vigilance among these subjects at 3 months.

Research protocols attempting to determine the impact of CPAP therapy on neurocognitive outcomes have been hampered by a variety of methodological factors. In an effort to address many of these limitations, a large multicenter study (APPLES) randomly assigned 1105 subjects diagnosed with OSA to either active CPAP or sham CPAP.[74] CPAP use for the active arm averaged 4.2 hours per night. At 2- and 6-month follow-up, subjective and objective sleepiness were significantly reduced in actively treated participants and most prominently among those with severe OSA (AHI >30). The primary measure of executive and frontal-lobe function (E/F) was improved at 2 months in the active CPAP group compared with sham CPAP, but no differences were noted among groups in regard to measures of L/M or attention and psychomotor function (A/P) at 2 or 6 months. Further stratification by markers of sleep apnea severity (AHI or oxygen desaturation) resulted in transient differences among study arms in the primary E/F and one secondary E/F variable.[74] The study may have been somewhat limited by the absence of a healthy control group and the overall intelligence of the participants, who may have had relatively high neurocognitive reserve. However, adjustment for IQ did not alter the findings. Despite the lack of robust neurocognitive improvements with CPAP therapy, it is possible that the neurocognitive benefits related to CPAP may require more than 6 hours of use per night[43] or perhaps may occur among a genetically unique subset of subjects.

Lin and colleagues[75] recently investigated the effect of good versus suboptimal CPAP compliance on neurocognitive measures (CANTAB). Subjects that used CPAP for more than 70% of nights over 3 months had improvements in decision making and response control domains compared with less adherent subjects.

The effects of CPAP therapy on neurocognitive function specifically among older adults have been studied and have demonstrated inconsistent benefit. Gutierrez Iglesias and colleagues[76] found CPAP treatment was beneficial for selective and divided attention, working memory, verbal and short-term memory, and visual long-term memory.

In the PROOF study, Crawford-Achour and colleagues[77] assessed the benefit of CPAP therapy on neurocognitive outcomes in those 65 years of age and older with severe OSA at baseline and at 10-year follow-up. Those subjects that received CPAP were very compliant with a mean usage of more than 6 hours per night. Compared with untreated controls, CPAP users demonstrated maintenance of memory and improvements in mental abilities. The limitations of this study are noteworthy as treated subjects were few (26% of sample), had worse OSA severity (higher AHI and ODI), were more symptomatic (higher ESS) at baseline, and were selected to receive therapy at the discretion of their primary care physician. Another study of CPAP therapy in older adults with OSA found improvements in daytime sleepiness at 3 months, particularly in those with increased CPAP use and higher scores on pretreatment ESS. These benefits were shown at 12 months but were not seen for other neurocognitive measures (MMSE, Trail Making Test-B, DSST, and simple and 4-choice reaction time), which remained unchanged at 12 months.[78]

CPAP therapy may provide cognitive benefits in patients with neurodegenerative disorders. In a recent study by Troussière and colleagues,[79] those subjects with mild-to-moderate Alzheimer disease and severe OSA who used CPAP had significantly less cognitive decline at 3-year follow-up compared with an otherwise matched non-CPAP group.

There is increasing evidence that CPAP therapy can reverse sleep apnea–related brain morphologic changes. The Canessa study, described previously, reported reversal of GM volume decrements after 3 months of CPAP treatment in specific hippocampal and frontal regions that correlated with improvements in memory, attention, and executive function.[41] Other investigators using brain MRS[44] found 6 months of CPAP

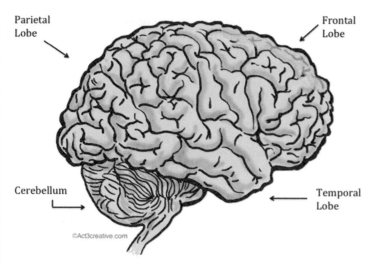

Fig. 1. Green area represents OSA effect on executive function that is localized to the frontal lobe. (Ron Hill/Act 3 LLC, www.act3 creative.com. *Data from* Castronovo V, Scifo P, Castellano A, et al. White matter integrity in obstructive sleep apnea before and after treatment. Sleep 2014;37(9):1465–75.)

therapy did not improve metabolite ratios in the frontal lobe but did eliminate significant differences for the hippocampus compared with controls. Although measures of vigilance and executive function showed some improvement with this length of CPAP treatment, cerebral metabolite concentrations did not correlate with neurocognitive test results.

The effects of 3 and 12 months of CPAP therapy on WM fiber integrity, as measured by DTI, and neurocognitive performance were assessed in 17 positive air pressure–naïve OSA subjects and 15 healthy controls.[43] Despite only limited changes noted in WM integrity among treated subjects at 3 months, there was near complete normalization in affected regions in CPAP-compliant subjects at 1 year. These changes paralleled neurocognitive test improvements in memory, attention, and executive function.

CONTINUOUS POSITIVE AIR PRESSURE WITHDRAWAL

Others have evaluated the consequences of acute and short-term CPAP withdrawal on neurocognitive outcomes. In a study by Filtness and colleagues,[80] 11 subjects who were deemed long-term (mean 7.8 years) CPAP compliant users underwent 2 daytime driving simulations, one following regular nighttime CPAP use and the other after sleeping one night without therapy. There were significantly more driving incidents, decreased latency to first incident, marked increase in α and θ electroencephalogram activity and increased subjective sleepiness the day following CPAP withdrawal. Two nights of CPAP withdrawal among participants with either mild to moderate or severe OSA were associated with reappearance of both subjective and objective

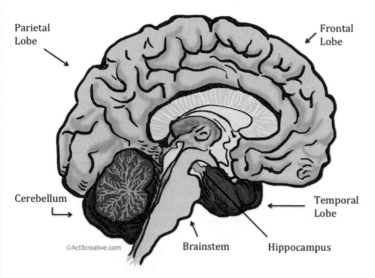

Fig. 2. Green area represents OSA effect on memory that is localized to the hippocampus. (Ron Hill/ Act 3 LLC, www.act3creative.com. *Data from* Castronovo V, Scifo P, Castellano A, et al. White matter integrity in obstructive sleep apnea before and after treatment. Sleep 2014;37(9):1465–75.)

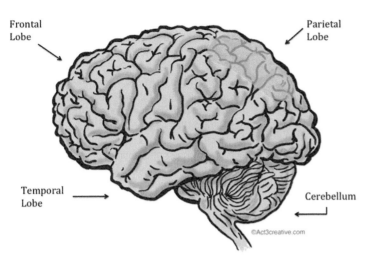

Frontal Lobe

Parietal Lobe

Temporal Lobe

Cerebellum

©Act3creative.com

Fig. 3. Green area represents OSA effect on abstract reasoning that is localized to the parietal lobe. (Ron Hill/Act 3 LLC, www.act3creative.com. *Data from* Castronovo V, Scifo P, Castellano A, et al. White matter integrity in obstructive sleep apnea before and after treatment. Sleep 2014;37(9):1465–75.)

sleepiness and altered vigilance testing to pre-treatment levels.[81] However, psychomotor performance measures of divided attention and vigilance were not significantly altered by 2 weeks of CPAP discontinuation in a study conducted by Kohler and colleagues.[82]

SUMMARY

Studies have shown that OSA can impair attention, verbal memory, executive function, and learning. Affected cognitive domains that localize to discrete regions of the brain, with documented structural changes, are shown in **Figs. 1–3**. There is a paucity of data examining OSA effects on delayed visual memory, visual perception, and visuospatial memory. Imaging modalities including MRI with VBM, DTI, MRS, and fMRI provide insight into the impact of OSA on brain structure and function. Magnetic resonance elastography is a relatively new technique to measure brain tissue integrity that could further expand this knowledge.[83] Mechanisms of cerebral remodeling include neuro-inflammation, oxidative stress, and sympathetic overactivation. CPAP use of at least 4 hours per night improves executive function at 2 months. CPAP use of 6 hours or more may provide additional neurocognitive improvement for vulnerable populations with decreased neurocognitive reserve in the setting of aging and comorbidities, such as cardiovascular disease, diabetes, mild cognitive impairment, and Alzheimer dementia. Genetic profiles may also help predict neurocognitive effects of CPAP. Further studies are needed to elucidate mechanisms of neurocognitive impairment and identify factors most likely to enhance the beneficial effects of CPAP on cognition for OSA patients.

REFERENCES

1. Young T, Palta M, Dempsey J, et al. The occurrence of sleep-disordered breathing among middle-aged adults. N Engl J Med 1993;328(17):1230–5.
2. Ancoli-Israel S, Kripke DF, Klauber MR, et al. Sleep-disordered breathing in community-dwelling elderly. Sleep 1991;14(6):486–95.
3. Young T, Peppard PE, Gottlieb DJ. Epidemiology of obstructive sleep apnea: a population health perspective. Am J Respir Crit Care Med 2002; 165(9):1217–39.
4. Peppard PE, Young T, Palta M, et al. Prospective study of the association between sleep-disordered breathing and hypertension. N Engl J Med 2000; 342(19):1378–84.
5. Marin JM, Carrizo SJ, Vicente E, et al. Long-term cardiovascular outcomes in men with obstructive sleep apnoea-hypopnoea with or without treatment with continuous positive airway pressure: an observational study. Lancet 2005;365(9464):1046–53.
6. Arzt M, Young T, Finn L, et al. Association of sleep-disordered breathing and the occurrence of stroke. Am J Respir Crit Care Med 2005;172(11):1447–51.
7. Peppard PE, Szklo-Coxe M, Hla KM, et al. Longitudinal association of sleep-related breathing disorder and depression. Arch Intern Med 2006;166(16): 1709–15.
8. Aronsohn RS, Whitmore H, Van Cauter E, et al. Impact of untreated obstructive sleep apnea on glucose control in type 2 diabetes. Am J Respir Crit Care Med 2010;181(5):507–13.
9. Karaca Z, Ismailogullari S, Korkmaz S, et al. Obstructive sleep apnoea syndrome is associated with relative hypocortisolemia and decreased hypothalamo-pituitary-adrenal axis response to 1 and 250 μg ACTH and glucagon stimulation tests. Sleep Med 2013;14(2):160–4.

10. Mulgrew AT, Nasvadi G, Butt A, et al. Risk and severity of motor vehicle crashes in patients with obstructive sleep apnoea/hypopnoea. Thorax 2008;63(6):536–41.

11. Ronald J, Delaive K, Roos L, et al. Health care utilization in the 10 years prior to diagnosis in obstructive sleep apnea syndrome patients. Sleep 1999; 22(2):225–9.

12. Bucks RS, Olaithe M, Eastwood P. Neurocognitive function in obstructive sleep apnoea: a meta-review. Respirology 2013;18(1):61–70.

13. Gagnon K, Baril AA, Gagnon JF, et al. Cognitive impairment in obstructive sleep apnea. Pathol Biol (Paris) 2014;62(5):233–40.

14. Sforza E, Roche F. Sleep apnea syndrome and cognition. Front Neurol 2012;3:87.

15. Batool-Anwar S, Kales SN, Patel SR, et al. Obstructive sleep apnea and psychomotor vigilance task performance. Nat Sci Sleep 2014;6:65–71.

16. Olaithe M, Skinner TC, Hillman D, et al. Cognition and nocturnal disturbance in OSA: the importance of accounting for age and premorbid intelligence. Sleep Breath 2015;19(1):221–30.

17. Findley LJ, Barth JT, Powers DC, et al. Cognitive impairment in patients with obstructive sleep apnea and associated hypoxemia. Chest 1986; 90(5):686–90.

18. Wong KK, Marshall NS, Grunstein RR, et al. Comparing the neurocognitive effects of 40 h sustained wakefulness in patients with untreated OSA and healthy controls. J Sleep Res 2008;17(3): 322–30.

19. Vakulin A, Catcheside PG, Baulk SD, et al. Individual variability and predictors of driving simulator impairment in patients with obstructive sleep apnea. J Clin Sleep Med 2014;10(6):647–55.

20. Karimi M, Hedner J, Zou D, et al. Attention deficits detected in cognitive tests differentiate between sleep apnea patients with or without a motor vehicle accident. Sleep Med 2015;16(4):528–33.

21. Gozal D, Capdevila OS, Kheirandish-Gozal L, et al. APOE epsilon 4 allele, cognitive dysfunction, and obstructive sleep apnea in children. Neurology 2007;69(3):243–9.

22. Wallace A, Bucks RS. Memory and obstructive sleep apnea: a meta-analysis. Sleep 2013;36(2):203–20.

23. Hoth KF, Zimmerman ME, Meschede KA, et al. Obstructive sleep apnea: impact of hypoxemia on memory. Sleep Breath 2013;17(2):811–7.

24. Manukhina EB, Downey HF, Mallet RT. Role of nitric oxide in cardiovascular adaptation to intermittent hypoxia. Exp Biol Med (Maywood) 2006;231(4): 343–65.

25. Goryacheva AV, Kruglov SV, Pshennikova MG, et al. Adaptation to intermittent hypoxia restricts nitric oxide overproduction and prevents beta-amyloid toxicity in rat brain. Nitric Oxide 2010;23(4):289–99.

26. Ramos AR, Tarraf W, Rundek T, et al. Obstructive sleep apnea and neurocognitive function in a Hispanic/Latino population. Neurology 2015;84(4): 391–8.

27. Young T, Hutton R, Finn L, et al. The gender bias in sleep apnea diagnosis. Are women missed because they have different symptoms? Arch Intern Med 1996;156(21):2445–51.

28. Edwards KM, Kamat R, Tomfohr LM, et al. Obstructive sleep apnea and neurocognitive performance: the role of cortisol. Sleep Med 2014;15(1):27–32.

29. Vaessen TJ, Overeem S, Sitskoorn MM. Cognitive complaints in obstructive sleep apnea. Sleep Med Rev 2015;19:51–8.

30. Bixler EO, Vgontzas AN, Lin HM, et al. Prevalence of sleep-disordered breathing in women: effects of gender. Am J Respir Crit Care Med 2001;163(3 Pt 1):608–13.

31. Lau EY, Ip MS, Lee TM. Neurocognitive and psychosocial outcomes of obstructive sleep apnoea in Hong Kong Chinese. Hong Kong Med J 2014; 20(Suppl 7):19–23.

32. Kilpinen R, Saunamaki T, Jehkonen M. Information processing speed in obstructive sleep apnea syndrome: a review. Acta Neurol Scand 2014;129(4): 209–18.

33. Lal C, Strange C, Bachman D. Neurocognitive impairment in obstructive sleep apnea. Chest 2012;141(6):1601–10.

34. Bawden FC, Oliveira CA, Caramelli P. Impact of obstructive sleep apnea on cognitive performance. Arq Neuropsiquiatr 2011;69(4):585–9.

35. Landry S, Anderson C, Andrewartha P, et al. The impact of obstructive sleep apnea on motor skill acquisition and consolidation. J Clin Sleep Med 2014;10(5):491–6.

36. Djonlagic I, Saboisky J, Carusona A, et al. Increased sleep fragmentation leads to impaired off-line consolidation of motor memories in humans. PLoS One 2012;7(3):e34106.

37. Olaithe M, Bucks RS. Executive dysfunction in OSA before and after treatment: a meta-analysis. Sleep 2013;36(9):1297–305.

38. Borges JG, Ginani GE, Hachul H, et al. Executive functioning in obstructive sleep apnea syndrome patients without comorbidities: focus on the fractionation of executive functions. J Clin Exp Neuropsychol 2013;35(10):1094–107.

39. Idiaquez J, Santos I, Santin J, et al. Neurobehavioral and autonomic alterations in adults with obstructive sleep apnea. Sleep Med 2014;15(11):1319–23.

40. Blackwell T, Yaffe K, Laffan A, et al. Associations between sleep-disordered breathing, nocturnal hypoxemia, and subsequent cognitive decline in older community-dwelling men: the osteoporotic fractures in men sleep study. J Am Geriatr Soc 2015;63(3): 453–61.

41. Canessa N, Castronovo V, Cappa SF, et al. Obstructive sleep apnea: brain structural changes and neurocognitive function before and after treatment. Am J Respir Crit Care Med 2011;183(10):1419–26.

42. Torelli F, Moscufo N, Garreffa G, et al. Cognitive profile and brain morphological changes in obstructive sleep apnea. Neuroimage 2011;54(2):787–93.

43. Castronovo V, Scifo P, Castellano A, et al. White matter integrity in obstructive sleep apnea before and after treatment. Sleep 2014;37(9):1465–75.

44. O'Donoghue FJ, Wellard RM, Rochford PD, et al. Magnetic resonance spectroscopy and neurocognitive dysfunction in obstructive sleep apnea before and after CPAP treatment. Sleep 2012;35(1):41–8.

45. Kielb SA, Ancoli-Israel S, Rebok GW, et al. Cognition in obstructive sleep apnea-hypopnea syndrome (OSAS): current clinical knowledge and the impact of treatment. Neuromolecular Med 2012; 14(3):180–93.

46. Yaffe K, Laffan AM, Harrison SL, et al. Sleep-disordered breathing, hypoxia, and risk of mild cognitive impairment and dementia in older women. JAMA 2011;306(6):613–9.

47. Mallory GB Jr, Fiser DH, Jackson R. Sleep-associated breathing disorders in morbidly obese children and adolescents. J Pediatr 1989;115(6):892–7.

48. Wing YK, Hui SH, Pak WM, et al. A controlled study of sleep related disordered breathing in obese children. Arch Dis Child 2003;88(12):1043–7.

49. Silvestri JM, Weese-Mayer DE, Bass MT, et al. Polysomnography in obese children with a history of sleep-associated breathing disorders. Pediatr Pulmonol 1993;16(2):124–9.

50. Marcus CL, Curtis S, Koerner CB, et al. Evaluation of pulmonary function and polysomnography in obese children and adolescents. Pediatr Pulmonol 1996; 21(3):176–83.

51. Marcus CL, Brooks LJ, Draper KA, et al. Diagnosis and management of childhood obstructive sleep apnea syndrome. Pediatrics 2012;130(3):576–84.

52. Grigg-Damberger M, Ralls F. Cognitive dysfunction and obstructive sleep apnea: from cradle to tomb. Curr Opin Pulm Med 2012;18(6):580–7.

53. Bourke R, Anderson V, Yang JS, et al. Cognitive and academic functions are impaired in children with all severities of sleep-disordered breathing. Sleep Med 2011;12(5):489–96.

54. Jackman AR, Biggs SN, Walter LM, et al. Sleep-disordered breathing in preschool children is associated with behavioral, but not cognitive, impairments. Sleep Med 2012;13(6):621–31.

55. Landau YE, Bar-Yishay O, Greenberg-Dotan S, et al. Impaired behavioral and neurocognitive function in preschool children with obstructive sleep apnea. Pediatr Pulmonol 2012;47(2):180–8.

56. Biggs SN, Bourke R, Anderson V, et al. Working memory in children with sleep-disordered breathing: objective versus subjective measures. Sleep Med 2011;12(9):887–91.

57. Hannon TS, Rofey DL, Ryan CM, et al. Relationships among obstructive sleep apnea, anthropometric measures, and neurocognitive functioning in adolescents with severe obesity. J Pediatr 2012;160(5):732–5.

58. Esposito M, Antinolfi L, Gallai B, et al. Executive dysfunction in children affected by obstructive sleep apnea syndrome: an observational study. Neuropsychiatr Dis Treat 2013;9:1087–94.

59. Miano S, Paolino MC, Urbano A, et al. Neurocognitive assessment and sleep analysis in children with sleep-disordered breathing. Clin Neurophysiol 2011;122(2):311–9.

60. Ferini-Strambi L, Marelli S, Galbiati A, et al. Effects of continuous positive airway pressure on cognition and neuroimaging data in sleep apnea. Int J Psychophysiol 2013;89(2):203–12.

61. Veasey SC. Piecing together phenotypes of brain injury and dysfunction in obstructive sleep apnea. Front Neurol 2012;3:139.

62. Harper RM, Kumar R, Ogren JA, et al. Sleep-disordered breathing: effects on brain structure and function. Respir Physiol Neurobiol 2013;188(3):383–91.

63. Zhang X, Ma L, Li S, et al. A functional MRI evaluation of frontal dysfunction in patients with severe obstructive sleep apnea. Sleep Med 2011;12(4): 335–40.

64. Gozal D. CrossTalk proposal: the intermittent hypoxia attending severe obstructive sleep apnoea does lead to alterations in brain structure and function. J Physiol 2013;591(2):379–81.

65. Sapin E, Peyron C, Roche F, et al. Chronic intermittent hypoxia induces chronic low-grade neuroinflammation in the dorsal hippocampus of mice. Sleep 2015;38(10):1537–46.

66. Smith SM, Friedle SA, Watters JJ. Chronic intermittent hypoxia exerts CNS region-specific effects on rat microglial inflammatory and TLR4 gene expression. PLoS One 2013;8(12):e81584.

67. Sales LV, Bruin VM, D'Almeida V, et al. Cognition and biomarkers of oxidative stress in obstructive sleep apnea. Clinics (Sao Paulo) 2013;68(4):449–55.

68. Nair D, Dayyat EA, Zhang SX, et al. Intermittent hypoxia-induced cognitive deficits are mediated by NADPH oxidase activity in a murine model of sleep apnea. PLoS One 2011;6(5):e19847.

69. Ramesh V, Nair D, Zhang SX, et al. Disrupted sleep without sleep curtailment induces sleepiness and cognitive dysfunction via the tumor necrosis factor-alpha pathway. J Neuroinflammation 2012;9:91.

70. Goya TT, Silva RF, Guerra RS, et al. Increased muscle sympathetic nerve activity and impaired executive performance capacity in obstructive sleep apnea. Sleep 2016;39(1):25–33.

71. Fatouleh RH, Hammam E, Lundblad LC, et al. Functional and structural changes in the brain associated

with the increase in muscle sympathetic nerve activity in obstructive sleep apnoea. Neuroimage Clin 2014;6:275–83.

72. Gay P, Weaver T, Loube D, et al. Evaluation of positive airway pressure treatment for sleep related breathing disorders in adults. Sleep 2006;29(3):381–401.

73. Antic NA, Catcheside P, Buchan C, et al. The effect of CPAP in normalizing daytime sleepiness, quality of life, and neurocognitive function in patients with moderate to severe OSA. Sleep 2011;34(1):111–9.

74. Kushida CA, Nichols DA, Holmes TH, et al. Effects of continuous positive airway pressure on neurocognitive function in obstructive sleep apnea patients: the apnea positive pressure long-term efficacy study (APPLES). Sleep 2012;35(12):1593–602.

75. Lin SW, Chou YT, Kao KC, et al. Immediate and long-term neurocognitive outcome in patients with obstructive sleep apnea syndrome after continuous positive airway pressure treatment. Indian J Otolaryngol Head Neck Surg 2015;67(Suppl 1):79–85.

76. Gutierrez Iglesias B, Jacas Escarceller C, Bardes Robles I, et al. Effectiveness of 6-months continuous positive airway pressure treactment in OSAS-related cognitive deficit in older adults. Behav Neurol 2013; 26(3):191–4.

77. Crawford-Achour E, Dauphinot V, Martin MS, et al. Protective effect of long-term CPAP therapy on cognitive performance in elderly patients with severe OSA: the PROOF study. J Clin Sleep Med 2015;11(5):519–24.

78. McMillan A, Bratton DJ, Faria R, et al. Continuous positive airway pressure in older people with obstructive sleep apnoea syndrome (PREDICT): a 12-month, multicentre, randomised trial. Lancet Respir Med 2014;2(10):804–12.

79. Troussière AC, Charley CM, Salleron J, et al. Treatment of sleep apnoea syndrome decreases cognitive decline in patients with alzheimer's disease. J Neurol Neurosurg Psychiatry 2014;85(12):1405–8.

80. Filtness AJ, Reyner LA, Horne JA. One night's CPAP withdrawal in otherwise compliant OSA patients: marked driving impairment but good awareness of increased sleepiness. Sleep Breath 2012;16(3):865–71.

81. Young LR, Taxin ZH, Norman RG, et al. Response to CPAP withdrawal in patients with mild versus severe obstructive sleep apnea/hypopnea syndrome. Sleep 2013;36(3):405–12.

82. Kohler M, Stoewhas AC, Ayers L, et al. Effects of continuous positive airway pressure therapy withdrawal in patients with obstructive sleep apnea: a randomized controlled trial. Am J Respir Crit Care Med 2011;184(10):1192–9.

83. Kruse SA, Rose GH, Glaser KJ, et al. Magnetic resonance elastography of the brain. Neuroimage 2008; 39(1):231–7.

Personalized Medicine for Obstructive Sleep Apnea Therapies
Are We There Yet?

Bradley A. Edwards, PhD[a],*, Shane Landry, PhD[a],
Simon A. Joosten, MBBS, BMedSc, FRACP, PhD[b,c],
Garun S. Hamilton, MBBS, FRACP, PhD[b,c]

KEYWORDS

• Apnea • Phenotyping • Combination therapy

KEY POINTS

- Despite the existence of several treatments for obstructive sleep apnea (OSA), it is difficult for clinicians to know which therapy to recommend for a particular individual because they are either poorly tolerated or only resolve OSA in a proportion of patients.
- Recent evidence has highlighted that OSA is a multifactorial disorder, whereby each individual has OSA due to a combination of different pathophysiologic traits.
- Given this evidence, the concept of personalized medicine and the need for individualized therapy for OSA patients is now receiving a wealth of attention.
- Tools have now been developed to quantify deficits in specific physiologic traits contributing to OSA in a given individual.
- The development of such tools provides clinicians with a new way to systematically determine what treatment options are best suited for individual patients, paving the way toward personalizing the treatment of OSA.

Obstructive sleep apnea (OSA) is a highly prevalent sleep disorder with serious cardiovascular[1–3] and neurocognitive consequences.[4] Importantly, the currently available treatments have been shown to improve both the physiologic and the metabolic consequences of OSA and possibly even increase survival in those individuals in whom the intervention effectively treats the disorder. However, a major concern for both patients and clinicians is that in many cases the current treatments (discussed later) are either poorly tolerated (both initially and long-term adherence) or only resolve OSA in a proportion of patients. Therefore, understanding OSA pathophysiology

B.A. Edwards and S. Landry contributed equally to this work.

Disclosure Statement: Dr B.A. Edwards is supported by the National Health and Medical Research Council (NHMRC) of Australia's CJ Martin Overseas Biomedical Fellowship (1035115). Dr S. Landry is supported by the NHMRC NeuroSleep Centre of Research Excellence. G.S. Hamilton has received equipment to support research from Resmed and Philips Respironics.

[a] Sleep and Circadian Medicine Laboratory, Department of Physiology, School of Psychological Sciences and Monash Institute of Cognitive and Clinical Neurosciences, Monash University, 264 Ferntree Gully Road, Notting Hill 3168, Australia; [b] Monash Lung and Sleep, Monash Medical Centre, 246 Clayton Road, Clayton 3168, Victoria, Australia; [c] Department of Medicine, School of Clinical Sciences, Faculty of Medicine, Nursing and Health Sciences, Monash University, Clayton 3800, Victoria, Australia

* Corresponding author. Sleep and Circadian Medicine Laboratory, Monash University, Ground Floor BASE Facility, 264 Ferntree Gully Road, Clayton, Victoria, Australia.

E-mail address: bradley.edwards@monash.edu

Sleep Med Clin 11 (2016) 299–311
http://dx.doi.org/10.1016/j.jsmc.2016.05.003
1556-407X/16/$ – see front matter © 2016 Elsevier Inc. All rights reserved.

and developing efficacious treatments are clinical imperatives.

CURRENT TREATMENT OPTIONS FOR OBSTRUCTIVE SLEEP APNEA PATIENTS
Continuous Positive Airway Pressure

Continuous positive airway pressure (CPAP) is the current gold-standard treatment for OSA and works by pneumatically splinting open the upper airway to the point that airway obstruction is not possible. CPAP therapy is exceedingly effective in abolishing OSA and improves hypoxemic and sleep quality parameters.[5–7] Furthermore, it has been shown to improve daytime sleepiness and quality of life as well as reduce hypertension and the risk of fatal and nonfatal cardiovascular events.[8–10] For these reasons, clinicians usually recommend CPAP as the first-line treatment for OSA. Despite its effectiveness, CPAP is poorly tolerated by many individuals, with up to 50% of patients unable to tolerate or adhere to therapy beyond 3 months.[11,12] For those that refuse or cannot tolerate this treatment, clinicians often consider trialing alternative treatments/interventions such as mandibular advancement splints (MAS), upper airway surgical procedures, or weight loss.

Mandibular Advancement Splints

MAS devices work by repositioning the tongue and bringing the mandible forward, thereby tightening the soft tissue and muscles of the upper airway and increasing the lateral cross-sectional dimensions and overall volume of the airway.[13] Between ~48% and 64% of patients can be effectively treated with a MAS device (defined as reducing the apnea-hypopnea index [AHI] to <5 events/h), although this varies substantially between studies (in part due to the definition used for treatment success).[14] Although in general MAS therapy is less effective in reducing the AHI compared with CPAP, the improvement in other important patient health outcomes (ie, daytime sleepiness, neurobehavioral, and blood pressure) with MAS therapy appears to be equivalent to CPAP.[15,16] A potential reason for the equivalent effects of CPAP and MAS on these health outcomes may be attributed to a higher adherence to MAS therapy offsetting the greater treatment efficacy of CPAP.[15]

Upper Airway Surgery

Although less commonly used compared with CPAP or MAS, various surgical procedures are also used clinically for the treatment of OSA. Most often these are last resort options, typically only initiated once a patient has demonstrated noncompliance with CPAP or MAS. The most common surgical treatment of OSA is a procedure called an uvulopalatopharyngoplasty or UPPP,[17] which involves the removal of the tonsils and adenoids as well as a "tightening" of the soft palate. However, there are several other procedures surgeons consider, each targeting different structures in the airway, including: nasal surgery, tonsillectomy, various palatal procedures, tongue base reduction and repositioning surgeries, maxillomandibular advancements (MMA), and in rare cases, tracheostomy.[18] Nonetheless, similar to MAS therapy, the treatment success of these procedures varies considerably in the literature. This variability may be attributed to the type of procedure, characteristics of the patients undergoing surgery, and definitions of treatment success.[19]

Weight Loss

Obesity is a leading risk factor for OSA.[20] Accordingly, weight loss via lifestyle interventions (diet, exercise, or both) for overweight or obese OSA patients is commonly recommended by clinicians, not only to lessen the severity of OSA but also to offset the wealth of obesity-related health problems. Systematic review and meta-analysis of intensive weight loss interventions suggest that these can significantly reduce both the body mass index (BMI) and the AHI; however, resolution of OSA is only achieved in a minority of individuals.[21,22] Surgical weight loss procedures are typically used in cases of severe obesity and have been shown to have a greater efficacy in reducing BMI and AHI compared with lifestyle interventions.[23] Such procedures result in reducing the AHI by an average of 71%; however, complete resolution of OSA is still uncommon (less than 38%), with many patients demonstrating a residual AHI in the moderate severity range.[24]

Summary

Notably, a common finding among the non-CPAP interventions is that they resolve OSA in only a portion of patients, and the success rate between studies varies dramatically.[14,24,25] Importantly, all of the current treatments for OSA use an overly simplistic "one-size-fits-all" approach that fails to take into account the multiple "phenotypes" now recognized to comprise OSA. Given that the concept of precision or personalized medicine is gaining in popularity for the treatment of a variety of diseases, there is now a great deal of momentum to develop an individualized approach to treating OSA, whereby newer treatment strategies personalized to an OSA patient's requirements are used. However, in order to deliver such an approach, an appreciation of the multiple causes of OSA must first be described.

OBSTRUCTIVE SLEEP APNEA IS A MULTIFACTORIAL DISORDER

Although OSA has often been thought of as a disorder that is caused by unfavorable upper airway anatomy, which leads to a more collapsible airway during sleep, there is now a wealth of evidence demonstrating that the causes of OSA are multifactorial. Specifically, recent evidence has identified several nonanatomic factors (or traits) that also play an important role in OSA pathogenesis.[26] These factors include (1) an oversensitive ventilatory control system (ie, ventilatory control instability or high loop gain), (2) a low respiratory arousal threshold, and (3) poor pharyngeal muscle responsiveness or effectiveness during sleep. Importantly, the relative contribution of each of these traits (**Fig. 1**) varies substantially between individuals.[26,27] Thus, OSA occurs for different reasons in different people.

Despite the multifactorial nature of OSA, the current standard treatment options (CPAP, MAS, upper airway surgery) are all directed at improving upper airway anatomy only and have variable efficacy (**Fig. 1**). The variable response to these anatomically directed treatments likely results from 2 potential failures of the therapy. First, the treatment may not be powerful enough to correct gross anatomic deficits; second, the treatments do not address nonanatomic contributors to OSA (loop gain, arousal threshold, muscle responsiveness). Given that nonanatomic mechanisms play an important role in the majority (69%) of OSA patients,[26] there has been an intense research effort into identifying therapies (many of which are highlighted in later discussion) that could be used to alter these traits.

Alternative Therapies Targeting the Nonanatomic Traits

High loop gain
A key physiologic trait contributing to OSA severity in approximately one-third of OSA patients is a hypersensitive ventilatory control system, also referred to as a high "loop gain."[28–30] Loop gain is an engineering term that describes the sensitivity of the negative feedback system controlling

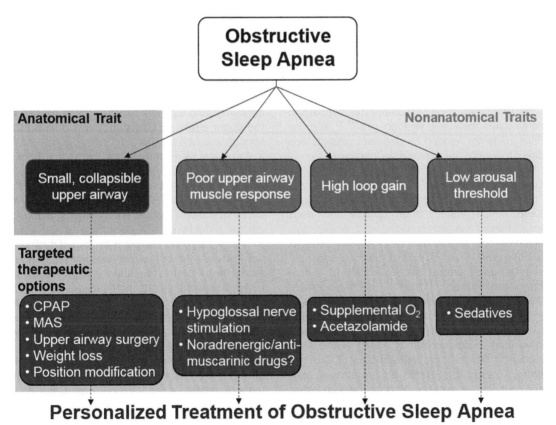

Personalized Treatment of Obstructive Sleep Apnea

Fig. 1. Personalizing the treatment of OSA using therapies targeted toward the underlying mechanisms.

ventilation. It is defined as the size of a corrective ventilatory response divided by the size of the ventilatory disturbance that elicits the correction; a large response to a small disturbance represents a system with a high loop gain. Importantly, the higher the loop gain, the greater the instability in the system, such that a small disturbance in breathing (ie, a hypopnea) results in large corrective increases in ventilation, which in turn leads to an associated decrease in ventilation and ventilatory drive. These oscillations in ventilation and ventilatory drive predispose the airway to further collapse in phases where ventilatory drive is low and excitatory inputs to the upper airway dilator muscles are correspondingly reduced. Therapies aimed at lowering loop gain have therefore become an exciting new treatment option.[31,32] Although treatments such as oxygen therapy[31] and the respiratory stimulant acetazolamide[32] have been able to lower loop gain by ~40%, this reduction has translated into resolving OSA in only ~20% of patients. Interestingly, those enrolled in these oxygen and acetazolamide trials were unselected OSA patients, and this likely explains the low response rates. That is, despite lowering loop gain by 40%, previous studies have (1) not targeted treatment specifically towards subjects with a high loop gain and (2) usually include subjects with other abnormalities that mediate ongoing OSA, such as a poor upper airway anatomy. Indeed, a severely compromised anatomy has been found previously to explain failure of loop gain–targeted therapies.[33] A key direction for future work on loop gain–lowering therapies is to target the treatments to patients likely to respond. To achieve this, simple and noninvasive measures of loop gain[34,35] and the other traits are needed to preselect patients and direct them into the appropriate therapies.

Low arousal threshold

The hallmark of OSA is pharyngeal collapse during sleep, which raises carbon dioxide and leads to increased ventilatory drive and increasingly negative pharyngeal pressure. As the pharynx is collapsing, these respiratory stimuli can activate the upper airway dilator muscles to restore pharyngeal patency, thus protecting against OSA.[36–40] However, adequate upper airway dilator muscle activation and restoration of sufficient airflow can only occur if sufficient ventilatory drive can build up during sleep without an arousal.[33,36,41] In approximately 50% of OSA patients,[42] respiratory events are terminated early due to a low respiratory arousal threshold, preventing the opportunity for sufficient ventilatory drive to accumulate and restore pharyngeal patency during sleep. In this subset of patients,

strategies to raise the arousal threshold could potentially resolve OSA[43] by allowing enough time to pass such that adequate ventilatory drive accumulates and stimulates upper airway dilator muscles to maintain airway patency. As such, several studies have used sedatives in an attempt to raise the arousal threshold, thereby allowing patients more time to recruit pharyngeal muscles during sleep and achieve stable breathing. Although studies administering eszopiclone and trazodone in unselected patients have increased the arousal threshold,[43–47] these have typically only produced modest improvements in OSA severity, with varying results among studies. Again, this is likely because only a proportion of patients have a major pathogenic contribution from a low arousal threshold. The challenge for providing true personalized treatment for OSA is to develop accurate noninvasive measures of the arousal threshold, to enable better targeting of treatments such as sedatives.

Poor upper airway muscle responsiveness

At least one-third of OSA patients demonstrate reduced activation of upper airway dilator muscles in response to the increasingly negative airway collapsing pressures.[26] Such individuals are therefore less able to compensate by mechanically reopening the airway and correspondingly restore ventilation during airway collapse.[38,48] Direct electrical stimulation to these muscles, particularly the genioglossus, can decrease the collapsibility of the airway and increase pharyngeal airflow.[49] Modern commercial devices are surgically implanted and similarly improve the activation of the upper airway musculature by stimulating the hypoglossal nerve. This form of stimulation specifically targets the efferent nerve fibers, which innervate the genioglossus and other upper airway dilator muscles while minimizing sensory (afferent nerve) stimulation.[50] Clinical trials of hypoglossal nerve stimulation devices have demonstrated significant reductions in the AHI between 50% and 57% as well as improvements in oxygen desaturation indices and subjective sleepiness. Furthermore, these treatment-related improvements are largely maintained at 12-month follow-up.[51]

In addition to electrically stimulating the muscles of the upper airway, promising results in animal studies have demonstrated that upper airway muscle activity can be pharmacologically manipulated during sleep, such that the potassium channel blocker AVE0118 can increase the responsiveness of the upper airway dilator muscles to negative airway collapsing pressures and hence prevent airway collapse.[52] Furthermore, the suppression of genioglossus activity in rapid-eye-movement sleep can be pharmacologically reversed via muscarinic receptor antagonism at the hypoglossal motor pool.[53] However, to date there has been limited investigation into methods to pharmacologically reverse the decrease in upper airway dilator muscle activity that occurs in sleeping humans. Recent evidence has now shown for the first time in healthy humans that the drug Desipramine is capable of both inhibiting the reduction in upper airway muscle activity that occurs during sleep onset and improving airway collapsibility.[54] Although promising, it is yet to be tested in patients with OSA.

Combinations of Therapies

With the exception of CPAP therapy, each of the alternative treatments for OSA (whether they are used in mainstream clinical practice or are relatively novel) demonstrates variable efficacy and effectiveness across patients. Part of the variability in response is likely attributable to the fact that most patients with OSA demonstrate abnormalities in multiple pathogenic factors.[26] Importantly, each of the previously described treatments is targeted at improving only one pathogenic trait, whereas the other traits are not addressed. Many patients may therefore be more effectively treated if their therapy consists of a combination of interventions targeting multiple pathogenic causes of OSA. Nevertheless, to date, very few attempts have been made to treat OSA with combination therapies.

Dieltjens and colleagues[55] demonstrated an additional reduction in AHI when patients wearing a MAS device were also encouraged to sleep in the lateral position. Similarly, Oliven and colleagues[56] assessed the impact of a combination of electrical stimulation of the genioglossus with MAS (targeting muscle responsiveness and anatomy/collapsibility, respectively) on airway collapsibility in 14 OSA patients under anesthesia. Although the investigators did not assess the impact of these interventions on the AHI or other markers of OSA severity, their findings indicate that there was an additive improvement in airway anatomy/collapsibility when compared with the individual manipulations. Last, Inoue and colleagues[57] assessed the combined effect of acetazolamide and UPPP (targeting loop gain and anatomy/collapsibility) on OSA severity and showed that this combination led to a greater reduction in the AHI than either of the individual treatments alone. Although this study was only conducted in 5 patients with severe OSA, taken together with the other studies described, they provide strong support for the concept that combination therapy may be viable in treating OSA.

PERSONALIZED MEDICINE FOR OBSTRUCTIVE SLEEP APNEA

For most cases, the status quo for OSA management consists of a diagnostic sleep study followed by a trial of CPAP therapy if OSA is confirmed. If patients do not tolerate CPAP, treatment reverts to one of several potential alternative therapies, with treatment selection based on many situational factors and with no guarantee of success. Currently, there is very little done in the way of personalizing OSA therapy in the clinic, with the few currently utilized approaches described below (**Table 1**).

Currently Applied/Available Methods to Personalize or Predict Therapeutic Response

Supine predominant obstructive sleep apnea and supine avoidance therapy

It has long been recognized that OSA patients suffer a worsening of respiratory events in the supine sleeping position.[58] Clinical definitions for what constitutes supine predominant OSA have evolved over time, with early studies using a ratio of supine to nonsupine AHI of greater than 2:1.[59–61] More recently, a low/normal AHI in the lateral position has been incorporated into this definition.[62] The AHI is known to have a night-to-night variability,[63–65] and this is pertinent to the treatment of supine-related OSA in that, first, in order for treatment to be worthwhile, the problem needs to be present from night to night and, second, the lateral AHI needs to be reliably low from night to night. Current evidence suggests that supine predominant OSA is a repeatable entity in men (more so than in women) when the ratio of supine to nonsupine AHI is greater than or equal to 4:1, and that the lateral AHI has good repeatability in these patients.[66]

Treatment of supine predominant OSA has largely relied on the principle of making supine sleep uncomfortable. The "tennis ball technique" has received disproportionate clinical attention given that it is not particularly effective and has poor long-term adherence.[67,68] Other techniques involving pillows or bolsters preventing movement to the supine position come with the potential side effect of shoulder and hip discomfort, given that patients are often stranded on one side all night. Currently, the most effective devices are those that allow free movement and use vibration as a way of warning patients when they are lying in the supine position.[69] Importantly, long-term adherence data and randomized controlled trials exploring the cardiovascular effects of positional treatments are currently lacking.

Table 1
The strengths and limitations of the available personalized approaches to treating obstructive sleep apnea

Personalization Approaches	Information/Benefits	Limitations
Supine dominant OSA	• Characterizes the degree to which OSA is limited to supine position • Easily obtained from routine PSG	• Requires sufficient positional sleep • Repeatability can vary
MAS titration devices	• Easily implementable in clinic • Predicts MAS success • Provides degree of MAS protrusion	• Does not inform reason for MAS failure • Provides no information about nonanatomic traits
DISE	• Characterizes the anatomic deficiency • Determines site of collapse • May inform either the type of surgical procedure required or likelihood of MAS success	• Costly • Requires anesthesiologist and surgeon • Requires drug-induced sedation • May not exactly replicate what happens to the airway during sleep, and therefore, may not accurately predict treatment response • Provides no details about nonanatomic traits

Mandibular advancement titration and prediction algorithms

Remote-controlled mandibular positioner devices are now becoming commercially available. Such devices allow mandibular advancement to be progressively increased during a polysomnographic sleep study. This technology effectively allows the degree of mandibular protrusion to be titrated in a similar fashion to CPAP. Not only does this allow the degree of protrusion of a MAS device to be personalized based on objective polysomnographic data but it also allows efficacy of MAS treatment to be assessed on the individual patient level. Importantly, the outcomes of this form of titration study have shown good accuracy in predicting therapeutic success with MAS.[70–72] To date, several investigators have used both clinical and polysomnographic predictors of MAS success and have found that patients who gain the greatest benefit are often younger, are less obese, have a smaller neck circumference, display a lower baseline AHI, and have positional OSA.[14,73–75] However, the prediction models generated by these studies do not have sufficient accuracy to be directly translated into clinical practice, and hence, alternative prediction methods are likely to be required.

Drug-induced sleep endoscopy

Given that there is an increasing awareness of the heterogeneity of the sites and structures involved in airway collapse in OSA patients, drug-induced sleep endoscopy (DISE) is a procedure that has been used to determine the site of airway collapse.[76] This procedure involves using a strong sedative to cause a sleeplike state in the patient, while a surgeon passes a fiber-optic endoscope through the patient's nasal cavity to assess pharyngeal structures for evidence and site of obstruction. This technique is used to help guide which forms of surgery should be the most efficacious and whether multilevel surgery will likely be needed. For example, patients with isolated velum collapse may have better outcomes following UPPP. When DISE has been paired with simulation bite at the patients maximally comfortable protrusion of the mandible, DISE has been shown to predict the response to MAS therapy.[77] Other investigators have used DISE to demonstrate that MAS therapy works most effectively in patients with tongue-base collapse,[78] but not in those with isolated velum or epiglottic collapse.[79] However, DISE is most often used as a preoperative assessment rather than a screening or diagnostic tool. It also remains to be proven that DISE accurately reflects how the airway responds during natural sleep. Therefore, it is unlikely, in part due to cost constraints for the patient, that DISE will ever be implemented at a routine clinical level.

Summary

Several techniques exist for predicting the success of currently available treatments before their commencement; however, the predictive ability is either not good enough to be rolled out to large populations of unselected patients or the technique is too costly and cumbersome to be widely available. Therefore, treatment choice is currently made largely by a "therapeutic trial" before success can be determined. Importantly, clinicians make treatment recommendations without knowledge of the physiologic cause of a given individual's OSA. Although some of the existing techniques provide information about the degree of anatomic vulnerability, currently physicians receive no information about the influence of the nonanatomic traits that contribute to OSA, which is likely to be important when predicting the efficacy of non-CPAP interventions.

Personalized Treatment for Obstructive Sleep Apnea: A Physiologically Driven Treatment Model

The understanding of OSA pathophysiology suggests that personalized and targeted interventions (or combinations of interventions) to treat OSA on an individual level could be provided. In this model, physicians would make clinical recommendations based on the patient's history, clinical presentation, and polysomnographic as well as pathophysiologic information. The physician is then able to suggest a range of treatment recommendations based on their ability to treat the underlying cause of a given patient's OSA. The ability to elucidate a patient's individual pathophysiology could help the clinician predict which treatment or treatments may provide the best outcomes and may greatly increase efficacy and long-term adherence.

The transition to this personalized approach to treating OSA will require strategic change to current diagnostic and treatment practices. To succeed with this approach, the field of sleep medicine will need to:

1. Develop an individualized modeling approach that can describe the phenotypic traits and how they interact to promote (or protect against) OSA.
2. Develop clinically validated and practical methods to measure the pathophysiology on an individual patient level.
3. Identify targeted therapies to alter these traits and knowledge about their effect size, so that this information can be used to accurately predict those likely to benefit from a specific therapy or combination of therapies.
4. Conduct large-scale clinical trials to demonstrate the efficacy and long-term effectiveness of this personalized treatment model.

A predictive model for assessing the effectiveness of targeted therapeutic interventions

Wellman and colleagues[36,37] have recently developed, validated, and refined a new approach for measuring the 4 physiologic traits that involve manipulating CPAP and assessing the consequent changes in ventilation. Information on each trait can be diagrammatically modeled to demonstrate, with good sensitivity (80%) and specificity (100%), how all of the traits interact to either promote or protect against the development of OSA in any given patient[27] (**Fig. 2**A). Interpretation of these models can allow the determination of pivotal traits causing OSA, which importantly allows researchers and clinicians to make strategic choices as to which traits could be modified to alleviate an individual's OSA. Specifically, by using the growing literature demonstrating how each of the non-CPAP therapies modifies the physiologic traits and improves OSA (**Table 2**), this modeling approach allows predictions to be made as to whether a given patient will respond to a particular therapy or combination of therapies without the need for trialing the therapy (**Fig. 2**B–D). The investigators' findings suggested that ~25% of patients might be successfully treated by manipulating one trait—personalized to their particular abnormality. Importantly, the investigators showed that combinations of therapies targeting multiple traits would be predicted to successfully treat most OSA patients (50%–80%) without CPAP.

Clinically implementable methods for measuring the physiology responsible for obstructive sleep apnea

The gold-standard method for measuring the 4 physiologic traits described above uses difficult and time-consuming protocols involving complicated manipulations of CPAP pressure.[37] Although it is conceivable that a sleep technician could be trained to perform such procedures during a routine CPAP implementation study, it requires the use of specialized equipment to measure the patient's minute ventilation as well as a CPAP machine that is capable of producing pressures less than 4 cmH_2O (a limitation of commercial CPAP machines). Clearly, this particular method of OSA trait measurement is technically beyond the scope of most clinical settings.

As such, recent progress has been made to noninvasively quantify several of the pathophysiologic traits using data collected from a routine diagnostic clinical polysomnography (PSG). Terrill and colleagues[34] have developed a technique that allows the sensitivity of a patient's ventilatory control system (ie, loop gain) to be computationally quantified using standard electroencephalogram, sleep staging, and nasal pressure signals. This technique uses the easily measureable changes in ventilation that occur during obstructive apnea events and fits a simple ventilatory control model to the respiratory

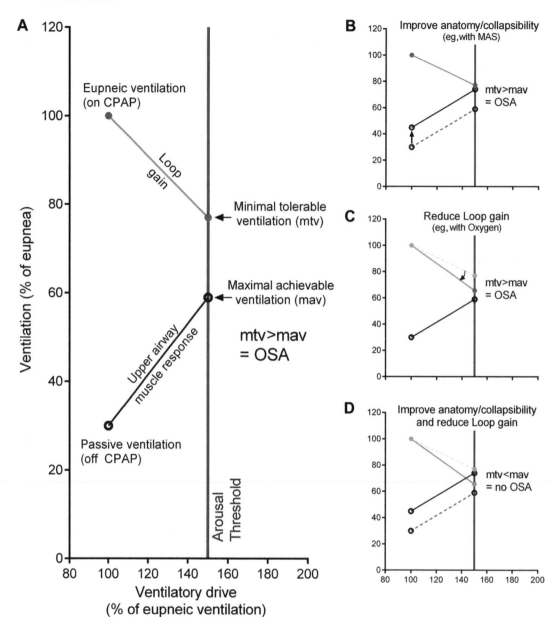

Fig. 2. Modeling the OSA pathophysiology and using this information to predict which therapy (or therapies) will successfully treat the patient. (*A*) An example of a model output for an individual patient illustrating how their 4 physiologic traits interact to produce OSA. Passive ventilation describes the amount of ventilation achievable when the upper airway muscles are passive and is a measure of the collapsibility of the upper airway. As ventilatory drive increases, so too does ventilation based on the individual's upper airway muscle responsiveness (slope of the *blue line*), until the individual reaches their maximum achievable ventilation (mav), after which further increases in ventilatory drive results in an arousal (ie, arousal threshold, *red line*). Eupneic ventilation represents an individual's ventilatory requirement during sleep (ie, ventilation = ventilatory drive). As ventilation decreases, ventilatory drive increases according to an individual's loop gain (slope of the *green line*). The point at which this line crosses the arousal threshold represents the minimally tolerable ventilation (mtv) during sleep. The difference between the mtv and mav, which is referred to as the physiologic "gap," quantifies the ventilatory insufficiency and thereby predicts whether stable breathing or OSA will emerge. A positive "gap" (ie, mtv > mav), as shown in (*A*), predicts the presence of OSA because the ventilation needed to avoid arousal cannot be achieved through the activated airway. Using the published literature on how much particular therapies can alter the traits can therefore be incorporated into the model to predict the treatment success of the particular therapy. In this individual, improving anatomy/collapsibility with a MAS (*B*), or reducing loop gain with oxygen (*C*), would not be sufficient to eliminate OSA. However, the combination of a MAS device and oxygen therapy (*D*) would be predicted to resolve this individual's OSA. For more details on the modeling approach, see Owens and colleagues.[27]

Table 2
Noncontinuous positive airway pressure therapies and their effect on the traits and obstructive sleep apnea severity

Intervention	Primary Affected Trait	Effect Size on Trait	Effect on AHI	Cure Rate (%)
Current treatments				
MAS	Anatomy/collapsibility	↓6.4 cmH$_2$O[80]	↓9.3 events/h[81]	30–85[14]
Upper airway surgery	Anatomy/collapsibility	↓3.3 cmH$_2$O[82,a]	↓15 events/h (33%)[19]	Not reported
Weight loss				
Lifestyle intervention	Anatomy/collapsibility	↓5.5 cmH$_2$O[83,b]	↓12–16 events/h[21,22]	10–63[21,22]
Bariatric surgery	Anatomy/collapsibility	Has not been assessed	↓71%[24]	44[24]
Alternative treatments				
Positional therapy	Anatomy/collapsibility	↓3.9 cmH$_2$O[84]	↓7–11 events/h[69,85,c]	61%[c]
Upper airway muscle stimulation	Anatomy/collapsibility (upper airway muscle response?)	↓2.0 cmH$_2$O[56]	↓18 events/h (50%)[51]	53
Oxygen	Loop gain	↓51%[31]	↓18 events/h (33%)[31]	17[31]
Acetazolamide	Loop gain	↓41%[32]	↓22 events/h (47%)[32]	16[32]
Trazodone	Arousal threshold	↑32%–48%[44,45]	↓10 events/h (26%)[47]	23[47]
Eszopiclone/zopiclone	Arousal threshold	↑29%[43]	↓7 events/h (22%)[43]	17[43,46]

For each treatment listed (whether used currently in clinical practice or has been tested in a research setting), the table reports which of the 4 primary traits the treatment targets and by how much (ie, effect size) it can alter that trait. The table also reports the effect that manipulating the trait has on altering OSA severity (in unselected populations) and the percentage cure rates (defined as an AHI <10 events/h) if reported. Note that the effect size of therapies improving anatomy/collapsibility is quantified by assessing the changes in the pharyngeal critical closing pressure (P$_{crit}$), that is, the pressure at which the airway collapses under "passive" conditions.

^{a} The improvement in P$_{crit}$ and AHI with upper airway surgery corresponds specifically to a UPPP procedure.[82]
^{b} The improvement in P$_{crit}$ with weight loss induced via a lifestyle intervention is achieved with a corresponding reduction in BMI by 17.4%.
^{c} The effect on AHI and cure rate was determined from studies conducted in patients with supine-predominant OSA only.

disturbance and the observed overshoot in ventilation occurring at the termination of the apnea/hypopnea. Sleep studies can therefore be used to quantify the loop gain of a particular individual, which could enable clinicians to target loop gain without the need for complicated experiments. In addition, a clinical tool has recently been developed that enables a patient's respiratory arousal threshold to be calculated using the combination of standard PSG statistics (AHI, degree of oxygen desaturation, and number of hypopneas compared with apneas) that might be able to be used to screen patients for those likely to respond to pharmacologic manipulation of the arousal threshold.[42]

In addition to these techniques, there is now also an intensive research effort to determine noninvasive ways to quantify the other traits (anatomy/collapsibility and upper airway muscle responsiveness). A recent review[86] has highlighted

how information about these traits could potentially be obtained via measures embedded within a diagnostic PSG, although studies will still need to be conducted to demonstrate their clinical utility.

Necessary clinical trials
Future trials are needed to establish the efficacy of this personalized therapy approach in the management of OSA. First, clinical trials are needed to establish that knowledge of the physiologic traits can predict treatment responses. Second, additional studies will be required to demonstrate long-term effectiveness—that is, does this form of personalized, physiologically driven, treatment approach improve the adverse health consequences of OSA (eg, daytime sleepiness, hypertension) and produce better patient outcomes than the status quo?

SUMMARY

For clinicians working with OSA patients, CPAP remains the first-line therapy. However, there are clear shortcomings to this "one-size-fits-all" approach. Many patients cannot tolerate CPAP and are left to work through CPAP-alternative treatments in an ad-hoc fashion, with variable treatment response rates. The current treatment paradigm for OSA demands that improvements be made to our approach, and the way to advance the field is through a personalized approach to treatment.

In recent years, major advances have been made in the understanding of OSA pathogenesis. It is now appreciated that both anatomic and nonanatomic (loop gain, arousal threshold, muscle responsiveness) factors interact to contribute to OSA in a given patient, and that the degree of contribution varies dramatically from one patient to another. Furthermore, many of the traits that contribute to OSA can be manipulated pharmacologically, opening the path for personalized treatment.

The current major barrier to implementing a physiologically driven personalized treatment approach is the ability to measure the physiology simply and noninvasively in a clinical setting and deliver the information in a digestible format to clinicians. Some methods exist to do this, but more work is needed. Once the physiologic traits can routinely be measured, large clinical studies will be needed to measure the efficacy and long-term clinical effectiveness of using this approach, applied to both currently available and future novel treatments. Although currently not quite there yet, we are at the threshold of an exciting new era of OSA treatment, and personalized treatment of OSA will soon become a reality.

REFERENCES

1. Shahar E, Whitney CW, Redline S, et al. Sleep-disordered breathing and cardiovascular disease: cross-sectional results of the Sleep Heart Health Study. Am J Respir Crit Care Med 2001;163:19–25.
2. Peppard PE, Young T, Palta M, et al. Prospective study of the association between sleep-disordered breathing and hypertension. N Engl J Med 2000; 342:1378–84.
3. Nieto FJ, Young TB, Lind BK, et al. Association of sleep-disordered breathing, sleep apnea, and hypertension in a large community-based study. Sleep Heart Health Study. JAMA 2000;283:1829–36.
4. Redline S, Strauss ME, Adams N, et al. Neuropsychological function in mild sleep-disordered breathing. Sleep 1997;20:160–7.
5. Sullivan CE, Issa FG, Berthon-Jones M, et al. Reversal of obstructive sleep apnoea by continuous positive airway pressure applied through the nares. Lancet 1981;1:862–5.
6. Issa FG, Sullivan CE. The immediate effects of nasal continuous positive airway pressure treatment on sleep pattern in patients with obstructive sleep apnea syndrome. Electroencephalogr Clin Neurophysiol 1986;63:10–7.
7. Kakkar RK, Berry RB. Positive airway pressure treatment for obstructive sleep apnea. Chest 2007;132: 1057–72.
8. Engleman HM, Martin SE, Kingshott RN, et al. Randomised placebo controlled trial of daytime function after continuous positive airway pressure (CPAP) therapy for the sleep apnoea/hypopnoea syndrome. Thorax 1998;53:341–5.
9. Kohler M, Stoewhas AC, Ayers L, et al. Effects of continuous positive airway pressure therapy withdrawal in patients with obstructive sleep apnea: a randomized controlled trial. Am J Respir Crit Care Med 2011;184:1192–9.
10. Marin JM, Carrizo SJ, Vicente E, et al. Long-term cardiovascular outcomes in men with obstructive sleep apnoea-hypopnoea with or without treatment with continuous positive airway pressure: an observational study. Lancet 2005;365:1046–53.
11. Kribbs NB, Pack AI, Kline LR, et al. Objective measurement of patterns of nasal CPAP use by patients with obstructive sleep apnea [see comments]. Am Rev Respir Dis 1993;147:887–95.
12. Engelman H, Wild MR. Improving CPAP use by patients with the sleep apnea/hypopnea syndrome (SAHS). Sleep Med Rev 2003;71:81–99.
13. Chan ASL, Sutherland K, Schwab RJ, et al. The effect of mandibular advancement on upper airway structure in obstructive sleep apnoea. Thorax 2010;65:726–32.
14. Sutherland K, Vanderveken OM, Tsuda H, et al. Oral appliance treatment for obstructive sleep apnea: an update. J Clin Sleep Med 2014;10:215–27.
15. Phillips CL, Grunstein RR, Darendeliler MA, et al. Health outcomes of continuous positive airway pressure versus oral appliance treatment for obstructive sleep apnea: a randomized controlled trial. Am J Respir Crit Care Med 2013;187:879–87.
16. Bratton DJ, Gaisl T, Wons AM, et al. CPAP vs mandibular advancement devices and blood pressure in patients with obstructive sleep apnea a systematic review and meta-analysis. JAMA 2015;314:2280–93.
17. Fujita S. UPPP for sleep apnea and snoring. Ear Nose Throat J 1984;63:227–35.
18. Smith DF, Cohen AP, Ishman SL. Surgical management of OSA in adults. Chest 2015;147:1681–90.
19. Caples SM, Rowley JA, Prinsell JR, et al. Surgical modifications of the upper airway for obstructive sleep apnea in adults: a systematic review and meta-analysis. Sleep 2010;33:1396–407.

20. Young T, Peppard PE, Taheri S. Excess weight and sleep-disordered breathing. J Appl Physiol (1985) 2005;99:1592–9.

21. Araghi MH, Chen YF, Jagielski A, et al. Effectiveness of lifestyle interventions on obstructive sleep apnea (OSA): systematic review and meta-analysis. Sleep 2013;36:1553–62.

22. Mitchell LJ, Davidson ZE, Bonham M, et al. Weight loss from lifestyle interventions and severity of sleep apnoea: a systematic review and meta-analysis. Sleep Med 2014;15(10):1173–83.

23. Ashrafian H, Toma T, Rowland SP, et al. Bariatric surgery or non-surgical weight loss for obstructive sleep apnoea? A systematic review and comparison of meta-analyses. Obes Surg 2015;25:1239–50.

24. Greenburg DL, Lettieri CJ, Eliasson AH. Effects of surgical weight loss on measures of obstructive sleep apnea: a meta-analysis. Am J Med 2009;122:535–42.

25. Browaldh N, Nerfeldt P, Lysdahl M, et al. SKUP3 randomised controlled trial: polysomnographic results after uvulopalatopharyngoplasty in selected patients with obstructive sleep apnoea. Thorax 2013;68:846–53.

26. Eckert DJ, White DP, Jordan AS, et al. Defining phenotypic causes of obstructive sleep apnea. Identification of novel therapeutic targets. Am J Respir Crit Care Med 2013;188:996–1004.

27. Owens RL, Edwards BA, Eckert DJ, et al. An integrative model of physiological traits can be used to predict obstructive sleep apnea and response to non positive airway pressure therapy. Sleep 2015;38:961–70.

28. Wellman A, Jordan AS, Malhotra A, et al. Ventilatory control and airway anatomy in obstructive sleep apnea. Am J Respir Crit Care Med 2004;170:1225–32.

29. Salloum A, Rowley JA, Mateika JH, et al. Increased propensity for central apnea in patients with obstructive sleep apnea: effect of nCPAP. Am J Respir Crit Care Med 2010;81(2):189–93.

30. Loewen A, Ostrowski M, Laprairie J, et al. Determinants of ventilatory instability in obstructive sleep apnea: inherent or acquired? Sleep 2009;32:1355–65.

31. Wellman A, Malhotra A, Jordan AS, et al. Effect of oxygen in obstructive sleep apnea: role of loop gain. Respir Physiol Neurobiol 2008;162:144–51.

32. Edwards BA, Sands SA, Eckert DJ, et al. Acetazolamide improves loop gain but not the other physiological traits causing obstructive sleep apnoea. J Physiol 2012;590:1199–211.

33. Xie A, Teodorescu M, Pegelow DF, et al. Effects of stabilizing or increasing respiratory motor outputs on obstructive sleep apnea. J Appl Physiol (1985) 2013;115:22–33.

34. Terrill PI, Edwards BA, Nemati S, et al. Quantifying the ventilatory control contribution to sleep apnoea using polysomnography. Eur Respir J 2015;45:408–18.

35. Nemati S, Edwards BA, Sands SA, et al. Model-based characterization of ventilatory stability using spontaneous breathing. J Appl Physiol (1985) 2011;111:55–67.

36. Wellman A, Eckert DJ, Jordan AS, et al. A method for measuring and modeling the physiological traits causing obstructive sleep apnea. J Appl Physiol (1985) 2011;110:1627–37.

37. Wellman A, Edwards BA, Sands SA, et al. A simplified method for determining phenotypic traits in patients with obstructive sleep apnea. J Appl Physiol (1985) 2013;114:911–22.

38. Patil SP, Schneider H, Marx JJ, et al. Neuromechanical control of upper airway patency during sleep. J Appl Physiol (1985) 2007;102:547–56.

39. Gold AR, Bleecker ER, Smith PL. A shift from central and mixed sleep apnea to obstructive sleep apnea resulting from low-flow oxygen. Am Rev Respir Dis 1985;132:220–3.

40. McGinley BM, Schwartz AR, Schneider H, et al. Upper airway neuromuscular compensation during sleep is defective in obstructive sleep apnea. J Appl Physiol (1985) 2008;105:197–205.

41. Younes M. Role of respiratory control mechanisms in the pathogenesis of obstructive sleep disorders. J Appl Physiol 2008;105:1389–405.

42. Edwards BA, Eckert DJ, McSharry DG, et al. Clinical predictors of the respiratory arousal threshold in patients with obstructive sleep apnea. Am J Respir Crit Care Med 2014;190:1293–300.

43. Eckert DJ, Owens RL, Kehlmann GB, et al. Eszopiclone increases the respiratory arousal threshold and lowers the apnoea/hypopnoea index in obstructive sleep apnoea patients with a low arousal threshold. Clin Sci (Lond) 2011;120:505–14.

44. Heinzer RC, White DP, Jordan AS, et al. Trazodone increases arousal threshold in obstructive sleep apnoea. Eur Respir J 2008;31:1308–12.

45. Eckert DJ, Malhotra A, Wellman A, et al. Trazodone increases the respiratory arousal threshold in obstructive sleep apnea patients with a low arousal threshold. Sleep 2014;37:811–9.

46. Carter SG, Berger MS, Carberry JC, et al. Zopiclone increases the arousal threshold without impairing genioglossus activity in obstructive sleep apnea. Sleep 2015;39(4):757–66.

47. Smales ET, Edwards BA, Deyoung PN, et al. Trazodone effects on obstructive sleep apnea and non-REM arousal threshold. Ann Am Thorac Soc 2015;12:758–64.

48. Jordan AS, Wellman A, Heinzer RC, et al. Mechanisms used to restore ventilation after partial upper

airway collapse during sleep in humans. Thorax 2007;62:861–7.

49. Oliven A, Tov N, Geitini L, et al. Effect of genioglossus contraction on pharyngeal lumen and airflow in sleep apnoea patients. Eur Respir J 2007;30:748–58.

50. Gerek M, Binar M. Physiology of hypoglossal nerve stimulation. Oper Tech Otolaryngol - Head Neck Surg 2015;26:105–7.

51. Certal VF, Zaghi S, Riaz M, et al. Hypoglossal nerve stimulation in the treatment of obstructive sleep apnea: a systematic review and meta-analysis. Laryngoscope 2015;125:1254–64.

52. Wirth KJ, Steinmeyer K, Ruetten H. Sensitization of upper airway mechanoreceptors as a new pharmacologic principle to treat obstructive sleep apnea: investigations with AVE0118 in anesthetized pigs. Sleep 2013;36:699–708.

53. Grace KP, Hughes SW, Horner RL. Identification of the mechanism mediating genioglossus muscle suppression in REM sleep. Am J Respir Crit Care Med 2013;187:311–9.

54. Taranto-Montemurro L, Edwards BA, Sands SA, et al. Desipramine increases genioglossus activity and reduces upper airway collapsibility during non-REM sleep in healthy subjects. Am J Respir Crit Care Med 2016. [Epub ahead of print].

55. Dieltjens M, Vroegop AV, Verbruggen AE, et al. A promising concept of combination therapy for positional obstructive sleep apnea. Sleep Breath 2015;19:637–44.

56. Oliven R, Tov N, Odeh M, et al. Interacting effects of genioglossus stimulation and mandibular advancement in sleep apnea. J Appl Physiol (1985) 2009;106:1668–73.

57. Inoue Y, Takata K, Sakamoto I, et al. Clinical efficacy and indication of acetazolamide treatment on sleep apnea syndrome. Psychiatry Clin Neurosci 1999;53:321–2.

58. Patient's wife cures his snoring. Chest J 1984;85:582-c. Available at: http://journal.publications.chestnet.org/article.aspx?articleID=1056106.

59. Cartwright RD. Effect of sleep position on sleep apnea severity. Sleep 1984;7:110–4.

60. Pevernagie DA, Stanson AW, Sheedy PF 2nd, et al. Effects of body position on the upper airway of patients with obstructive sleep apnea. Am J Respir Crit Care Med 1995;152:179–85.

61. Oksenberg A, Silverberg DS, Arons E, et al. Positional vs nonpositional obstructive sleep apnea patients: anthropomorphic, nocturnal polysomnographic, and multiple sleep latency test data. Chest 1997;112:629–39.

62. Mador MJ, Kufel TJ, Magalang UJ, et al. Prevalence of positional sleep apnea in patients undergoing polysomnography. Chest 2005;128:2130–7.

63. Bittencourt LR, Suchecki D, Tufik S, et al. The variability of the apnoea-hypopnoea index. J Sleep Res 2001;10:245–51.

64. Chediak AD, Acevedo-Crespo JC, Seiden DJ, et al. Nightly variability in the indices of sleep-disordered breathing in men being evaluated for impotence with consecutive night polysomnograms. Sleep 1996;19:589–92.

65. Levendowski DJ, Zack N, Rao S, et al. Assessment of the test-retest reliability of laboratory polysomnography. Sleep Breath 2009;13:163–7.

66. Joosten SA, O'Donoghue FJ, Rochford PD, et al. Night-to-night repeatability of supine-related obstructive sleep apnea. Ann Am Thorac Soc 2014;11:761–9.

67. Bignold JJ, Deans-Costi G, Goldsworthy MR, et al. Poor long-term patient compliance with the tennis ball technique for treating positional obstructive sleep apnea. J Clin Sleep Med 2009;5:428–30.

68. Skinner MA, Kingshott RN, Filsell S, et al. Efficacy of the 'tennis ball technique' versus nCPAP in the management of position-dependent obstructive sleep apnoea syndrome. Respirology 2008;13:708–15.

69. Bignold JJ, Mercer JD, Antic NA, et al. Accurate position monitoring and improved supine-dependent obstructive sleep apnea with a new position recording and supine avoidance device. J Clin Sleep Med 2011;7:376–83.

70. Remmers J, Charkhandeh S, Grosse J, et al. Remotely controlled mandibular protrusion during sleep predicts therapeutic success with oral appliances in patients with obstructive sleep apnea. Sleep 2013;36:1517–25.

71. Dort LC, Hadjuk E, Remmers JE. Mandibular advancement and obstructive sleep apnoea: a method for determining effective mandibular protrusion. Eur Respir J 2006;27:1003–9.

72. Tsai WH, Vazquez JC, Oshima T, et al. Remotely controlled mandibular positioner predicts efficacy of oral appliances in sleep apnea. Am J Respir Crit Care Med 2004;170:366–70.

73. Sutherland K, Takaya H, Qian J, et al. Oral appliance treatment response and polysomnographic phenotypes of obstructive sleep apnea. J Clin Sleep Med 2015;11:861–8.

74. Holley AB, Lettieri CJ, Shah AA. Efficacy of an adjustable oral appliance and comparison with continuous positive airway pressure for the treatment of obstructive sleep apnea syndrome. Chest 2011;140:1511–6.

75. Lee CH, Jung HJ, Lee WH, et al. The effect of positional dependency on outcomes of treatment with a mandibular advancement device. Arch Otolaryngol Head Neck Surg 2012;138:479–83.

76. Croft CB, Pringle M. Sleep nasendoscopy: a technique of assessment in snoring and obstructive

sleep apnoea. Clin Otolaryngol Allied Sci 1991;16: 504–9.

77. Vroegop AVMT, Vanderveken OM, Dieltjens M, et al. Sleep endoscopy with simulation bite for prediction of oral appliance treatment outcome. J Sleep Res 2013;22:348–55.

78. Ng AT, Qian J, Cistulli PA. Oropharyngeal collapse predicts treatment response with oral appliance therapy in obstructive sleep apnea. Sleep 2006;29: 666–71.

79. Vanderveken OM, Maurer JT, Hohenhorst W, et al. Evaluation of drug-induced sleep endoscopy as a patient selection tool for implanted upper airway stimulation for obstructive sleep apnea. J Clin Sleep Med 2013;9:433–8.

80. Ng AT, Gotsopoulos H, Qian J, et al. Effect of oral appliance therapy on upper airway collapsibility in obstructive sleep apnea. Am J Respir Crit Care Med 2003;168:238–41.

81. Sharples LD, Clutterbuck-James AL, Glover MJ, et al. Meta-analysis of randomised controlled trials of oral mandibular advancement devices and continuous positive airway pressure for obstructive sleep apnoea-hypopnoea. Sleep Med Rev 2016; 27:108–24.

82. Schwartz AR, Schubert N, Rothman W, et al. Effect of uvulopalatopharyngoplasty on upper airway collapsibility in obstructive sleep apnea. Am Rev Respir Dis 1992;145:527–32.

83. Schwartz AR, Gold AR, Schubert N, et al. Effect of weight loss on upper airway collapsibility in obstructive sleep apnea. Am Rev Respir Dis 1991;144: 494–8.

84. Joosten SA, Edwards BA, Wellman A, et al. The effect of body position on physiological factors that contribute to obstructive sleep apnea. Sleep 2015; 38(9).

85. Loord H, Hultcrantz E. Positioner - a method for preventing sleep apnea. Acta Otolaryngol 2007;127(8): 861–8.

86. Sands SA, Owens RL, Malhotra A. New approaches to diagnosing sleep-disordered breathing. Sleep Med Clin 2016;11(2):143–52.

Managing Comorbid Illness in Obstructive Sleep Apnea
What Can We Learn from Other Diseases?

Walter D. Conwell, MD[a,*], Sheila C. Tsai, MD[a,b]

KEYWORDS

- Obstructive sleep apnea • CPAP therapy • Hypersomnia • Comorbid disease

KEY POINTS

- Obstructive sleep apnea (OSA) is associated with numerous comorbid conditions.
- OSA often acts synergistically with coexisting illness, resulting in an increase in morbidity and mortality.
- Symptoms of sleep apnea may mimic those of other disorders.
- It is important to screen for OSA in patients with associated disorders.
- In patients with comorbid disorders, treatment of OSA is often an adjunct to primary therapy, and as such, it is important to initiate treatment for both disorders.

INTRODUCTION

As the importance of sleep is increasingly being recognized, the implications of untreated obstructive sleep apnea (OSA) on overall health are also being realized. Medical providers are managing an ever-growing number of medical conditions, many of which can be associated with OSA. These conditions encompass all organ systems, and if untreated, increase morbidity and mortality. In order to effectively manage these disorders physicians must be educated about disease associations, diligent in screening efforts to identify comorbid conditions, and thoughtful in therapeutic management. Therefore, in OSA syndrome, it is important to treat both the sleep disorder and the comorbid condition, because while OSA may be a key driving force in perpetuating disease, there may be other contributors to disease. It is important to manage patients comprehensively and to understand that treatment of sleep apnea leads to improvements in not only sleep symptoms but also overall health. In this article, associations between OSA and various comorbid conditions will be discussed; rationale for screening for OSA in these conditions will be reviewed, and treatment considerations, which may affect the management of OSA or its comorbid conditions, will be addressed.

CARDIOVASCUAR DISORDERS

Numerous cardiovascular disorders have been associated with OSA. Activation of the sympathetic nervous system during sleep and intermittent hypoxia may be primary mechanisms behind the development and persistence of cardiovascular disease. There is a large body of evidence

The authors have nothing to disclose.
[a] Department of Medicine, University of Colorado Denver School of Medicine, 13001 East 17th Place, Aurora, CO 80045, USA; [b] Department of Medicine, National Jewish Health, 1400 Jackson Street, Denver, CO 80206, USA
* Corresponding author. 1400 Jackson Street, Denver, CO 80206.
E-mail address: walter.conwell@ucdenver.edu

supporting the association between sleep apnea and cardiovascular complications such as hypertension, atrial fibrillation, and congestive heart failure. Research also supports the benefit of treatment of sleep apnea on these coexisting conditions. Not infrequently, patients with these conditions may be relatively asymptomatic, particularly in the setting of systemic hypertension. Likewise, there may be little symptomatology associated with the OSA. Therefore, it is crucial to educate the patient on the association between sleep apnea and cardiovascular disorders and on the importance of treating each of these disorders to maximize medical benefit.

Overview

Hypertension
OSA is a risk factor for the development of systemic hypertension. The likelihood of developing hypertension increases in a dose–response fashion, with the severity of OSA.[1] Patients with OSA are also at increased risk of developing resistant hypertension.[2] Successful treatment of sleep apnea may lead to improvement in blood pressure control, which may reduce long-term cardiovascular complications.[3]

Atrial fibrillation
There is an increased prevalence of OSA in patients with cardiac dysrhythmias, particularly atrial fibrillation (AF). Studies have shown AF in 21% to 80% of OSA patients, and patients with AF and untreated OSA are less likely to maintain sinus rhythm after cardioversion.[4] However, patients with AF and OSA may not report symptoms of excessive daytime sleepiness, which may lead to underdiagnosis of sleep apnea.[5]

Congestive heart failure
Up to 75% of patients with congestive heart failure (CHF) have sleep-disordered breathing, with up to 50% having central sleep apnea/cheyne-stokes respiration (CSA-CSR).[6] The prevalence of CSA-CSR increases with the severity of cardiac dysfunction.[7,8] Pharyngeal edema may contribute to the development of OSA in patients with CHF.[9]

Management Goals

Patients with hypertension, AF, and CHF should be screened for OSA signs and symptoms. There should be a low threshold for diagnostic testing, which should include polysomnography, if appropriate. If OSA is identified, treatment should be initiated in order to prevent long-term cardiovascular complications and improve quality of life. Patients should be educated on the potential benefits of sleep apnea therapy on cardiovascular health.

Treatment Considerations

Treatment should be initiated for hypertension, AF, CHF or other cardiovascular disorders in conjunction with treatment for OSA. Because OSA is associated with increased sympathetic nervous system (SNS) activation, it may be beneficial to choose therapies that can blunt SNS and renin-angiotensin-aldosterone system activity.[10]

In patients with sleep apnea and hypertension, dosing antihypertensive medications in the evening has been shown to improve daytime blood pressure control and increase the proportion of patients that experiences nocturnal dipping, when compared with dosing in the morning.[11] Continuous positive airway pressure (CPAP) may reduce the occurrence of paroxysmal AF and increase the success rate of cardioversion.[12,13] There is evidence that treating OSA may improve cardiac function and quality of life. However, the evidence for treating CSA-CSR is controversial. Data from two large, multi-center trials evaluating the efficacy of PAP modalities in CHF patients have suggested a decrease in survival with PAP therapy in patients with CSA-CSR.[14,15] Treating the CHF may improve CSA-CSR, and therefore, optimizing medical management of CHF is important. The significance of CSA-CSR in CHF is controversial. It has been proposed to be a marker of CHF control or may be a compensatory mechanism. If CSA-CSR is identified, discuss the potential risks versus benefits of PAP treatment with the patient.

Monitoring Therapy

Reassess adequacy of medical management of hypertension, AF, CHF and other cardiovascular disorders/complications on a regular basis. Monitor compliance with OSA therapy and re-evaluate OSA severity if there is a worsening of OSA or comorbid disease symptoms. In light of potential harm with PAP therapy in patients with CHF, careful monitoring and frequent review of symptomatology are encouraged.

PULMONARY DISORDERS

There is compelling evidence supporting the association between OSA and numerous pulmonary disorders including asthma, chronic obstructive pulmonary disease (COPD), and chronic hypoventilation related to obesity hypoventilation syndrome (OHS) and neuromuscular disorders (NMDs). The proposed pathophysiologic mechanisms that underlie these interactions are numerous and include neuromechanical reflex bronchoconstriction, worsening gastroesophageal reflux, local/systemic inflammation, and decreased ventilatory drive.[16,17] These conditions may also share risk factors with OSA such as obesity and tobacco smoking. Importantly, there is good evidence that treatment of OSA may be beneficial in the management of these comorbid pulmonary conditions.

Overview

Obstructive lung disease
Approximately 8% and 10% of the population suffer from asthma and COPD, respectively. The prevalence of OSA within patients with COPD has been reported to be between 5% and 85%. The true prevalence could be the same as in the general population.[18] However when both disorders coexist, patients usually experience more severe sleep-related hypoxemia. These patients also tend to have more severe hypercarbia both during sleep and during wake.[17]

Interstitial lung disease
OSA is now known to be a common comorbidity in patients with idiopathic pulmonary fibrosis (IPF). Recent studies have shown a prevalence of 59% to 88% in patients with IPF aged 60 to 69 years. There may be a bidirectional relationship whereby OSA may contribute to the progression of IPF by worsening gastroesophageal reflux disease (GERD) and through oxidative stress, and IPF may contribute to OSA through a decrease in lung volumes and a loss of tethering forces on the upper airway.[19]

Chronic hypoventilation
OSA is common in patients with neuromuscular disorders. These patients may suffer from upper airway muscle hypotonia, pharyngeal neuropathy, bulbar dysfunction, and anatomic factors.[20] With regard to obesity hypoventilation syndrome, it is estimated that 0.15% to 0.4% of the population suffers from OHS, and approximately 90% of those patients with OHS also have OSA.[17,18] Finally, OSA may be more common than CSA in patients on long-term opioid therapy. One study reported an OSA prevalence of 35.2% and a CSA prevalence of 14.1% in patients in a methadone maintenance treatment program.[21]

Management Goals

Screen patients with asthma, COPD, obesity, neuromuscular disorders, and chronic opioid therapy for signs and symptoms of OSA. Have a low threshold for diagnostic testing, which would include a polysomnography, if appropriate. If OSA is identified, initiate treatment in order to prevent long-term respiratory and cardiovascular complications and to improve quality of life.

Educate the patient on the potential benefits of sleep apnea therapy on respiratory health.

Treatment Considerations

Initiate treatment for obstructive lung disease, interstitial lung disease, and chronic hypoventilation in conjunction with treatment for OSA. Although pharmacologic treatment of obstructive lung disease may improve nocturnal breathing, prolonged use of inhaled corticosteroids may lead to changes in upper airway fat distribution and place some patients at risk for increased upper airway collapsibility.[22] CPAP therapy may decrease exacerbations, hospitalization rates, and mortality in patients with OSA and obstructive lung disease.[23] Treatment with CPAP has been shown to increase quality of life, sleep quality, and functional capacity; additionally, it may improve mortality in patients with IPF. It may therefore be complementary to pharmacologic therapy for IPF.[24] Successful medical treatment of some neuromuscular disorders (eg, myasthenia gravis) can lead to marked improvement in comorbid sleep-disordered breathing.[25] Although PAP therapy can improved quality of life and survival in patients with NMD, therapy can also lead to sleep disruption via a number of mechanisms,[20] such as air leaks, ineffective breathing, autotriggering, prolonged insufflation, central apnea, and glottic closure. Patients with daytime hypercarbia or persistent nocturnal hypoxemia and/or hypercarbia may benefit from transition to nocturnal BiPAP therapy.[26]

Monitoring Therapy

Reassess the adequacy of medical management of obstructive lung disease, interstitial lung disease, and chronic hypoventilation on a regular basis. Monitor compliance with OSA therapy and re-evaluate OSA severity if there is a worsening of OSA or comorbid disease symptoms. Assess potential benefits of BiPAP versus CPAP therapy.

PSYCHIATRIC

Psychiatric disorders have been associated with OSA. Two disorders (depression, posttraumatic stress disorder) for which there is sufficient evidence for both association and cotreatment will be reviewed. Population-based studies have found an increased rate of OSA in patients with major depressive disorder (MDD) with a range of 7.4% to 44%. Numerous studies have shown improvement in depressive symptoms with OSA treatment.[27] However, it is not clear if these benefits are superior to other antidepressant therapy.[28] A recent meta-analysis showed that PAP therapy was not superior to sham PAP in reducing depression symptoms, suggesting that other treatment-associated factors, such as frequent patient interaction, may be of benefit in management.[29] Population-based studies have also found an increased rate of OSA of up to 50% in patients with post-traumatic stress disorder (PTSD). Adherence to CPAP therapy in these patients has been associated with a decrease in nightmare frequency.[27]

Overview

There is a strong association between major depressive disorder and OSA. Increased rates of depression are noted in patients with OSA. OSA symptoms (sleepiness, fatigue) may mimic depressive symptoms. Increased rates of OSA have also been found in patients with PTSD.

Management Goals

Understand the association between sleep apnea and depression. Recognize similarities in symptom presentation between depression and OSA. Screen for OSA in patients with psychiatric disorders, in particular in those with depression and PTSD.

Treatment Considerations

If OSA is identified, treat this sleep disorder in order to prevent mood deterioration and to clarify whether symptoms are caused by the patient's underlying mood disorder or his or her sleep disorder. OSA treatment may decrease nightmares in PTSD.

Initiate treatment for depression and PTSD in conjunction with treatment for OSA. Be aware that some antidepressants have been associated with weight gain, which may worsen the severity of sleep apnea.[30] Other antidepressants have been associated with weight loss. Although PAP therapy may be beneficial in nightmare control, patients with PTSD are often less compliant with PAP therapy.[27]

Monitoring Therapy

Reassess adequacy of mental health management on a regular basis. Adjust, and potentially decrease, pharmacologic management as psychiatric symptoms change. Monitor compliance with OSA therapy and re-evaluate OSA severity if there is a worsening of OSA or comorbid disease symptoms.

NEUROLOGIC DISORDERS

Neurologic disorders have also been associated with OSA. These disorders include, but are not limited to, cerebrovascular accidents (CVAs) and cognitive decline or dementia. Numerous studies have shown an association between OSA and CVA; however, the significance of the risk has been debated. Potential mechanisms include the effect of OSA on hypertension, cerebral blood flow, endothelial function, and alterations in the clotting and inflammatory pathways. CVAs may also contribute to the development of obstructive and/or central sleep apnea in some patients.[31] There is emerging evidence that treatment of sleep apnea improves outcomes in stroke or transient ischemic attacks (TIAs), and cohort studies have shown a decrease in risk of stroke in patients treated with PAP therapy.[32] Based on this, the American Heart Association recommends evaluation for sleep apnea in those with ischemic stroke or TIA and lists sleep apnea as a potentially modifiable risk.[33]

The prevalence of OSA and mild cognitive impairment/dementia increases with age. Disturbances in intellectual and executive function may result from intermittent hypoxemia, while issues with vigilance, attention, and memory are attributed to sleep disruption.[34] It has been shown that both elderly men and women with moderate-to-severe OSA (apnea-hypopnea index [AHI] >15) have about a 1.85 odds of developing mild cognitive impairment (MCI) and dementia.[35,36] This cognitive decline may be delayed with CPAP therapy.[36] Furthermore, in a review of PAP therapy, it has been shown to improve attention and vigilance.[37]

Overview

An increased risk of stroke exists in patients with untreated OSA. Sleep apnea is highly prevalent in patients following a stroke. Moderate-to-severe sleep apnea is associated with an increased risk of developing at least MCI and dementia.

Management Goals

Screen patients who may be at risk for CVA for OSA and consider diagnostic testing if appropriate. Screen patients with cognitive decline for sleep disorders, especially sleep apnea. Evaluate factors such as sleep apnea, which may be contributing to or exacerbating neurologic conditions.

Treatment Considerations

CPAP therapy may decrease morbidity and mortality following stroke, and it may attenuate cerebrovascular risks. Sleep apnea therapy may delay the onset of cognitive decline.

Monitoring Therapy

Monitor compliance with OSA therapy and re-evaluate OSA and cerebrovascular symptoms. Assess cognitive function periodically.

ENDOCRINE DISORDERS

Endocrine disorders have been associated with OSA. Hypothyroidism, type 2 diabetes, hypogo-nadism, and postmenopausal state have all been associated with OSA. Often this relationship is bidirectional. Symptoms of hypothyroidism may be difficult to distinguish from those of OSA. Fatigue and sleepiness are prominent features of hypothyroidism.[38] Up to half of hypothyroid patients have sleep-disordered breathing, compared with 29% in control patients.[39] OSA may be a consequence of hypothyroidism. Hypothyroidism can contribute to OSAS due to excess weight gain, decreased ventilatory drive, and myopathy. Goiter may cause mechanical obstruction. In some studies, thyroid hormone replacement has improved sleep-disordered breathing in hypothyroid patients with OSA.[40]

Large population-based studies, such as the Sleep Health Heart Study and the Wisconsin Sleep Cohort, have shown an association between the severity of OSA and the prevalence of insulin resistance and diabetes.[41,42] OSA may contribute to diabetes by causing oxidative stress, increasing inflammatory cytokines, and altering the hypothalamic-pituitary-adrenal axis. Treatment with PAP therapy may improve insulin sensitivity and over the long-term may reduce HbA1c.[43,44] Postmenopausal women have an increased prevalence of OSA when compared with premenopausal women, and when OSA occurs it is often more severe.[45] Although hormonal changes associated with the transition to menopause increase the risk for OSA, treatment with exogenous hormonal therapy has not been shown to consistently improve objective measures of OSA severity.[46] Although sleep apnea was once believed to be a risk factor for hypogonadism, recent studies have shown that this association can be mostly explained by comorbid obesity.[47] The presence of untreated severe OSA was previously deemed to be an absolute contraindication to testosterone replacement therapy. However, more recent studies have suggested only a mild and transient worsening of sleep-disordered breathing[48–50] with testosterone replacement. In addition, CPAP therapy has not been shown to consistently increase testosterone levels in men with hypogonadism and OSA. However, weight loss may improve to testosterone levels.[50,51]

Overview

OSA has been associated with a number of endocrine disorders, including hypothyroidism, diabetes, and hypogonadism. This relationship is often bidirectional. Obesity and weight gain may be a unifying factor.

Although sleep complaints are common in postmenopausal women, consider sleep apnea as a potential contributor/exacerbator of sleep issues. Hypothyroidism and untreated OSA may have similar symptomatology.

Management Goals

Screen patients with endocrine disorders for OSA and consider diagnostic testing if appropriate.Screen patients with low testosterone levels who are considering testosterone replacement therapy for OSA. Patients with hypersomnia should be evaluated for sleep apnea in addition to thyroid disorders.Consider lifestyle modification through diet and exercise in an effort to treat both the sleep disorder and the endocrine abnormality.

Treatment Considerations

Treatment with PAP therapy may improve insulin sensitivity and reduce HbA1C.[43,44]

Initiate treatment for menopausal symptoms in conjunction with treatment for OSA. Although PAP therapy is effective in postmenopausal women, advanced age and female gender are predictive factors for noncompliance.[52] Exogenous testosterone is associated with worsening of OSA. Reassess adequacy of hormonal management on a regular basis.

Monitoring Therapy

Endocrine abnormalities may improve with treatment of sleep apnea. Sleep apnea may improve with treatment of endocrine abnormalities. Monitor compliance with therapy and re-evaluate symptoms periodically.

SLEEP DISORDERS

Patients with OSA often have comorbid sleep conditions, and the management of other sleep disorders can be confounded by the presence of obstructive sleep apnea. Therefore, as part of a comprehensive sleep evaluation, patients should be screened for common sleep disorders including OSA, insomnia, and restless legs syndrome (RLS).

Table 1
A summary of the effect of untreated obstructive sleep apnea on comorbid medical conditions and the potential impact of positive airway pressure therapy on these conditions

Disorder	Effect of Untreated OSA on Comorbid Condition	Effect of OSA Treatment on Comorbid Condition
Hypertension	OSA worsens hypertension in a dose related fashion.	CPAP therapy may lead to a small decrease in mean arterial pressure.
Atrial Fibrillation	Patients with OSA are more likely to develop AF and are less likely to stay in sinus rhythm after cardioversion.	CPAP may reduce the occurrence of paroxysmal AF and increase the success rate of cardioversion.
Congestive Heart Failure	The prevalence of sleep disordered breathing increases with the severity of ventricular dysfunction.	Treating OSA may improve cardiac function and quality of life.
Obstructive Lung Disease	Patients with the OLD-OSA overlap syndrome tend to have worse hypoxia and hypercarbia	CPAP therapy may decrease exacerbations, hospitalization rates, and mortality
Interstitial Lung Disease	The prevalence of OSA in patients with IPF, is greater than in the general population.	Treatment with CPAP has been shown to increase quality of life, sleep quality, functional capacity, and may improve mortality in patients with IPF.
Chronic Hypoventilation	The prevalence of OSA in patients with NMD, OHS and chronic opioid use, is greater than in the general population.	PAP therapy may improve quality of life and survival in patients with NMD and OHS.
Depression	The prevalence of OSA in patients with depression, is greater than in the general population; symptoms of untreated OSA may mimic depressive symptoms	PAP therapy improves depressive symptoms but is not clearly superior to antidepressant therapy; other treatment associated factors, such as frequent patient interaction, may be of benefit in management.
Post-traumatic stress disorder	The prevalence of OSA in patients with PTSD is greater than in the general population.	CPAP therapy may improve nightmare control.
Cerebral vascular accident	OSA increases the risk of CVA.	CPAP therapy may decrease the risk of stroke.
Cognitive impairment/ Dementia	OSA increases the odds of developing MCI and dementia in the elderly	CPAP therapy may delay the onset of MCI in elderly men and women with OSA
Hypothyroidism	Hypothyroidism may contribute to OSA development in some patients; sleepiness and fatigue may be symptoms of hypothyroidism and OSA	CPAP has not been shown to affect thyroid function; however, thyroid hormone replacement may improve OSA
Type 2 diabetes mellitus	There is an association between the severity of OSA and the prevalence of insulin resistance and diabetes	CPAP therapy may improve insulin sensitivity and, over the long term, may reduce HbA1c
Hypogonadism	Sleep apnea may be a risk factor for hypogonadism, although recent studies have shown that this association may be mostly explained by comorbid obesity	CPAP therapy has been shown to improve testosterone levels in some men with hypogonadism; however, results are not consistent; weight loss may improve testosterone levels as well as sleep apnea.

(continued on next page)

Disorder	Effect of Untreated OSA on Comorbid Condition	Effect of OSA Treatment on Comorbid Condition
Table 1 (*continued*)		
Menopause	Postmenopausal women have an increased prevalence of OSA when compared to premenopausal women, and when OSA occurs it is often more severe	CPAP therapy has not been shown to improve menopausal symptoms however it is effective in treating OSA in this population.
RLS	Untreated OSA may worsen RLS symptoms.	CPAP therapy may improve RLS symptoms
Insomnia	Untreated OSA may worsen insomnia	Combined treatment with CBT-I and CPAP may improve insomnia

Overview

Restless legs syndrome

OSA is common in patients presenting to sleep centers with the chief complaint of RLS, with 1 study reporting a prevalence of 55%.[53] The risk of OSA in these patients is related to older age, male gender, elevated body mass index (BMI), and the presence of OSA symptoms.[53] Treatment with CPAP therapy may improve RLS symptoms.[54]

Insomnia

Between 39% and 58% of patients with OSA experience comorbid insomnia, and between 29% and 67% of insomnia patients have an AHI greater than 5; however, those with insomnia may not report sleep apnea symptoms.[55] Patients may complain of sleep onset, sleep maintenance, or terminal insomnia.[56] The presence of occult OSA may confound the treatment of insomnia, and some sedatives may worsen the severity of OSA.[57]

Management Goals

Screen patients with RLS and insomnia for OSA signs and symptoms. If OSA is identified, initiate treatment in an effort to improve RLS and insomnia symptoms and decrease morbidity and mortality.

Treatment Considerations

Initiate treatment for RLS and insomnia in conjunction with treatment for OSA. Combination therapy with cognitive behavioral therapy for insomnia (CBT-I) and PAP therapy may result in better control of insomnia symptoms than either therapy alone.[55] Understand that certain medications used to treat insomnia may worsen sleep-disordered breathing. Benzodiazipines reduce upper airway muscle tone and increase the arousal threshold, thereby resulting in an increase in

number of obstructive events and increased duration of events.[58] GABAergic nonbenzodiazepine agents do not affect the severity of sleep apnea.[55]

Monitoring Therapy

Reassess adequacy of RLS and insomnia management on a regular basis. Monitor compliance with OSA therapy and reassess symptoms periodically. Review medications periodically since some hypnotics may worsen OSA.

SUMMARY

This article, discussed the association of OSA with numerous comorbid medical conditions. Symptoms of sleep apnea may mimic those of other comorbid conditions, such as insomnia, hypothyroidism, and depression. In some cases, there is a bidirectional relationship between sleep apnea and the comorbid condition. Often, untreated sleep apnea may be a significant pathophysiologic contributor to these disorders. Its presence may worsen outcomes from the primary disease, such as in the overlap syndrome with obstructive lung disease. Therefore, it is important to screen for sleep apnea symptoms, to have a low threshold to perform diagnostic testing, to treat OSA if present, and to closely monitor symptoms. PAP therapy for sleep apnea is often not primary therapy in management of comorbid illness but is a useful adjunct with potentially significant benefits. **Table 1** summarizes the impact of untreated sleep apnea on comorbid illnesses and the potential effects of PAP therapy on the comorbid medical condition.

REFERENCES

1. Peppard PE, Young T, Palta M, et al. Prospective study of the association between sleep-disordered

breathing and hypertension. N Engl J Med 2000; 342(19):1378–84.

2. Harding SM. Resistant hypertension and untreated severe sleep apnea: slowly gaining insight. J Clin Sleep Med 2014;10(8):845–6.

3. Shafazand S, Patel S. Effect of CPAP on blood pressure in patients with obstructive sleep apnea and resistant hypertension. J Clin Sleep Med 2014; 10(3):341–3.

4. Lavergne F, Morin L, Armistead J, et al. Atrial fibrillation and sleep-disordered breathing. J Thorac Dis 2015;7(12):E575–84.

5. Altmann DR, Ullmer E, Rickli H, et al. Clinical impact of screening for sleep related breathing disorders in atrial fibrillation. Int J Cardiol 2012;154(3):256–8.

6. Sharma B, Owens R, Malhotra A. Sleep in congestive heart failure. Med Clin North Am 2010;94(3): 447–64.

7. Oldenburg O, Lamp B, Faber L, et al. Sleep disordered breathing in patients with symptomatic heart failure. Eur J Heart Fail 2007;9:251–7.

8. Levy LM, Pepin J-L, Tamisier R, et al. Prevalence and impact of central sleep apnea in heart failure. Sleep Med Clin 2007;2:615–21.

9. Bucca CB, Brussino L, Battisti A, et al. Diuretics in obstructive sleep apnea with diastolic heart failure. Chest 2007;132(2):440–6.

10. Ziegler MG, Milic M, Sun P. Antihypertensive therapy for patients with obstructive sleep apnea. Curr Opin Nephrol Hypertens 2011;20(1):50–5.

11. Kasiakogias A, Tsioufis C, Thomopoulos C, et al. Evening versus morning dosing of antihypertive dugs in hypertensive patients with sleep apnea: a cross-overs study. J Hypertens 2015;33(2):393–400.

12. Abe H, Takahashi M, Yaegashi H, et al. Efficacy of continuous positive airway pressure on arrhythmias in obstructive sleep apnea patients. Heart Vessels 2010;25(1):63–9.

13. Kanagala R, Murali NS, Friedman PA, et al. Obstructive sleep apnea and the recurrence of atrial fibrillation. Circulation 2003;107(20):2589–94.

14. Bradley TD, Logan AG, Kimoff RJ, et al. Continuous positive airway pressure for central sleep apnea and heart failure. N Engl J Med 2005;353(19):2025–33.

15. Cowie MR, Woehrie H, Wegscheider K, et al. Adaptive servo ventilation for central sleep apnea in systolic heart failure. N Engl J Med 2015;373:1095–105.

16. Alkhalil M, Schulman E, Getsy J. Obstructive sleep apnea syndrome and asthma: what are the links? J Clin Sleep Med 2009;5:71–8.

17. Verbraecken J, McNicholas W. Respiratory mechanics and ventilator control in overlap syndrome and obesity hypoventilation. Respir Res 2013;14:132.

18. Khatri SB, Ioachimescu OC. The intersection of obstructive lung disease and sleep apnea. Cleve Clin J Med 2016;83(2):127–40.

19. Schiza S, Mermigkas C, Margaritopoulos G, et al. Idiopathic pulmonary fibrosis and sleep disorders: no longer strangers in the night. Eur Respir Rev 2015;24:327–39.

20. Aboussouan L. Sleep-disorder breathing in neuromuscular disease. Am J Respir Crit Care Med 2015;191(9):979–89.

21. Sharkey K, Kurth M, Anderson B. Obstructive sleep apnea is more common than central sleep apnea in methadone maintenance patients with subjective sleep complaints. Drug Alcohol Depend 2010;108: 77–83.

22. Teodorescu M, Xie A, Sorkness C, et al. Effects of inhaled fluticasone on upper airway during sleep and wakefulness in asthma: a pilot study. J Clin Sleep Med 2014;10(2):183–93.

23. Marin JM, Soriano JB, Carrizo SJ, et al. Outcomes in patients with chronic obstructive pulmonary disease and obstructive sleep apnea: the overlap syndrome. Am J Respir Crit Care Med 2010;182:325–31.

24. Mermigkis C, Bouloukaki I, Antoniou K, et al. Obstructive sleep apnea should be treated in patients with idiopathic pulmonary fibrosis. Sleep Breath 2015;19:385–91.

25. Morgenstern M, Singas E, Zleik B, et al. Resolution of severe obstructive sleep apnea after treatment of anti-muscle kinase receptor-positive myasthenia gravis despite 60-pound weight gain. J Clin Sleep Med 2014;10:813–4.

26. McEvoy RD, Pierce RJ, Hillman D, et al. Nocturnal non-invasive nasal ventilation in stable hypercapnic COPD: a randomised controlled trial. Thorax 2009; 64:561–6.

27. Gupta M, Simpson F. Obstructive sleep apnea and psychiatric disorders: a systematic review. J Clin Sleep Med 2015;11(2):165–75.

28. Povitz M, Bolo CE, Heitman SJ, et al. Effect of treatment of obstructive sleep apnea on depressive symptoms: systematic review and meta-analysis. PLoS Med 2014;11(11):e1001762.

29. Gupta M, Simpson F, Lyons D. The effect of treating obstructive sleep apnea with positive airway pressure on depression and other subjective symptoms: as systematic review and meta-analysis. Sleep Med Rev 2016;28:51–64.

30. Serretti A, Mandelli L. Antidepressants and body weight: a comprehensive review and meta-analysis. J Clin Psychiatry 2010;71(10):1259–72.

31. Somers V, White D, Amin R, et al. Sleep apnea and cardiovascular disease. J Am Coll Cardiol 2008; 52(8):686–717.

32. Kim Y, Koo YS, Lee HY, et al. Can continuous positive airway pressure reduce the risk of stroke in obstructive sleep apnea patients? A systematic review and meta-analysis. PLoS One 2016;11(1):e0146317.

33. Kernan WN, Ovbiagele B, Black HR, et al, on behalf of the American Heart Association Stroke Council,

Council on Cardiovascular and Stroke Nursing, Council on Clinical Cardiology, and Council on Peripheral Vascular Disease. Guidelines for the prevention of stroke in patients with stroke and transient ischemic attack: a guideline for healthcare professionals from the American Heart Association/ American Stroke Association. Stroke 2014;45: 2160–236.

34. Sateia MJ. Neuropsychological impairment and quality of life in obstructive sleep apnea. Clin Chest Med 2003;24(2):249–59.

35. Yaffe K, Laffan A, Harrison S, et al. Sleep disordered breathing, hypoxia, and risk of mild cognitive impairment and dementia in older women. JAMA 2011; 306(6):613–9.

36. Osorio R, Gumb T, Pirraglia E, et al. Sleep-disordered breathing advances cognitive decline in the elderly. Neurology 2015;84(19):1964–71.

37. Aloia MS, Arnedt JT, Davis JD, et al. Neuropsychological sequelae of obstructive sleep apnea-hypopnea syndrome: a critical review. J Int Neuropsychol Soc 2004;10(5):772–85.

38. Grunstein RR, Sullivan CE. Sleep apnea and hypothyroidism: mechanisms and management. Am J Med 1988;85:775–9.

39. Jha A, Sharma SK, Tandon N, et al. Thyroxine replacement therapy reverses sleep-disordered breathing in patients with primary hypothyroidism. Sleep Med 2006;7:55–61.

40. Resta O, Carratù P, Carpagnano GE, et al. Influence of subclinical hypothyroidism and T4 treatment on the prevalence and severity of obstructive sleep apnoea syndrome (OSAS). J Endocrinol Invest 2005;28:893–8.

41. Punjabi NM, Shahar E, Redline S, et al, Sleep Heart Health Study Investigators. Sleep-disordered breathing, glucose intolerance, and insulin resistance: the Sleep Heart Health Study. Am J Epidemiol 2004;160(6):521–30.

42. Reichmuth KJ, Austin D, Skatrud JB, et al. Association of sleep apnea and type II diabetes: a population-based study. Am J Respir Crit Care Med 2005;172(12):1590–5.

43. Pamidi S, Wroblewski K, Stepien M, et al. Eight hours of nightly continuous positive airway pressure treatment of obstructive sleep apnea improves glucose metabolism in patients with prediabetes. Am J Respir Crit Care Med 2015;192(1):96–105.

44. Gallegos L, Dharia T, Gadegbeku AB. Effect of continuous positive airway pressure on type 2 diabetes mellitus and glucose metabolism. Hosp Pract (1995) 2014;42(2):31–7.

45. Andersen ML, Bittencourt LRA, Antunes IB, et al. Effects of progesterone on sleep: a possible pharmacological treatment for sleep-breathing disorders? Curr Med Chem 2006;13(29):3575–82.

46. Tal J, Suh S, Dowdle C, et al. Treatment of insomnia, insomnia symptoms, and obstructive sleep apnea during and after menopause: therapeutic approaches. Curr Psychiatry Rev 2015;11(1):63–83.

47. Barrett-Connor E, Thuy-Tien D, Stone K. The association of testosterone levels with overall sleep quality, sleep architecture, and sleep-disordered breathing. J Clin Endocrinol Metab 2008;93(7):2602–9.

48. Bhasin S, Cunningham GR, Hayes FJ, et al. Testosterone therapy in men with androgen deficiency syndromes: an Endocrine Society clinical practice guideline. J Clin Endocrinol Metab 2010;95(6): 2536–59.

49. Hoyos CM, Killick R, Yee BJ, et al. Effects of testosterone therapy on sleep and breathing in obese men with severe obstructive sleep apnoea: a randomized placebo- controlled trial. Clin Endocrinol (Oxf) 2012; 77(4):599–607.

50. Killick ROO, Wang D, Hoyos CM. Obstructive sleep apnea: the effects of testosterone on ventilatory responses in men with obstructive sleep apnea : a randomised, placebo-controlled trial. J Sleep Res 2013;22(3):331–6.

51. Grossmann M. Low testosterone in men with type 2 diabetes: significance and treatment. J Clin Endocrinol Metab 2011;96:2341–53.

52. Pelletier-Fleury N, Rakotonanahary D, Fleury B. The age and other factors in the evaluation of compliance with nasal continuous positive airway pressure for obstructive sleep apnea syndrome. A Cox's proportional hazard analysis. Sleep Med 2001;2(3): 225–32.

53. Lin S, Chen Y, Kao K, et al. Diseases in patients coming to a sleep center with symptoms related to restless legs syndrome. PLoS One 2013;8:e71499.

54. Rodrigues D, Esraa A, Pratesi R. Outcome of restless legs severity after continuous positive air pressure (CPAP) treatment in patients affected by the association of RLS and obstructive sleep apneas. Sleep Med 2006;7:235–9.

55. Luyster F, Buysee D, Strollo P. Comorbid insomnia and obstructive sleep apnea: challenges for clinical practice and research. J Clin Sleep Med 2010;6: 196–204.

56. Krell SB, Kapur VK. Insomnia complaints in patients evaluated for obstructive sleep apnea. Sleep Breath 2005;9:104–10.

57. Lavie P. Insomnia and sleep-disordered breathing. Sleep Med 2007;8:S21–5.

58. Dolly FR, Block AJ. Effect of flurazepam on sleep-disordered breathing and nocturnal oxygen desaturation in asymptomatic subjects. Am J Med 1982;73: 239–43.

Continuous Positive Airway Pressure Therapy for Obstructive Sleep Apnea
Maximizing Adherence Including Using Novel Information Technology–based Systems

Bretton Hevener, BS, RPSGT*, William Hevener, RPSGT

KEYWORDS

- Sleep-disordered breathing • Sleep apnea • OSA • Untreated sleep apnea • Adherence
- Compliance • Positive airway pressure • PAP • CPAP

KEY POINTS

- Sleep apnea is a form of sleep-disordered breathing that is associated with an increase in disease comorbidities, mortality risks, health care costs, and traffic accidents.
- Sleep apnea is most commonly treated with positive airway pressure (PAP).
- PAP can be difficult for patients to tolerate.
- This leads to initial and long-term noncompliance.

Approximately 42 million American adults have sleep-disordered breathing.[1] This disease prevalence is similar to both asthma and diabetes combined.[1] Obstructive sleep apnea (OSA) is the most common form of sleep-disordered breathing. OSA occurs when the muscles in the back of the throat fail to keep the airway open, despite efforts to breathe. OSA occurs in all age groups and both sexes.[2] Untreated OSA is associated with an increase in disease comorbidities, mortality risks, health care costs, and traffic accidents.[1] Although it is estimated that 75% of severe sleep-disordered breathing cases remain undiagnosed,[1] over the past 5 to 10 years, the sleep industry's focus has shifted from diagnosing sleep apnea to managing the patient's sleep apnea treatment. There are multiple methods to treat sleep apnea, and medically appropriate methods should be embraced. However, positive airway pressure (PAP), a treatment that uses mild air pressure to keep the airways open, is the most common method currently used to treat sleep apnea.

In 2004, a quantitative review of 50 years of research on variations in patients' adherence to medical recommendations showed adherence rates of approximately 70% for most medical conditions.[3] The poorest rates of adherence were related to human immunodeficiency virus and sleep disorders.[3] PAP compliance or adherence is commonly defined as using the therapy for an average of 4 hours a night for at least 70% of the nights queried. Most insurance companies follow Centers for Medicare and Medicaid Services (CMS) guidelines and define PAP compliance or adherence as the use of PAP 4 or more hours per night on 70% of nights during any consecutive

Neither author has any commercial of financial interest or funding source.
Sleep Data Services LLC, Sleep Data Diagnostics Inc, 4420 Hotel Circle Court, Suite 240, San Diego, CA 92108, USA
* Corresponding author.
E-mail address: bhevener@sleepdata.com

Sleep Med Clin 11 (2016) 323–329
http://dx.doi.org/10.1016/j.jsmc.2016.04.004

30-day period during the initial 90 days of use.[4] Empiric studies suggest that PAP compliance ranges from 30% to 60%.[5]

Most insurance companies require compliance with PAP treatment to cover ongoing reimbursements for the device and related disposable supplies. Reimbursement rates have been steadily declining for some time. This decrease in reimbursement and the increase in adherence outcomes require the industry to take a businesslike approach in order to sustain service businesses. Therefore, the business of PAP compliance has been created. An applicable holistic business approach to transform industry's focus is to apply the organizational model of people, process, and technology. Using the data that have been gathered and the skills of the people in sleep medicine, new technology and processes can be applied to efficiently and effectively solve the PAP adherence problem.

In order to create PAP adherence, one must embrace everything known about creating behavioral change. There are some consistent components of the behavioral change process that are included in accepted theory-based methods, like the comprehensive Transtheoretical Model of Health Behavior (**Fig. 1**) or Optum's more recent model, The ASM Model (awareness, skill building, and maintenance).[6,7] There are a plethora of published experiences where researchers have applied these behavioral change models to health conditions like smoking cessation, weight control, treatment adherence, and others. These models can be studied to see how PAP patients may move through or between the stages of behavioral change. Then, the behavioral change processes can be applied to facilitate an increase in PAP adherence within the sleep apnea patient population. As these processes are applied, population cohorts that are positively affected by the interventions and other cohorts that are not will be discovered. These experiences can then be used to apply a more customized approach at the right time, providing an efficient and effective standardized methodology to create increased understanding, tolerance of PAP therapy, and adherence to PAP therapy within a population.

Patients who have been diagnosed with sleep apnea and who have been prescribed continuous positive airway pressure (CPAP) or bilevel therapy will begin a process of behavioral change that it is hoped will lead to adherence to PAP therapy. In some patients, lasting change occurs overnight; in some, change takes much longer, and unfortunately, some never change or are unable to maintain change.

According to the Transtheoretical Model, the first stage is the precontemplation change.

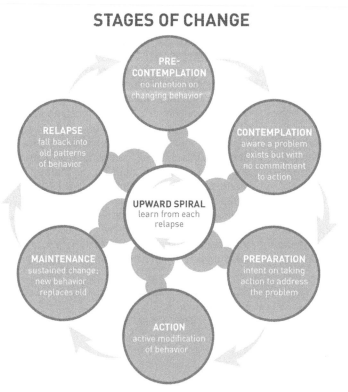

STAGES OF CHANGE

PRE-CONTEMPLATION no intention on changing behavior

CONTEMPLATION aware a problem exists but with no commitment to action

RELAPSE fall back into old patterns of behavior

UPWARD SPIRAL learn from each relapse

MAINTENANCE sustained change; new behavior replaces old

PREPARATION intent on taking action to address the problem

ACTION active modification of behavior

Fig. 1. Transtheoretical model of behavioral change.

Essentially, in this stage, the patient is not acknowledging that there is a problem behavior that needs to be changed and is not intending to take any actions.[7] This group avoids activities and even thoughts about their high-risk behavior. When addressing a PAP patient in this stage, the authors have found a few techniques that assist in moving patients through this stage. Most of these techniques found to be effective to date are related to creating awareness of the health consequences of untreated sleep apnea. It can be even more effective if the awareness is personalized. A common theme seen across several articles on PAP adherence show that education has a significant impact on awareness. The patient's awareness creates a significant improvement on PAP adherence. In a randomized controlled trial of patients with both OSA and cardiovascular disease, patients were assigned to receive either positively or negatively framed education about untreated sleep apnea.[8] Objective adherence measurements following 30 days of home CPAP therapy showed CPAP use was greater in the group receiving the negatively framed message.[8] It has also been demonstrated that showing a patient a video of himself or herself having a sleep apneic event creates a sense of personal urgency and a significant increase in PAP adherence.[9] This empiric evidence shows that PAP compliance programs must have materials in various media form: verbal, written (hardcopy and electronic), and videos on the effects of a variety of different medical conditions, psychological or behavioral conditions, and even the evidence of the increase in accidents or decrease in workplace productivity as it relates to sleep apnea in order to be relevant to a specific patient. The motivation that can be created through this awareness can accelerate the patient into the next stages of behavioral change.

The second stage of the Transtheoretical Model is contemplation. Now the patient is actively thinking about the need to change a behavior. Often the patient is doing a pro/con analysis. Sometimes the analysis is momentary, and the patient moves on from this stage relatively quickly. Other times, this patient can enter a cycle of chronic contemplation. It may be necessary to support the patient in creating their inventory of pros and cons. A structured way to do this is to begin to use a technique called motivational interviewing (MI) to guide patients through this process.[10] Motivational interviewing has been proven to improve treatment engagement, program retention, and outcome in individuals who seek treatment for substance abuse.[11] In addition, programs using MI have shown improvements in

weight loss, increase in exercise behaviors, and adherence to diabetes treatments.[12] The sleep community is using this increasingly popular behavioral change technique to address behavioral changes to improve outcomes for patients complaining of sleep deprivation symptoms and insomnia symptoms and to improve PAP adherence to therapy. When a patient begins the inventory process, it may be discovered that the motivating factor is not due to the effect of sleep apnea on a medical condition, but instead poor performance at the workplace due to sleepiness. Once this is discovered, the practitioner can begin to guide the patient through relevant information in order to stack the pros and cons in a more influential manner. The intent is to create a platform of open-ended questions where the patient can talk himself or herself into using PAP therapy. Creating an inventory of pro-change arguments will eventually tip the status quo balance toward the desired behavior change (**Box 1**). According to experts in MI, as the scale tips, the next step is to key into or elicit a kind of talk called "change talk."[10] There are 6 kinds of change talk: desire, ability, reasons, need, commitment, and taking steps.[10]

MI can be continued to be used to move into the next stage of the Transtheoretical Model. This stage is the preparation stage. Preparation is the

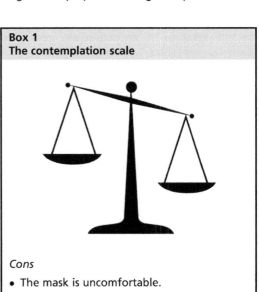

Box 1
The contemplation scale

Cons
- The mask is uncomfortable.
- My spouse will not find me attractive.

Pros
- I could try it to see if I have more energy to spend with my spouse.
- I may be more productive at work.
- I need to get my high blood pressure under control.

stage where patients are planning to take action in the immediate future.[6] It can be started by asking the patients how they would take action to begin using PAP therapy. His or her plan can be supplemented with information that will support success with their plan of action. A patient's initial action may be to schedule an appointment with the sleep physician, sleep center, or durable medical equipment company. Because the process of behavioral change is fluid, the patients can move back and forth between stages; it is important to have administrators at this facility who are trained or experienced in the common pro-and-con arguments for the use of PAP therapy to treat sleep apnea. These personnel will often encounter financial objections and clinical fears before the clinical personnel. Listening, informing, and guiding patients will often overcome resistance and navigate them through the administrative actions required by health plan and insurance networks toward therapy engagement and eventually adherence. It is important to remember that the process of behavior change is fluid and that poor customer service can create a con argument that will tip the scale back to status quo.

The preparation stage is also about mustering determination. Mustering determination is done through extrinsic motivation and intrinsic motivation. Intrinsic motivation is the motivation to engage in a behavior that arises from within the patient because it is intrinsically rewarding. Extrinsic motivation involves engaging in a behavior in order to earn external rewards or avoid punishments. The support of family and friends create an atmosphere of extrinsic motivation that facilitates behavioral change. The support of family and friends was noted in a 2012 study that showed collaboration with a patient's wife led to increased compliance with CPAP.[13] Other behavioral change research has validated this theory by showing that participants who felt self-determined, or intrinsically motivated, were more likely to perform well than those lacking an internalized motivation.[14] Intrinsic rewards involve creating positive emotions within the patient. Activities can generate these intrinsic feelings when they give a sense of meaning, a sense of progress, or competence (**Table 1**).

After gathering an inventory of intrinsic motivations and creating an action plan with the patient, the patient is ready to enter the action stage of behavior change. Although action is only 1 of the 6 stages of the Transtheoretical Model, this is the area in which the sleep industry as a whole has done much of its work for the past 30 years. The ASM Model of Optum may have a more appropriate naming of this stage, "skill-building."[7]

Table 1	
Examples of intrinsic and extrinsic motivations	
Extrinsic Motivations	**Intrinsic Motivations**
A bed partner who complains that he or she is unable to sleep in the same bedroom due to loud disturbing snoring.	A personal concern of an early death due to untreated sleep apnea.
A physician who tells the patient he or she needs to use PAP therapy to treat sleep apnea.	A feeling of accomplishment after sleeping an entire night using the PAP device.
A screening questionnaire that yields results suggestive of sleep apnea.	An improvement in sleep apnea symptoms after using PAP therapy.

During the action stage, tasks are provided. It is important that the tasks are well set. As each task is accomplished, skills will be built and intrinsic motivation will be generated from the patient's increasing self-confidence.

Many important issues can create hurdles in the realm of CPAP use. There are social issues, financial issues, interface issues, therapeutic pressure and modality issues, and treatment efficacy issues. Clinicians and patients will benefit by honesty about challenges patients may face during adaptation to therapy. Patients should not feel like they are they alone or inferior to others in their struggle to use the device. They should also be made to feel as if they can accomplish PAP adherence. All this can be quite a dance in the patient-practitioner relationship. Before a patient is sent home with PAP therapy, he or she should try on several masks to figure out which one will fit them best. Masks have many manufacturers that cover a variety of sizes and fits. However, there are 3 categories of mask styles to choose from. It is important that the clinician uses their experience to inform the patient about these styles. The full face mask generally has a larger footprint than the others. As a larger mask, it can be heavier than a mask in either of the other 2 categories. In addition, there are many more contact points with the skin, leading to more concern for mask leaks or skin irritations. This mask operates well at any therapeutic pressure. The nasal mask is designed to only cover the nose. Because of this, it is smaller in footprint than the full face mask and often lighter on the face. This mask allows the patient to breathe through the nose only. This mask also does well at all pressures. The newest mask style category is the nasal pillow mask. This mask is the smallest of the 3 designs. It fits into the nares or just around the end of the nose only, rather than over the entire nose. It has the smallest footprint of the group and also is the lightest on the face. This mask style allows breathing through the nose only. This mask does best at low- and mid-range pressures. However, on the occasional patient, it does well at high pressures too. A chin strap can be added to help keep the mouth closed when using either a nasal mask or nasal pillow mask.

Mask fit is crucial to successful adaptation and adherence to therapy. To that effect, the clinician should be sure to consider all things relevant, such as oral venting, facial structural abnormalities, therapeutic pressure needs, and the patient's preference on mask footprint size and fit style. Although mask fit is an important clinical decision, it is an opportunity to create intrinsic motivation. The clinician should inform the patient's mask choice by providing education on the masks and by providing a few appropriate masks for the patient to choose from. It is important not to overestimate the importance of providing only a few select masks. Although research has shown that choices from large assortments are advantageous when individuals value freedom, are variety-seekers, or have a very clear idea of their preferences and ideal attribute combinations, research has also shown that too much choice can overload decision-makers and lead to outcomes such as frustration or indecision.[15] A choice between 2 or 3 masks gives the patient control and ownership in this adaptation process.

Once alone and using PAP therapy at home, the patient may experience some common feelings associated with PAP adaptation. The mask may feel more uncomfortable that it did when they were in the office, or, after using the mask for some time, it may irritate the patient's skin in a particular spot. The therapeutic PAP pressure may feel like it is too hard to breathe out against. The mask or air pressure may create a feeling of claustrophobia. The air flow may feel as if it is drying out the patient's airway. The hose may feel as if it is constantly getting tangled as a patient tosses and turns to achieve comfort. Patients may feel as if they are unable to sleep or are waking up more often with the PAP than they were without it. All of these issues lead to a feeling of therapy failure or perceived lack of benefit from treatment. Early intervention and support are crucial during this phase. Positive or negative experiences with PAP therapy within the first days of treatment can predict future PAP adherence.[16] Those who need assistance with a problem tend to be focused on primarily, but it is important that an efficient method is in place to acknowledge the successes of those who struggle less with therapy. The acknowledgement of accomplishments will build positive experiences to counteract negative ones. Now is the time that the practitioner creates experiences to disrupt the patient's normal sleep experience. Over time, sleeping with untreated apnea will become the uncomfortable experience, and sleeping with PAP therapy will be preferred.

Once a patient is using PAP, he or she enters the behavioral change stage, maintenance. The maintenance stage is when the patient and his or her support team work to create a sustained behavioral change and to prevent relapse. Relapse in the case of PAP adherence is defined as not using the therapy device. It is important that the patient is informed and that they understand that sleeping without CPAP for even one night results in the return of symptoms and other manifestations of untreated OSA.[17] Patients in the maintenance stage are using PAP therapy with regularity or at least significant regularity. The patient has settled on a mask, and they most often believe at some level it is helping their symptoms. However, many patients still struggle with the idea of putting on therapy at night and sometimes take it off after a few hours. The patient may leave it off for naps, or when they get a cold, or they may consider it burdensome to travel with their equipment. Patients in this stage can often meet the 90-day insurance compliance requirements and are on their way toward the complete behavior change of CPAP adherence. However, this is a stage where patients often backslide. Based on temptation and self-efficacy data, researchers estimate that the maintenance stage generally lasts between 6 months and 5 years.[6] In regards to sleep apnea, there is minimal research regarding long-term compliance with therapy. Current estimates of PAP adherence after 1 year of use is approximately 50%.[3] Empiric research shows that when supportive interventions using education, consistent follow-up, and feedback are used, compliance rates as high as 85% at 6 months can be cultivated.[18] However, these models are often labor intensive and therefore costly.

This stage is where data and technology can have a significant effect on PAP adherence for both the patient and the business entity responsible for it. An incredible amount of technological advancements related to PAP devices, data communication, and patient management tools plays a significant role in improving patient PAP therapy compliance.

Internal provider facing software has been a tool for providers for some time now. Resmed's Airview (formerly known as EasyCare Online and ResTraxx), Resmed's U-Sleep, Philips Respironics EncoreAnywhere, and Fisher & Paykel's InfoSmart are cloud-based sleep apnea management platforms that allow providers to be able to manage patient data collected from data card download or via wireless modem data transfer. These databases, especially when paired with wireless technology, provide a reduction in labor for both the provider and the patient. Compliance reports can be acquired with a database query. Pressure changes can be performed online and communicated to the patient's device via modem communications. EncoreAnywhere, InfoSmart, and U-Sleep have features that assist in population management. Work lists can be created to provide useful information, such as usage cohorts, modem-reporting problems, elevated apnea hypopnea index (AHI), and elevated mask leaks. This data can be very useful when it comes to prioritizing patients who need a call or a visit at any given moment. No longer are expensive payroll dollars needed to call patients on a standard timeline to check in and see if they are having adherence problems. Instead, providers can use exception management to reach out to the right person at the right time. Recent research suggests a 59% reduction in costly coaching calls using ResMed's U-Sleep platform and a telehealth program to achieve similar compliance results as a "high-touch" standard model of care with scheduled contacts.[19] Resmed's AirView and Philips Respironics EncoreAnywhere have taken exception management to another level by introducing exception buckets into their patient management platform. These buckets capture patients who need assistance at scheduled intervals. Philips Respironics EncoreAnywhere has an algorithm, the Adherence Profiler, that determines the possibility of coaching to success and then scores each patient. This feature provides an ability to manage by exception in a way that reduces cost and improves adherence outcomes care.

Device manufacturers have also created patient facing self-management applications from the data coming in. Philips Respironics SleepMapper and ResMed's myAir applications are both outstanding patient facing resources to keep the patient involved in their own care and success. Both have features that support the methods taught by the Transtheoretical Behavioral Change Model, such as educational libraries to improve awareness, goal setting for action plan creation, notification through e-mail for congratulations or encouragement to improve confidence, and

notifications to address support issues associated with mask leak, low usage, and elevated AHI. SleepMapper even has a component of MI built in. These platforms are giving patients understanding and control of their own sleep apnea health care. A retrospective study of 15,000 patients from the EncoreAnywhere database has shown that patients who used SleepMapper had a 78% adherence rate based on CMS guidelines.[20] Patients who did not use SleepMapper had a 56% rate of adherence.[20] This same retrospective study showed that the SleepMapper application had a positive effect on patients who struggled with therapy but used the application versus those that did not.[20] In this cohort, 33% of the patients who engaged with the SleepMapper application were able to achieve adherence at 90 days compared with only 11% achievement in those who did not engage in SleepMapper.[20]

ResMed has provided a retrospective analysis of data in their AirView and myAir database. These data suggest several interesting adherence characteristics that can be used to create awareness and processes to improve adherence.[21] A cohort of patients in this database was categorized as "strugglers."[21] This analysis went on to say that female struggles took longer than male struggles to achieve CMS adherence.[21] The analyses also provided data that indicate that patients who used therapy for greater than 180 days have higher adherence rates and longer time periods of use than patients who have used therapy for 90 to 180 days,[21] suggesting that rates of behavioral change are significant after 6 months of PAP adherence.

A time series analysis of PAP adherence data for a cohort of patients suffering from moderate to severe sleep apnea yielded the distinct adherence patterns for 7 usage phenotypes: Good Users, Slow Improvers, Slow Decliners, Variable Users, Occasional Attempters, Early Dropouts, and Non-users.[16] These usage phenotypes may provide another level to exception management. The exception management motto can develop to "Right person, right time, with the most effective approach."

Data have been collected for years. As patient management databases are merging with patient medical record databases, the data be analyzed to continue to develop practices to improve therapy adherence rates in the sleep apnea population. Manufacturers and vendors are beginning to integrate their databases. ResMed and Philips Respironics have integrated their CMS compliance data with the home medical equipment/durable medical equipment billing software Brightree and the integrated sleep management software platform Somnoware. Sleep centers are beginning to create databases or add device data to their own databases. The potential of the intelligence that can be gained regarding sleep apnea patient phenotypes and therapy adherence begs further development and evaluation. Unlike many of the other medical conditions that are struggling with the problem of patient adherence to treatments, the sleep apnea field now has a plethora of data and various platforms and experienced researchers to query that data. Other medical fields may soon be taking the findings and applying them to solve their own treatment adherence concerns.

REFERENCES

1. ResMed: sleep apnea facts and figures. 2010. Available at: http://www.quinlansmedical.com/pdf/sleep_apnea_facts_figures.pdf. Accessed February 27, 2016.

2. Sleep apnea. National sleep foundation. Available at: https://sleepfoundation.org/sleep-disorders-problems/sleep-apnea. Accessed February 12, 2016.

3. Ballard RD, Gay PC, Strollo PJ. Interventions to improve compliance in sleep apnea patients previously non-compliant with continuous positive airway pressure. J Clin Sleep Med 2007;3(7):706–12.

4. Department of health and human services centers for Medicare & Medicaid services. Continuous and bi-level positive airway pressure (CPAP/BPAP) devices: complying with documentation & coverage requirements. 2013. Available at: https://www.cms.gov/Outreach-and-Education/Medicare-Learning-Network-MLN/MLNProducts/downloads/PAP_DocCvg_Factsheet_ICN905064.pdf. Accessed February 3, 2016.

5. Weaver TE, Sawyer AM. Adherence to continuous positive airway pressure treatment for obstructive sleep apnea: implications for future interventions. Indian J Med Res 2010;131:245–58.

6. Prochaska JO, Velicer WF. The transtheoretical model of health behavior change. Am J Health Promot 1997;12(1):38–48.

7. Modeling behavior change for better health. 2013. Optum. Available at: http://www.optum.co.uk/content/dam/optum/resources/whitePapers/101513-ORC-WP-modeling-behavior-change-for-the-better.pdf. Accessed February 3, 2016.

8. Trupp RJ, Corwin EJ, Ahijevych KL, et al. The impact of educational message framing on adherence to continuous positive airway pressure therapy. Behav Sleep Med 2011;9(1):38–52.

9. After watching disturbing videos, CPAP usage soars. Denver (CO): 2014. Available at: https://www.nationaljewish.org/about/mediacenter/pressreleases/2014-News/CPAP-Usage-Soars?feed=3a1c70d4-03ba-44e3-b0cf-acfb03e1d48a. Accessed February 3, 2016.

10. Rollnick S, Miller W, Butler C. Motivational interviewing in healthcare, helping patients change behavior. New York: The Gilford Press; 2008.

11. Carroll KM, Ball SA, Nich C, et al. Motivational interviewing to improve treatment engagement and outcome in individuals seeking treatment for substance abuse: a multisite effectiveness study. Drug Alcohol Depend 2006;81(3):301–12.

12. Christie D, Channon S. The potential for motivational interviewing to improve outcomes in the management of diabetes and obesity in paediatric and adult populations: a clinical review. Diabetes Obes Metab 2014;16:381–4.

13. DiNapoli CM. Strategies to improve continuous positive airway pressure compliance: a review. New York: Weill Cornell Medical College Center for Sleep Medicine; 2014.

14. Osbaldiston R, Sheldon KM. Promoting internalized motivation for environmentally responsible behavior: a prospective study of environmental goals. J Environ Psychol 2003;23:349–57.

15. Inbar Y, Botti S, Hanko K. Decision speed and choice regret: when haste feels like waste. J Exp Social Psychol 2011;47:533–40.

16. Aloia MS, Arnedt JT, Stanchina M, et al. How early in treatment is PAP adherence established? Revisiting night-to-night variability. Behav Sleep Med 2007;5(3):229–40.

17. Kribbs NB, Pack AI, Kline LR, et al. Effects of one night without nasal CPAP treatment on sleep and sleepiness in patients with obstructive sleep apnea. Am Rev Respir Dis 1993;147(5):1162–8.

18. Sin DD, Mayer I, Man GC, et al. Long-term compliance rates to continuous positive airway pressure in obstructive sleep apnea. Chest 2002;121:430–5.

19. Munafo D, Hevener W, Crocker M, et al. A telehealth program for CPAP adherence reduces labor and yield similar adherence and efficacy when compared to the standard of care. Sleep Breath 2016;20(2):777–85.

20. Hardy W, Powers J, Jasko JG., et al. 2014. SleepMapper. A mobile application and website to engage sleep apnea patients in PAP therapy and improve adherence to treatment. Philips Respironics. Available at: http://cdn.sleepreviewmag.com/sleeprev/2014/06/SleepMapper-Adherence-White-Paper.pdf. Accessed February 3, 2016.

21. Lynch S, Blase A, Wimms A, et al. Retrospective descriptive study of CPAP adherence associated with use of the ResMed myAir application. Sydney (Australia):: ResMed Science Center, ResMed Ltd; 2015. Available at: http://www.resmed.com/us/dam/documents/products/data-management/myair/1018839_myair_white-paper_amer_eng.pdf.

Surgical Approaches to Obstructive Sleep Apnea

Stuart G. MacKay, BSc(Med), FRACS*, Lyndon Chan, MBBS, FRACS

KEYWORDS

• OSA surgery • OSA • CPAP failure • Multilevel surgery • Effectiveness • Evidence

KEY POINTS

- Contemporary obstructive sleep apnea (OSA) surgery is a key salvage treatment option for patients who have failed device use (ie, continuous positive airway pressure [CPAP] or mandibular advancement splint [MAS]).
- Nasal surgery should be considered a prephase option to facilitate subsequent CPAP or MAS or airway surgery.
- Newer variants of modified palatal and tongue surgeries are increasingly supported for their ability to achieve improved outcomes with less sacrifice of functional tissue.
- New modalities such as cranial nerve stimulation show significant promise.
- The current status of high-level literature supports a role for contemporary airway surgery in OSA, but ongoing level I and level II studies are still necessary.

INTRODUCTION

Surgery in adult obstructive sleep apnea (OSA) has undergone significant advancement in recent years and continues to evolve. It is a modality of treatment used in the context of failed device use, specifically, failed continuous positive airway pressure (CPAP) or mandibular advancement splint (MAS). In this context, the role of surgery is as salvage therapy to improve outcomes[1–3] or to facilitate better tolerance of device use. Other treatments such as weight loss, adjuvant nasal therapy (medical ± prephase nasal surgery), and positional devices may be combined with airway surgery. Both pediatric OSA, being a separate entity to adult OSA, and bariatric surgery are discussed and are considered elsewhere. In general, patients with OSA are managed with in-hospital monitoring perioperatively, but where ambulatory considerations are realistic, they are highlighted in this article.

DEFINITION OF OBSTRUCTIVE SLEEP APNEA SURGERY

Adult OSA surgery includes an array of operative procedures to open or stabilize the upper airway and is outlined in **Box 1**. It is much more than just uvulopalatopharyngoplasty (UPPP) or maxillo-mandibular surgery as a fall back. Procedures are rarely isolated or directed to a single level of the airway and are often concurrent or staged. Prephase nasal surgery is used to facilitate return to device use with better adherence, or before multilevel surgery.

PHILOSOPHY OF SURGERY

In real clinical context, patients who fail primary device use therapy would remain otherwise untreated without salvage options such as upper airway OSA surgery.[4] Many such patients are usually desperate for an alternative, at least to reduce

Conflicts of Interest: The authors have no commercial or financial conflicts of interest related to this article. Associate Professor S.G. MacKay is a chief investigator on NHMRC Project App ID 1059510 as well as a recent recipient of a Garnett-Passe Rodney Williams Foundation Conjoint Grant.
Department of ENT Surgery, Illawarra ENT Head and Neck Clinic, Suite 1 & 2, 8-10 Victoria Street, Wollongong, New South Wales 2500, Australia
* Corresponding author.
E-mail address: sgmackay@ozemail.com.au

Sleep Med Clin 11 (2016) 331–341
http://dx.doi.org/10.1016/j.jsmc.2016.04.003

> **Box 1**
> **Sample of procedures used in obstructive sleep apnea surgery**
>
> *Traditional Procedures*
> - Tonsillectomy
> - Adenoidectomy
> - UPPP
> - Geniotubercle advancement
> - Hyoid suspension
> - Epiglottoplexy
> - Maxillomandibular advancement
>
> *More Contemporary Procedures*
> - Modified or variant UPPP
> - Expansion sphincteroplasty
> - Uvulopalatal flap
> - Lateral palatoplexy
> - Transpalatal advancement
> - Radiofrequency systems
> - Coblation channeling
> - Midline glossectomy
> - Submucosal lingualplasty
> - Lingual tonsillar reduction

symptom burden and improve quality of life, and to mitigate cardiovascular risk.

Contemporary ethos and summation of available evidence recognizes that OSA surgery allows at least partial treatment applied all the time, as opposed to CPAP, which although a complete treatment modality, may only be applied part of the time.[5] What constitutes effective CPAP use to ameliorate complications of OSA is still yet to be clarified.[6]

CLINICAL ASSESSMENT IN OBSTRUCTIVE SLEEP APNEA SURGERY, INCLUDING DYNAMIC AIRWAY ASSESSMENT

A comprehensive sleep history with focus on snoring, partner-witnessed apnea, disrupted sleep, sleep hygiene, sleep position, tiredness, sleepiness, nasal symptoms, weight, and its progression should be taken. Symptoms indicating other treatable diseases such as thyroid disorders, inflammatory conditions, and depression must be explored. This history needs to be put in the context of patient concerns, such as daytime somnolence, reduced executive function, or social and marital disruption, as well as clinician concerns for cardiovascular, motor vehicle, and industrial accident risk.

Examination includes documentation of body mass index (height and weight), neck circumference, and blood pressure. Maxillofacial assessment for significant maxillary hypoplasia, retrognathia, and unfavorable soft tissue anatomy is made. Nasal examination includes dynamic evaluation of nasal valve, anterior rhinoscopy, and nasendoscopy. The oral cavity and oropharynx are examined, and the Friedman tonsil and tongue-relative-to-palate grade is recorded.[7] Flexible nasendoscopy is performed in the erect and supine positions, combined with the modified Mueller maneuver and Woodson hypotonic method.[8–10] The airway is examined at multiple levels both in the natural position and with a jaw thrust maneuver, used to assess the magnitude of change in the airway. Sedation endoscopy may be used either in certain select cases, or in some clinician's practices, routinely.[11]

Clinical questionnaires generally include a measure of snoring (eg, Snoring Severity Scale[12]), a measure of sleepiness (eg, Epworth Sleepiness Scale [ESS][13]), a quality-of-life yardstick (eg, Functional Outcomes of Sleep Questionnaire-30 [FOSQ-30][14]), and in some practices predictive tools (eg, Berlin[15] or STOP-BANG[16]).

Formal in-laboratory polysomnography is preferred, but if unavailable, a sleep physician–requested and reviewed level II ambulatory study are performed preoperatively and after definitive surgical intervention.

PREPHASE NASAL SURGERY

Nasal obstruction affects 25% to 40% of CPAP users,[21] and the need for nasal airway patency in the treatment of OSA is well established. Depending on the underlying disorder, this may be achieved via medical therapies, surgery, immunotherapy, or a combination. Anatomic obstructions can be addressed with prephase nasal surgery with the intention of facilitating frontline OSA therapies.[22] Nasal surgery also significantly decreases pressure requirements and improves compliance in CPAP use.[17] In isolation, it may improve apnea hypopnea index (AHI) and the symptoms of OSA, and on the rare occasion, may even obviate further treatment.[20,23,24] However, it must be emphasized that these are not the objectives of nasal surgery, and the need for further treatment is usually required.

Surgical reduction of inferior turbinate size, usually with concomitant correction of septal deviations, remains the mainstays of improving nasal airway patency and has been shown to result in the greatest decrease in CPAP pressures.[17] Other procedures include dynamic nasal valve surgery, rhinoplasty, functional endoscopic sinus surgery, polypectomy, and adenoidectomy. The type of surgery required is individualized to each patient and may require a combination of procedures to achieve optimal nasal airway. The procedures are generally well tolerated, and complete healing usually occurs within 6 weeks, during which time CPAP may still be used. Complications of nasal surgery are infrequent, and serious adverse outcomes are rare. Simultaneous nasal and pharyngeal surgery should be avoided where possible because there is an associated higher complication rate,[25] but in select cases may be necessary.

The role of nasal surgery is outlined earlier, but more specific indications are listed in **Box 2** with the supporting literature. Ambulatory prephase nasal surgery can be considered,[26] but this needs careful deliberation in the context of severity of OSA and potential perioperative complications, anesthetic risk, as well as patient and clinician preferences.

CONTEMPORARY SURGICAL INTERVENTION PARADIGMS AND SELECTION

The first 2 indications for surgery in **Box 3** have been discussed at length.[4,27,28] The latter 2 (asterisks) are open to debate, particularly when considering patients who prefer surgery but refuse outright a trial of device use under sleep physician supervision. Primary surgery in patients with favorable anatomy (such as tonsillar hypertrophy and dynamic collapse) has been a topic of recent consideration in the literature.[29]

Fig. 1 demonstrates an overview of how adult OSA patients come to surgery. Patients undergoing surgical treatment will likely initially undergo phase 1 type procedures either as staged or as multilevel procedures. However, individual circumstances may mandate bypassing of phase 1 procedures and moving straight to phase 2 surgeries. Contemporary variations on traditional techniques are noteworthy; previous surgeries involving resection of palatal soft tissue should no longer be performed. Most surgeries involve

---

Box 2
Indications for prephase nasal surgery

- Failed tolerance or efficacy of device use[17]
- Significant complications of device use[17]
- Significant symptoms related to nasal mucosal abnormality itself[18]
- Significant correctable structural/dynamic nasal anatomy[17,19]
- A treatment modality to improve sleep disordered breathing (in select cases)[20]

Box 3
Indications for contemporary upper airway surgery in obstructive sleep apnea

- Failed compliance/tolerance of CPAP/MAS use
- Significant complications/side effects of device use
- Patient favors/desires surgery*
- Particularly favorable anatomy for surgery*

*Indications not absolute, requires further discussion.

---

soft tissue work to reposition the palate, and modified variants of UPPP that focus on superolateral velopharyngeal port opening without resecting functional tissues are now standard of care.[29–33] Some investigators recommend ambulatory UPPP in selected patients[34–36]; however, this should be approached with caution in patients with moderate to severe OSA. Transpalatal advancement in patients requiring anterior repositioning or where modified UPPP has been or is likely to be inadequate, and where the arch of the palate is not excessively high and narrow, has found its place in contemporary protocols.[37] Bulky lingual tonsils can be reduced with suction diathermy or coblation. Gentle reduction of a bulky tongue can be achieved by minimally invasive coblation channeling,[30] a procedure that is well tolerated, has good safety profile, and can undergo repeat treatments. Tongue bulk can also be reduced by a variety of predominantly mucosally preserving surgeries, such as submucosal lingualplasty or the coblation-assisted Lewis and MacKay operation, and are preferred over traditional resective operations,[38,39] although newer robotic techniques are gaining momentum despite some posterior tongue mucosal sacrifice.[40]

Maxillomandibular advancement, which can be performed in conjunction with a high sliding genioplasty, is usually reserved for those who have entered the surgical pathway and are refractory to phase 1 surgical procedures or those with significant retrognathia, micrognathia, and/or maxillary hypoplasia. It involves expansion of the skeletal framework that encompasses the upper airways at all levels. Expansion of the skeletal framework is achieved via multiple transoral osteotomies of the maxilla and mandible, then advancing the entire complex 10 to 14 mm and stabilizing with hardware. A review reported that this procedure yielded superior results when compared with soft tissue surgery[41]; however, comparisons were only made to single-level airway surgery, not the multilevel surgery seen in contemporary operative management that is

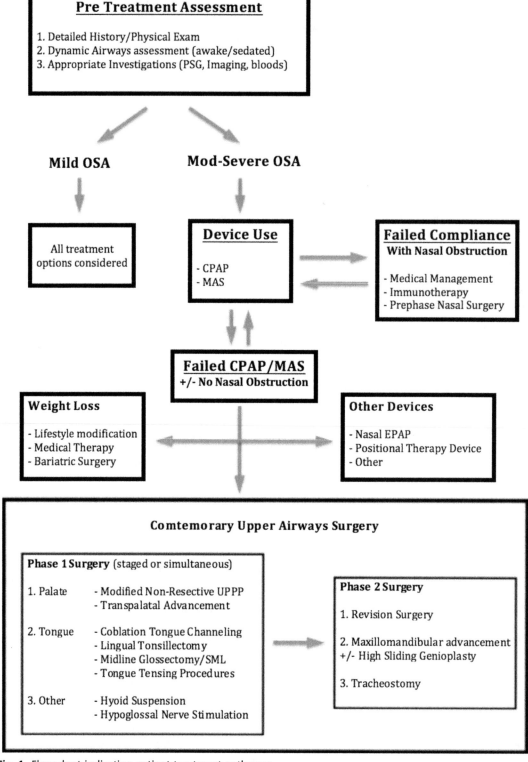

Fig. 1. Flow chart indicating patient treatment pathways.

currently performed in clinical practice. The same review also acknowledges that modern soft tissue palatal techniques may have better outcomes.[41] Recent meta-analysis shows that maxillomandibular surgery significantly reduces AHI and oxygen saturation nadir in most cases, with a "cure" achieved in 38.5% of patients.[42] However, these rates were lowered for the morbidly obese. Despite concern for complications, most patients report an improved quality of life[43] and consider it worthwhile.[44]

Tracheostomy is the ultimate procedure, because the upper airway is completely bypassed. A meta-analysis shows significant improvement in AHI, oxygen desaturation index, subjective sleepiness, and cardiovascular-related as well as overall mortality.[45] However, in both maxillomandibular advancement and tracheostomy, improvement may not apply to those over the age of 60 or those that are morbidly obese with obesity-hypoventilation syndrome and may even make their parameters worse.[46] Tracheostomy also has the inherent morbidities that come with an open-instrumented wound and is seldom a choice that most patients are willing to make.

Readers are encouraged to visit the Web site of the International Surgical Sleep Society for more information regarding the range of procedures considered to have treatment effect.[47]

COMPLICATIONS OF SURGERY

The presence of OSA is an independent risk factor for an increased complication rate and can mandate a higher level of perioperative care.[48,49] In airway reconstructive surgery, the spectrum of complications reflect the heterogeneity of the disease and surgical treatments available. The type and likelihood of complications have many influences, including factors related to the patient, anesthetic, perioperative care, surgical extent, and techniques used to address the patient-specific problem. Broadly, they can be divided into generic and procedure specific complications.

OSA-specific anesthetic considerations exist. Preoperative assessment and optimization are critical to avoid major perioperative cardiovascular and respiratory events. Mortality related to OSA surgery is rare; however, the need for overnight monitoring and higher level care, such as intensive care unit, is appropriate in most cases and should always be considered, especially in multilevel surgery and more severe OSA, but is not mandatory.[34] Potential airway obstruction must be anticipated. It may occur on induction of anesthesia or postoperatively, leading to inability to extubate, the need to reintubate, or necessitating

a tracheostomy. Fortunately, airway obstruction is an increasingly infrequent event, likely due to better understanding of OSA perioperative management, steroid use, and limiting respiratory depressants.[50,51]

Bleeding, infection, and pain resulting in odynophagia and consequential dehydration are ubiquitous risks in all OSA surgery. Bleeding is an uncommon but potentially major concern. Bleeding may occur directly into the upper aerodigestive tract or formation of a hematoma. Negation of bleeding diathesis and careful blood pressure control are achieved through activity modification and sometimes medication. All surgical wounds in the upper aerodigestive tract are inevitably colonized by pathogens, and antibiotics are generally prescribed for major airways procedures, although this may be contentious. Pain is by far the most notable issue from the patient perspective, particularly when tonsillectomy or lingual tonsillectomy forms a part of the procedure. For most, the pain peaks at day 4 to 7 and is managed by regular analgesia, and on occasion, steroids.

Palatal surgery is associated with velopalatal insufficiency and nasopharyngeal stenosis, but is less common and usually transient in contemporary nonresective operations. Globus, altered voice (in particular loss of guttural sounds), and palatal paraesthesia may also occur, usually transiently. Surgical procedures on the hard palate can cause mucosal flap necrosis, oronasal fistulae with an estimated incidence of 2% to 3%, and very rarely, eustachian tube dysfunction from loss of tensor veli palatini action.

Expansion of the retrolingual space is achieved via numerous methods. Tongue reduction procedures can injure the neurovascular bundle and cause hypoglossal nerve injury, dysgeusia, tongue paraesthesia, and globus. Geniotubercle advancement may result in mandibular fracture, mental nerve injury, disruption of the dental roots, genioglossal avulsion from the tubercle, cosmetic defect, and exposure/infection/failure of implanted hardware. Hyoid suspension has a preponderance for aspiration and dysphagia. Maxillomandibular advancement is the most morbid and extensive procedure; complications include altered cosmetics, dental malocclusion, paraesthesia, temporomandibular dysfunction, and hardware-related failures.

EFFECTIVENESS OF OBSTRUCTIVE SLEEP APNEA SURGERY: CURRENT STATUS OF LITERATURE: NONRANDOMIZED TRIALS

Over many years, high-level cohort studies have demonstrated a role for (salvage) airway surgery in adult OSA. Weaver and colleagues[1] followed 20,000 US War Veterans and actually found a survival advantage with surgery over CPAP provision (not CPAP application) at 4 years. Similarly, Marti and colleagues concluded that successful treatment with surgery (and indeed CPAP, MAS, and weight loss) reverted death risk to that of the general population.[2] A large Gothenburg cohort study of 370 patients (182 middle-aged men) demonstrated reduction in cardiovascular risk over 7 years in efficiently treated patients, where one of the treatment modalities was surgery.[3]

Other cohort studies confirming surgery can achieve important quality-of-life outcomes have been published in recent years, including articles by Rotenberg and colleagues[29] and Robinson and colleagues.[27] Both of these articles carry added importance given the use of real-life staged surgical interventions. In addition, recent literature confirms improvement in depression scores with surgery[52] and increase in baroreflex sensitivity with modified palatal and tongue reduction surgery.[53] The latter is particularly relevant in the context of awareness that depressed baroreflex sensitivity is a major contributor to cardiovascular morbidity/mortality in OSA.[54–56]

Some investigators have questioned the economic value of OSA surgery,[57] but a recent cost-effectiveness analysis has firmly established the benefit of palatopharyngeal reconstructive surgery using semi-Markov modeling.[58]

EFFECTIVENESS OF OBSTRUCTIVE SLEEP APNEA SURGERY: CURRENT STATUS OF LITERATURE AND CHALLENGES OF RANDOMIZED CONTROLLED TRIALS

Randomized controlled trials (RCTs) in surgery for OSA carry significant challenges related to methodology, design, and real-life execution. These challenges vary from how to define surgery and comparator groups, how to recruit patients, inclusion and exclusion criteria, maintaining a control group, generalizability of outcomes, and choice of outcome measures.

How to Define Obstructive Sleep Apnea Surgery

OSA surgery can be complex to characterize and is broadly defined as previously indicated. Procedures are often multilevel simultaneous or staged and based on comprehensive history, airway assessment, polysomnographic findings, and patient preferences.

In randomized trials, interventions may be single level only to reduce complexity, permit greater reproducibility, and avoid ethics ramifications.

Such single-level RCTs may achieve excellent results[33] but not reflect more commonly applied real-life multilevel surgeries. Staged surgical protocol[27,28,59] can be harder to apply in a high-level surgical RCT. In RCT level studies, individual surgeon-dictated variations in specific cases may be subjugated to achieve rigid, reproducible protocols that might be detrimental to patient outcome.

Patient Selection

Patients should desire surgery, and the surgeon must establish that it is an appropriate option in each case.[60] In a randomized surgery trial, inclusion and exclusion criteria may lead to variance in usual practice case-to-case modifications. Some studies recruit among vulnerable populations, such as children,[61] and may enroll subgroups who are less able to achieve "successful" surgery due to equipoise, because the population one wants to study may be less appropriate for the intervention.

Recruitment/Enrollment

Patients worried about complications of their disease may be concerned about being randomized away from surgery. If it remains their only option after CPAP/device use failure, they may avoid joining a trial. These patients and those that have private insurance might elect surgery outside of a trial, thereby skewing the study population.

Recruiting from private, community, and academic facilities may make RCT results more generalizable, and offering surgery to all control patients at study completion may help. Low-risk surgery can at least make the intervention closer to pill and placebo studies,[62] possibly increasing participation but again reducing real-life applicability.

Economics

Industry sponsorship is common in medication and device RCTs[63] but less frequent in surgical studies, and insurance companies may not fund operations if part of a trial, because it is considered "experimental." Less expensive procedures, such as radiofrequency to the palate and tongue,[64] might not reflect real world generalizability, but are ambulatory, reduce costs, and may demonstrate treatment effect.

These minor procedures are attractive to mitigate direct costs and inpatient fees,[62,64] which might be borne by the patient. Ambulatory sleep studies might also reduce costs, but they can also reduce reliability, compared with formal in-laboratory studies.[65]

Comparator Group

Placebo or "sham" CPAP devices may be applied as a comparator group intervention. "Sham" surgery is somewhat more difficult to institute in a trial and complex for Ethics committees to approve. Adult OSA surgery is usually applied in clinical practice when CPAP or oral appliances have failed,[27] and thereby, a common comparator group should be those with no treatment or conservative measures only. To ask a patient to randomize to or away from a treatment such as CPAP (a device) or medication is relatively acceptable, but to ask them to randomize to or away from a surgical intervention that carries immediate risk is vexed.[66] The patient must be willing to enroll and take the chance of being placed into a control group with no treatment. The result of untreated disease in OSA (when randomized to control arm) may result in significant morbidity and mortality.[54] Surgery trials might only achieve ethics approval if mild OSA is studied, given the risks to the control arm in severe disease.

Comparative effectiveness trials may not be practical, because surgery compared with another treatment is likely to need a large sample size to show a difference in effect. Such sample sizes are harder to achieve in surgical trials compared with device/medication trials. Efficacy measures favor CPAP over OSA surgery, creating added complexity in a surgery—CPAP trial.

Surgical RCTs comparing surgery with intent to treat and "sham" operations are neither practical nor ethical. Pain, anatomic rearrangements, and recovery will likely be perceived by patients, making patient blinding difficult. Randomization to a procedure that induces discomfort in a placebo arm without the benefit is also likely to be ethically inappropriate.

Outcome Measures

As indicated in the previous section on non-randomized evidence, long-term cohort studies suggest critical outcome measures, such as death,[1,2] cardiovascular risk,[3] and quality-of-life parameter measures,[27] are similar between CPAP and surgery. Effectiveness of CPAP use in the community differs to in-laboratory polysomnographic efficacy, detracting from conclusions that might be drawn from certain studies, unless mean disease alleviation is applied.[67]

Hence, objective measures may be discordant with symptom and quality-of-life improvement.[68] OSA RCTs comparing surgery to CPAP are likely to favor the latter if surrogate polysomnography parameters are used, and using death and cardiovascular measures might lengthen a trial beyond what is feasible.

Despite all of these challenges, published RCTs have demonstrated a role for surgery in OSA. A 4-year Scandinavian study showed significant AHI reduction with modified UPPP, and in real-life clinical practice, such surgery would often be combined with tongue reduction procedures or other interventions to conceivably achieve even better outcomes.[33]

An extension of this article also revealed important quality-of-life, sleepiness, and vigilance benefits.[69] Radiofrequency RCTs have identified key roles for treatment directed to turbinates[62] and the tongue and palate,[64] with the latter demonstrating impact on apnea and vigilance. Inspire Medical sponsored a study of the hypoglossal nerve stimulator with 126 patients experiencing a significant reduction in AHI from 29 to 9.[70] In the withdrawal component of the study, the problem of an untreated comparator arm was overcome by instigating a "stimulator turn-off/turn-on" policy.[71]

The same patients also demonstrated a significant improvement in ESS, FOSQ-30, FOSQ-10, and partner subjective snoring reports.[72] The benefits seen were maintained for at least 24 months. Other RCTs, including evaluating multilevel surgery across multiple centere, are in progress.

RCTs in OSA surgery are difficult to achieve for all the reasons outlined, but these challenges should not excuse the need to expand the volume of RCTs in this important field, nor should it overshadow the existing cohort level literature supporting a role for contemporary surgical intervention.

RECENT/CURRENT INNOVATIONS

Developments in recent years in OSA surgery can be broadly divided into newer technique variations, upper airway stimulation, and robotic surgery.

Newer technique variations have been covered earlier, particularly reconstructive and modified UPPPs and modified tongue reduction.

Upper airway stimulation has been evaluated over some years, but recent hypoglossal nerve stimulation (HGNS) trials have shown this to be an exciting evolution.[73] At this time, it is available only in the United States and other select countries. The current HGNS involves a surgically implanted complex of 3 components: an upper chest pulse generator, a cuffed electrode with stimulation lead on the hypoglossal nerve (or selective medial fibers), and an intercostal space sensor lead, to detect respiratory effort. Stated advantages of HGNS include probable "coupling" of retropalatal and retrolingual segments to afford reduction of multilevel collapse, ability to titrate to control of apnea and symptoms, and avoidance of endoluminal airway complications related to traditional upper airway surgery. Other similar, but less invasive devices are also being developed. Current literature supports an emerging role as a second-line therapy. Disadvantages include lifelong requirement of an implantable device and attachments, sleep disruption, and surgical risks, such as infection, hematoma, and cranial nerve injury.

Since Vicini and colleagues established the concept of using transoral robotic surgery in 2010,[40,74] advocates have highlighted its potential improved access to the base of tongue and lingual tonsil. Three-dimensional depth perception and robotic arms are used to reduce tissue bulk in this area, and a growing body of evidence supports its use.[40] Possible disadvantages include restricted financial access to equipment and lack of mucosal preservation.

FUTURE DIRECTIONS AND INNOVATIONS

As the body of literature evolves for contemporary multilevel airway surgery in CPAP failure, it is becoming important to test such surgery at higher levels of evidence. A National Health and Medical Research Council–funded randomized controlled clinical trial is underway in Australia assessing multilevel palatal and tongue surgery compared with best conservative medical care in device failure/rejection patients. It is hoped such trials will support a role for salvage surgery and encourage similar such investigations worldwide.

Physiologic phenotyping offers an exciting modality, if it can be combined with sound clinical and anatomic assessment, to improve patient selection for contemporary airway surgery. Preoperative patient advisement and predictability of improvement are the ultimate goals of surgical interventions, and correlation between particular polysomnographic parameters of disease, clinical findings, and outcomes will support such endeavors.

Finally, OSA airway modeling and simulation to allow subsequent assessment of newer biotechnology, smart polymers, and molecular alterations represent a possible future pathway for minimal surgical interventions to achieve stabilized airways in sleep, while avoiding disruption to normal upper aerodigestive tracts during wakefulness.

ACKNOWLEDGMENTS

The authors thank Ed Weaver, B. Tucker Woodson, and Susan Redline for their contributions regarding randomized controlled trials in OSA surgery and Sue Ellen Holmes for formatting.

REFERENCES

1. Weaver EM, Maynard C, Yueh B. Survival of veterans with sleep apnea: continuous positive airway pressure versus surgery. Otolaryngol Head Neck Surg 2004;130:659–65.
2. Marti S, Sampol G, Muñoz X, et al. Mortality in severe sleep apnoea/hypopnoea syndrome patients: impact of treatment. Eur Respir J 2002;20(6):1511–8.
3. Peker Y, Hedner J, Norum J, et al. Increased incidence of cardiovascular disease in middle-aged men with obstructive sleep apnea; a 7-year follow-up. Am J Respir Crit Care Med 2002;166:159–65.
4. Weaver EM. Judging sleep apnea surgery. Sleep Med Rev 2010;14(5):283–5.
5. Ravesloot MJL, de Vries N, Stuck BA. Treatment adherence should be taken into account when reporting treatment outcomes in obstructive sleep apnea. Laryngoscope 2014;124:344–5.
6. Crawford MR, Bartlett DJ, Coughlin SR, et al. The effect of continuous positive airway pressure usage on sleepiness in obstructive sleep apnoea: real effects or expectation of benefit? Thorax 2012;67:920–4.
7. Friedman M, Ibrahim H, Bass L. Clinical staging for sleep disordered breathing. Laryngoscope 2004;114(3):454–9.
8. Hsu PP, Tan BYB, Chan YH, et al. Clinical predictors in obstructive sleep apnea patients with computer-assisted quantitative videoendoscopic upper airway analysis. Laryngoscope 2004;114:791–9.
9. Hsu PP, Han HNC, Chan YH, et al. Quantitative computer-assisted digital-imaging upper airway analysis for obstructive sleep apnoea. Clin Otolaryngol Allied Sci 2004;29:522–9.
10. Woodson BT, Feroah T, Connolly LA, et al. A method to evaluate upper airway mechanics following intervention in snorers. Otolaryngology 1997;18(5):306–14.
11. Eichler C, Ulrich Sommer J, Stuck BA, et al. Does drug-induced endoscopy change the treatment concept of patients with snoring and OSA? Sleep Breath 2013;17(1):63–8.
12. Morris LG, Kleinberger A, Lee KC, et al. Rapid risk stratification for obstructive sleep apnea, based on snoring severity and body mass index. Otolaryngol Head Neck Surg 2008;139(5):615–8.
13. Johns MW. A new method for measuring daytime sleepiness: the Epworth sleepiness scale. Sleep 1991;14(6):540–5.
14. Weaver TE, Laizner AM, Evans LK, et al. An instrument to measure functional status outcomes for disorders of excessive sleepiness. Sleep 1997;20:835–43.

15. Netzer NC, Stoohs RA, Netzer CM, et al. Using the Berlin Questionnaire to identify patients at risk for the sleep apnea syndrome. Ann Intern Med 1999; 131:485–91.

16. Vasu TS, Doghramji K, Cavallazzi R, et al. Obstructive sleep apnea syndrome and postoperative complications: clinical use of the STOP-BANG questionnaire. Arch Otolaryngol Head Neck Surg 2010;136:1020–4.

17. Camacho M, Riaz M, Capasso R, et al. The effect of nasal surgery on continuous positive airway pressure device use and therapeutic treatment pressures: a systematic review and meta-analysis. Sleep 2015;38(2):279–86.

18. Georgalas C. The role of the nose in snoring and obstructive sleep apnea: an update. Eur Arch Otorhinolaryngol 2011;268(9):1365–73.

19. Friedman M, Tanyeri H, Lim J, et al. Effect of improved nasal breathing on OSA. Otolaryngol Head Neck Surg 2000;122(1):71–4.

20. Bican A, Kahrman A, Bora I, et al. What is the efficacy of nasal surgery in patients with obstructive sleep apnea? J Craniofac Surg 2010;21(6):1801–6.

21. Brander PE, Soirinsuo M, Lohela P. Nasopharyngeal symptoms in patients with obstructive sleep apnea syndrome. Effect of nasal CPAP treatment. Respiration 1999;66:128–35.

22. Epstein LJ, Kristo D, Strollo PJ, et al. Clinical guideline for the evaluation, management and long-term care of obstructive sleep apnea in adults. J Clin Sleep Med 2009;5:263–76.

23. Nakata S, Noda A, Yasuma F. Effects of nasal surgery on sleep quality in obstructive sleep apnea syndrome with nasal obstruction. Am J Rhinol 2008;22(1):59–63.

24. Park CY, Hong JH, Lee JH, et al. Clinical effect of surgical correction for nasal pathology on the treatment of obstructive sleep apnea syndrome. PLoS One 2014;9(6):e98765.

25. Mickelson S, Hakim I. Is pre-operative intensive care monitoring necessary after uvulopalatopharyngoplasty? Otolaryngol Head Neck Surg 1998;119(4):352–6.

26. Bhattacharyya N. Unplanned revisits and readmissions after ambulatory sinonasal surgery. Laryngoscope 2014;124:1983–7.

27. Robinson S, Chia M, Carney AS, et al. Upper airway reconstructive surgery long-term quality-of-life outcomes compared with CPAP for adult obstructive sleep apnea. Otolaryngol Head Neck Surg 2009; 141(2):257–63.

28. Mackay SG, Jefferson N, Marshall NS. Beyond uvulopalatopharyngoplasty for obstructive sleep apnoea: single surgeon case series of contemporary airway reconstruction. J Laryngol Otol 2013; 127(12):1184–9.

29. Rotenberg BW, Theriault J, Gottesman S. Redefining the timing of surgery for obstructive sleep apnea in anatomically favorable patients. Laryngoscope 2014;124:S1–9.

30. MacKay S, Carney S, Woods C, et al. Modified uvulopalatopharyngoplasty and coblation channeling of the tongue for obstructive sleep apnea: a multicentre Australian trial. J Clin Sleep Med 2013;9: 117–24.

31. Pang KP, Woodson BT. Expansion sphincter pharyngoplasty: a new technique for the treatment of obstructive sleep apnea. Otolaryngol Head Neck Surg 2007;137:110–4.

32. Cahali MB, Formigoni GG, Gebrim EM, et al. Lateral pharyngoplasty versus uvulopalatopharyngoplasty: a clinical, polysomnographic and computed tomography measurement comparison. Sleep 2004;27(5): 942–50.

33. Browaldh N, Nerfeldt P, Lysdahl M, et al. SKUP3 randomised controlled trial: polysomnographic results after uvulopalatopharyngoplasty in selected patients with obstructive sleep apnoea. Thorax 2013;68(9):846–53.

34. Kandasamy T, Wright E, Fuller J, et al. The incidence of early post-operative complications following uvulopalatopharyngoplasty: identification of predictive risk factors. J Otolaryngol Head Neck Surg 2013; 42(1):15.

35. Hathaway B, Johnston JT. Safety of uvulopalatopharyngoplasty as outpatient surgery. Otolaryngol Head Neck Surg 2006;134(4):542–4.

36. Bhattacharyya N. Revisits and readmissions following ambulatory uvulopalatopharyngoplasty. Laryngoscope 2015;125(3):754–7.

37. Woodson BT, Robinson S, Lim HJ. Transpalatal advancement pharyngoplasty outcomes compared with uvulopalatopharygoplasty. Otolaryngol Head Neck Surg 2005;133(2):211–21.

38. Mackay SG, Jefferson N, Grundy L, et al. Coblation-assisted Lewis and MacKay operation (CobLAMO): new technique for tongue reduction in sleep apnoea surgery. J Laryngol Otol 2013;127(12):1222–5.

39. Gunawardena I, Robinson S, Mackay S, et al. Submucosal lingualplasty for adult obstructive sleep apnea. Otolaryngol Head Neck Surg 2013;148(1):157–65.

40. Crawford JA, Montevechi F, Vicini C, et al. Transoral robotic sleep surgery: the obstructive sleep apnea–hypopnea syndrome. Otolaryngol Clin North Am 2014;47(3):397–406.

41. Caples SM, Rowley JA, Prinsell JR, et al. Surgical modifications of the upper airways for obstructive sleep apnea in adults: a systemic review and meta-analysis. Sleep 2010;33(10):1396–407.

42. Zaghi S, Holty JE, Certal V, et al. Maxillomandibular advancement for treatment of obstructive sleep apnea: a meta-analysis. JAMA Otolaryngol Head Neck Surg 2016;142(1):58–66.

43. Boyd SB, Walters AS, Waite P, et al. Long-term effectiveness and safety of maxillomandibular advancement for treatment of obstructive sleep apnea. J Clin Sleep Med 2015;11(7):699–708.

44. Goodday R, Bourque S. Subjective outcomes of maxillomandibular advancement surgery for treatment of obstructive sleep apnea syndrome. J Oral Maxillofac Surg 2012;70(2):417–20.

45. Camacho M, Certal V, Brietzke SE, et al. Tracheostomy as treatment for adult obstructive sleep apnea: a systematic review and meta-analysis. Laryngoscope 2014;124(3):803–11.

46. Camacho M, Teixeira J, Abdullatif J, et al. Maxillomandibular advancement and tracheostomy for morbidly obese obstructive sleep apnea: a systematic review and meta-analysis. Otolaryngol Head Neck Surg 2015;152(4):619–30.

47. Available at: http://www.surgicalsleep.org/isss-position-statement-on-sleep-surgery. Accessed May 16, 2016.

48. Vasu TS, Grewal R, Doghramji K. Obstructive sleep apnea syndrome and perioperative complications: a systematic review of the literature. J Clin Sleep Med 2012;8(2):199–207.

49. Adesanya AO, Lee W, Greilich NB, et al. Perioperative management of obstructive sleep apnea chest. Chest 2010;138(6):1489–98.

50. Pang KP, Siow JK, Tseng P. Safety of multilevel surgery in obstructive sleep apnea: a review of 487 cases. Arch Otolaryngol Head Neck Surg 2012;138(4):353–7.

51. Talei B, Cossu AL, Slepian R, et al. Immediate complications related to anesthesia in patients undergoing uvulopalatopharyngoplasty for obstructivesleep apnea. Laryngoscope 2013;123(11):2892–5.

52. Ishman SL, Benke JR, Cohen AP, et al. Does surgery for obstructive sleep apnea improve depression and sleepiness? Laryngoscope 2014;124(12):2829–36.

53. Huang CC, Lin WC, Chen HL, et al. Improvement of baroreflex sensitivity in patients with obstructive sleep apnea following surgical treatment. Clin Neurophysiol 2015;127(1):544–50.

54. Marin JM, Carrizo SJ, Vicente E, et al. Long-term cardiovascular outcomes in men with obstructive sleep apnoea-hypopnoea with or without treatment with continuous positive airway pressure: an observational study. Lancet 2005;365(9464):1046–53.

55. Partinen M, Jamieson A, Guilleminault C. Long-term outcome for obstructive sleep apnea syndrome patients. Mortality. Chest 1988;94(6):1200–4.

56. Ryan S, Ward S, Heneghan C, et al. Predictors of decreased spontaneous baroreflex sensitivity in obstructive sleep apnea syndrome. Chest 2007;131(4):1100–7.

57. Elshaug AG, Watt AM, Mundy L, et al. Over 150 potentially low-value health care practices: an Australian study. Med J Aust 2012;197(10):556–60.

58. Tan KB, Toh ST, Guilleminault C, et al. A cost-effectiveness analysis of surgery for middle-aged men with severe obstructive sleep apnea intolerant of CPAP. J Clin Sleep Med 2015;11(5):525–35.

59. Stewart S, Huang J, Mohorikar A, et al. AHI outcomes are superior after upper airway reconstructive surgery in adult CPAP failure patients. Otolaryngol Head Neck Surg 2016;154:553–7.

60. Field CJ, Robinson S, Mackay S, et al. Clinical equipoise in sleep surgery: investigating clinical trial targets. Otolaryngol Head Neck Surg 2011;145(2):347–53.

61. Marcus CL, Moore RH, Rosen CL, et al. A randomized trial of adenotonsillectomy for childhood sleep apnea. N Engl J Med 2013;368(25):2366–76.

62. Powell NB, Zonato AI, Weaver EM, et al. Radiofrequency treatment of turbinate hypertrophy in subjects using continuous positive airway pressure: a randomized, double-blind, placebo-controlled clinical pilot trial. Laryngoscope 2001;111(10):1783–90.

63. Miller FG, Shorr AF. Ethical assessment of industry-sponsored clinical trials: a case analysis. Chest 2002;121(4):1337–42.

64. Steward DL, Weaver EM, Woodson BT. Multilevel temperature-controlled radiofrequency for obstructive sleep apnea: extended follow-up. Otolaryngol Head Neck Surg 2005;132(4):630–5.

65. Portier F, Portman A, Czernichow P, et al. Evaluation of home versus laboratory polysomnography in the diagnosis of sleep apnea syndrome. J Resp Crit Care Med 2000;162(3):814–8.

66. Young JM, Solomon MJ, Harrison JD, et al. Measuring patient preference and surgeon choice. Surgery 2008;143(5):582–8.

67. Vanderveken OM, Dieltjens M, Wouters K, et al. Objective measurement of compliance during oral appliance therapy for sleep-disordered breathing. Thorax 2013;68(1):91–6.

68. Weaver EM, Woodson BT, Steward DL. Polysomnography indexes are discordant with quality of life, symptoms, and reaction times in sleep apnea patients. Otolaryngol Head Neck Surg 2005;132(2):255–62.

69. Browaldh N, Bring J, Friberg D. SKUP3 RCT; continuous study: changes in sleepiness and quality of life after modified UPPP. Laryngoscope 2015. http://dx.doi.org/10.1002/lary.25642.

70. Strollo PJ, Soose RJ, Maurer JT. Upper-airway stimulation for obstructive sleep apnea. N Engl J Med 2014;370:139–49.

71. Woodson BT, Gillespie MB, Soose RJ, et al. Randomized controlled withdrawal study of upper airway stimulation on OSA short- and long-term effect. Otolaryngol Head Neck Surg 2014;51(5):880–7.

72. Woodson BT, Soose RJ, Gillespie MB, et al, STAR Trial Investigators. Three-year outcomes of cranial nerve stimulation for obstructive sleep apnea: the

STAR trial. Otolaryngol Head Neck Surg 2016; 154(1):181–8.

73. Malhotra A. Hypoglossal-nerve stimulation for obstructive sleep apnea. N Engl J Med 2014; 370(2):170–1.

74. Vicini C, Dallan I, Canzi P, et al. Transoral robotic tongue base resection in obstructive sleep apnoea-hypopnoea syndrome: a preliminary report. ORL J Otorhinolaryngol Relat Spec 2010; 72:22–7.

Mandibular Advancement Splints

Ahmad A. Bamagoos, MBBS, MSc[a,b,c], Kate Sutherland, PhD[a,d],
Peter A. Cistulli, MBBS, PhD, MBA[a,d],*

KEYWORDS

- Obstructive sleep apnea treatment • Oral appliance • Mandibular advancement splint

KEY POINTS

- The overall effectiveness of mandibular advancement splint (MAS) and CPAP on general health outcomes, cognitive function, and quality of life appears to be similar, and this is likely explained by greater MAS usage mitigating the superiority of CPAP in reducing obstructive sleep apnea (OSA).
- The response variability to MAS is a major barrier for its implementation clinically.
- Several prediction tools have been proposed in the literature to enhance patient selection for MAS treatment. However, most are inadequate for routine clinical use.
- Phenotyping OSA patients may reveal characteristics that enable the prediction of response to MAS treatment and advance the path toward personalized medicine.

INTRODUCTION

Mandibular advancement splints (MAS), a form of oral appliances for the treatment of obstructive sleep apnea (OSA), are the leading alternative to the standard treatment, continuous positive airway pressure (CPAP). MAS are worn intraorally attached to the upper and lower dental arches to hold the mandible in a forward position. Current guidelines recommend MAS prescription as a second-line treatment for OSA patients who cannot tolerate or do not prefer CPAP treatment.[1]

MAS reduces upper airway collapsibility[2] with the major anatomic effect on the pharyngeal airway space being an increase in the velopharyngeal region, predominantly in the lateral dimension.[3,4] The anterior movement of the mandible and tongue facilitated by MAS presumably stretches soft tissue connections between the pharyngeal walls and the mandible,[5] preventing collapse of the tongue into the upper airway (UA) and increasing the caliber of the pharynx.

This article summarizes the current literature regarding the efficacy, effectiveness, adverse effects, and patient selection for MAS treatment.

EFFICACY AND HEALTH OUTCOMES OF MANDIBULAR ADVANCEMENT SPLINTS

MAS have demonstrated efficacy in reducing OSA with associated improvements in health outcomes. The reported mean reduction in

Disclosure: P.A. Cistulli holds an endowed academic Chair at the University of Sydney, created by funding from ResMed Inc. His department receives research support (equipment) from SomnoMed Ltd. He is a consultant and/or advisory board member for Zephyr Sleep Technologies, NovoNordisk, and Fisher and Paykel Healthcare. A.A. Bamagoos receives a scholarship funding for his PhD studies from King Abdulaziz University, Saudi Arabia. He also receives a top-up scholarship funding from NeuroSleep: NHMRC Centre of Research Excellence in Translational Sleep and Circadian Neurobiology.

[a] Department of Respiratory and Sleep Medicine, Royal North Shore Hospital, Reserve Road, St Leonards, New South Wales 2065, Australia; [b] Sleep Group, Charles Perkins Centre, Northern Clinical School, University of Sydney, Johns Hopkins Drive, Camperdown, New South Wales 2050, Australia; [c] Department of Physiology, Faculty of Medicine in Rabigh, King Abdulaziz University, Jeddah, Kingdom of Saudi Arabia; [d] Sleep Group, Charles Perkins Centre, Sydney Medical School, University of Sydney, Johns Hopkins Drive, Camperdown, New South Wales 2050, Australia

* Corresponding author. Department of Respiratory and Sleep Medicine, Royal North Shore Hospital, Level 8, Reserve Road, St Leonards, New South Wales 2065, Australia.
E-mail address: peter.cistulli@sydney.edu.au

Sleep Med Clin 11 (2016) 343–352
http://dx.doi.org/10.1016/j.jsmc.2016.04.002

apnea-hypopnea index (AHI) ranges between 24% and 72% (**Fig. 1**B), and mean proportion of OSA patients who resolve completely (AHI ≤5 events/h) with MAS treatment ranges between 29% and 71% (**Fig. 1**A).[6–13] Definition of OSA treatment success is a major factor that influences the reported efficacy. Most studies define successful OSA treatment as achieving a certain value of AHI, commonly AHI of no more than 5 or ≤10 events per hour, or a certain percentage of AHI reduction, commonly 50%. Others use more than 2 response classifications (eg, success, partial success, and failure). Studies also vary in incorporating symptomatic improvement, such as health outcomes, cognitive functions, and quality-of-life outcomes, to the definition of OSA treatment success. Hence, OSA treatment definition should be considered in evaluating the efficacy of MAS.

MAS reduce snoring[8,13,14] and improve polysomnographic indices of AHI, oxygen saturation (ODI), and sleep fragmentation compared with placebo devices (oral appliances that provide no mandibular advancement).[12–18] Excessive daytime sleepiness (EDS), measured both subjectively and objectively, is also reduced following MAS treatment.[8] MAS improve general and disease-specific measures of quality of life (QOL) assessed by questionnaire compared with placebo devices. For example, MAS improve the Functional Outcomes of Sleep Questionnaire (FOSQ),[13] the Profile of Mood States questionnaire (POMS),[19] and the Medical Outcome Survey: Short Form 36 (SF-36),[6,20] although 1 study reported no effect on SF-36.[13] Some cognitive functions, such as convergent thinking and psychomotor speed, show improvement with MAS treatment,[19,20] although most cognitive functions assessed do not demonstrate improvement with MAS treatment.[19] MAS improve diastolic and systolic 24-hour mean arterial blood pressure (especially in hypertensive patients)[21,22] and improve autonomic modulation during sleep.[23]

Long-term follow-up of MAS efficacy on OSA patients have indicated that reduction in AHI is sustained after 6 months up to 4 years of treatment.[9,24,25] Long-term efficacy was demonstrated in 1 study despite an overall increase in body mass index (BMI).[24] Positive health effects are also maintained with blood pressure reduction sustained 2.5 to 4.5 years after treatment.[24] Moreover, parameters of sleepiness, general health, and QOL continued to improve over time.[9,24] However, a recent study that followed patients for 16.5 years found that OSA may deteriorate despite continuous MAS use, and therefore regular follow-ups are required to maintain optimal MAS efficacy.[26]

MANDIBULAR ADVANCEMENT SPLINTS COMPARED WITH OTHER OBSTRUCTIVE SLEEP APNEA TREATMENT MODALITIES

CPAP is considered the first-line treatment for OSA.[1,27] It is highly efficacious in reducing sleep-disordered breathing and associated detrimental effects such as EDS and impaired cognitive function in the majority of patients.[28–31] Although highly efficacious, CPAP effectiveness in OSA treatment is limited by low patient adherence.[32] The proportion of OSA patents showing adequate adherence to CPAP (defined in most studies as CPAP use for ≥4 h/night and ≥5 nights per week) ranges between 46% and 89%.[33–36] Additionally, 25% of OSA patients refuse or discontinue CPAP use after 2 weeks of treatment.[33,37]

Comparison of MAS treatment to the gold standard CPAP treatment consistently shows CPAP to be more efficient in reducing respiratory events and completely resolving OSA (AHI ≤5 events/h) in a greater proportion of patients.[38–44] CPAP is also more efficient in reducing arousal index[38,40,45,46] and ODI,[38,42,43,46] although 1 study documented similar minimum arterial oxygen saturation ($minSaO_2$) in both treatments.[45]

Despite the superior efficacy of CPAP in improving polysomnographic indices compared to MAS, this does not seem to carry over into better health outcomes. The effects of MAS and CPAP on the outcomes of general health,

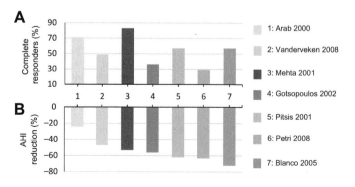

A

B

Fig. 1. Demonstrates (*A*) the percent of complete OSA responders (AHI ≤5 events/h) to MAS treatment; and (*B*) the percent of reduction in AHI on MAS compared with baseline, across studies using different MAS designs, inclusion criteria, and OSA treatment definitions.

1: Arab 2000
2: Vanderveken 2008
3: Mehta 2001
4: Gotsopoulos 2002
5: Pitsis 2001
6: Petri 2008
7: Blanco 2005

objective and subjective measures of EDS, and scales of anxiety and depression are consistently shown to be equivalent.[9,38,40–42,45,47,48] Additionally, MAS and CPAP are found to equally improve morning diastolic[38] and 24-hour mean arterial blood pressure,[45] and increase vasodilation in the short term.[49] Measures of cognitive functions also show equivalent improvement between MAS and CPAP treatments.[40,41] The effects of MAS and CPAP on QOL questionnaires were inconsistent in favoring either treatment. A few studies have shown CPAP superiority in improving QOL[40,41,45]; others found MAS to be superior,[38] and the reminder found CPAP and MAS to be equivalent in improving QOL.[42,50] In a long-term observational study, no difference between treatments was found in cardiovascular mortality.[51] The equivalence of MAS and CPAP in improving health outcomes despite the superiority of CPAP efficacy may be explained by the greater adherence and preference for MAS compared with CPAP, which may counteract any lower efficacy.

Comparisons of MAS treatment to other treatment modalities besides CPAP are limited. Only a few studies compared the efficacy of MAS treatment with that of surgical treatment for OSA. MAS were found to be superior to uvulopalatopharyngoplasty in reducing AHI and producing a greater proportion of complete responders (AHI $\leq$10 events/h) and sustained complete responders at 4 year after treatment.[52,53] However, improvement in QOL assessed by questionnaires was equivalent between MAS and UPPP at 1 year after treatment.[53,54] MAS have also been compared with maxillomandibular advancement procedure (MMA), which has the highest efficacy among other surgical procedures for OSA treatment.[55] MMA performs better than MAS in reducing AHI (reduction of 85% vs 47%) and producing greater proportion of complete responders (ie, AHI $\leq$10, 74% vs 30%).[56]

Although most studies evaluated MAS as an alternative to CPAP, a few suggest MAS as an adjunct treatment to reduce velopharyngeal resistance[57] and thereby the required therapeutic level of CPAP,[58] which can enhance patients' adherence to and reduce adverse effects of CPAP. A few studies also demonstrated that MAS treatment significantly reduces residual AHI and improves minSaO$_2$ 4 weeks, 6 months, and 2 years after UPPP.[59,60]

FACTORS INFLUENCING THE EFFICACY OF MANDIBULAR ADVANCEMENT SPLINTS
Design of Mandibular Advancement Splints

There is a wide variety of MAS designs available, which differ in several aspects such as customization and fabrication material. Custom-made MAS, the most common form of MAS, enable the personalization of MAS features, such as the amount of mandibular advancement and vertical opening, according to patients' dentition. Custom-made MAS come in either fixed 1-piece form (monobloc), which is relatively cheap and readily available, or adjustable two-piece form (separate upper and lower plates). Two-piece MAS enable a greater range of personalization, such as permissibility of lateral jaw movement, amount of dental retention, mechanisms of advancement, and mechanisms of coupling of the 2 plates.

The impact of MAS design on treatment efficacy has been investigated in studies comparing different MAS models. A few studies reported no difference in AHI reduction, EDS improvement, or adverse effects between monobloc and 2-piece MAS.[12,61] However, 1 retrospective study found a greater success rate of 2-piece MAS compared with monobloc MAS.[16] Comparison between different 2-piece MAS devices with different dental retention or advancement mechanisms did not find differences in treatment efficacy.[17,62] A recent cohort study found that adjoining a tongue protrusion component to customized MAS can induce greater AHI reduction compared with mandibular advancement alone.[63]

Noncustomized over-the-counter splints are a cheaper alternative. Studies of these devices are limited. One study showed that noncustomized MAS can reduce AHI by 26% to 36% compared with no treatment.[64] However, in direct comparison with customized MAS, noncustomised MAS failed to reduce AHI, and therefore patients' adherence to them does not exceed 20%.[65]

Adequate mandibular advancement is a key determinant in MAS treatment efficacy, and shows a dose-dependent effect on OSA treatment outcomes. For example, the amount of improvement and the proportion of participants who experienced improvement in upper airway (UA) closing pressure and overnight oxygen saturation increased with increasing mandibular advancement from baseline to 2, 4, and 6 mm advancement.[66] Additionally, the proportion of severe OSA participants who were successfully treated (AHI $\leq$10) was greater in participants who underwent 75% compared with 50% of the maximum possible advancement (52% vs 31%, respectively).[10] However, a couple of studies reported a similar success rate between 50% and 75% of mandibular advancement in mild-to-moderate OSA,[9,11] which may suggest a nonlinear relationship that requires titration to identify an optimum level of advancement for individual patients.

MAS also apply vertical opening to the mouth due to the vertical thickness of the fabrication material from which MAS are made. Greater vertical opening affects the patency of the UA negatively in most OSA patients,[67] although no negative effect was found on AHI.[7] Additionally, smaller vertical opening was preferred by most patients,[7] and therefore was considered to be more tolerable and beneficial.

Preference and Adherence to Mandibular Advancement Splints

Patients' preference and adherence are other major factors influencing the efficacy of MAS and therefore the adequacy of treatment. Several factors can contribute to patient preference including effectiveness, adverse effects, cost, convenience and portability, bed partner's preference, and social stigma.[68] Most studies compared patient adherence and preference to MAS with the gold standard treatment CPAP. Subjective self-reported adherence and preference were reported to be greater in MAS compared with CPAP,[9,43,44,50,69] although 1 trial documented similar patient preference towards both treatments,[41] and another documented a greater preference towards CPAP.[40] However, it has been recognized that self-reported CPAP usage is overestimated compared with objective monitoring,[38,42] and therefore a comparison of objective measures of adherence is required.

A few technologies have emerged to objectively measure patient adherence to MAS. Most of these depend on intraoral temperature sensors, and technology has advanced to reduce sensor dimensions and increase storage capacity.[70,71] Recently, thermal microsensors with good storage and readout capability have become commercially available.[72–74] The thermal microsensor chip is embedded into MAS, and the temperature readings are used to obtain an objective measure of hours of MAS usage. Initial reports of objective adherence data show a mean daily usage of MAS 3 months after treatment was 6.6 hours per night, with approximately 84% of participants being regular users ($\geq$4 hours per night and $\geq$5 days per week).[72] Long-term follow-up found that 89% of participants remained as regular users to MAS at 12 months after treatment.[73] This adherence rate is relatively high compared with CPAP, in which 58% to 78% of patients only are considered regular users.[75,76]

SIDE EFFECTS

Short-term side effects of MAS usually occur during the initial period of treatment. Common short-term adverse effects include sialorrhea, xerostomia, toothaches, gingival irritation, headaches, and temporomandibular joint (TMJ) pain.[77] Most adverse effects decline over time, and some resolve completely 6 to 12 months after treatment, including TMJ pain.[78,79]

Dental changes can also occur with MAS treatment and have been shown to progress over time.[80–82] Common dental changes include decrease in overbite and overjet, retroclination of the upper incisor and proclination of the lower incisors, reduction in the number of occlusal contacts, and increase in mandibular plane angle.[80,81,83–86] Dental changes are not necessarily negative and represent an improvement in approximately 45% of patients.[87] The frequency and intensity of side effects varies markedly between studies, majorly due to differences in MAS design and features, and differences in individuals' type of initial bite, general oral health, and hours of active MAS use.

PATIENT SELECTION

Treatment with MAS requires an extended period (2–3 months) of acclimatization to achieve the maximum therapeutic benefit. Therefore, MAS is not suitable for patients with comorbidities and severe daytime sleepiness, and specifically sleepy drivers who require immediate intervention. MAS are also not suitable for patients requiring major dental work, as MAS fitting may be disturbed due to changes in dental shape, and patients with major teeth loss, as MAS require a solid base to which it can anchor.

Another significant barrier for implementing MAS treatment clinically is the interindividual variability of OSA patient response to MAS. The reported average proportion of OSA patients who resolve completely (AHI $\leq$5 events/h) on MAS treatment ranges between 29% and 71%.[6–13,88] A recent cohort study that included 425 patients for analysis found that approximately one-third of these completely resolved on MAS; another third experienced more than 50% reduction in AHI, while the reminder of patients are considered failures, with less than 50% reduction in AHI.[89] The variability in response to MAS treatment between individuals is a major barrier for the implementation of MAS treatment in clinical practice. Therefore, much attention has been devoted to understand the reasons for treatment variability and to find predictors of successful treatment outcome. **Fig. 2** summarizes the positive and negative predictive values of different tools that have been used to predict response to MAS treatment.

Understanding patient characteristics related to successful MAS treatment has been explored in

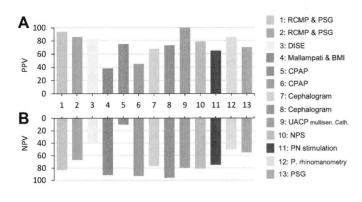

Fig. 2. Demonstrates (*A*) the positive predictive values; and (*B*) the negative predictive values, across studies using different tools to predict response to MAS treatment, MAS design, inclusion criteria, and OSA treatment definitions. BMI, body mass index; CPAP, continuous positive airway pressure; DISE, drug-induced sleep endoscopy; NPS, nasopharyngoscopy; P, posterior; PN, phrenic nerve; PSG, polysomnography; RCMP, remotely controlled mandibular positioner; UACP, upper airway closing pressure. (*Adapted from* Okuno K, Pliska BT, Hamoda M, et al. Prediction of oral appliance treatment outcomes in obstructive sleep apnea: a systematic review. Sleep Med Rev 2015;30:25–33.)

many studies. For example, anthropometric and demographic characteristics that have been related to treatment success include low BMI,[90–93] low mallampati score,[88] young age,[91,94] and female gender,[92] although 2 studies reported no difference in success rates between genders.[89,90] Polysomnographic measurements such as NREM sleep stage,[89] low AHI,[92,93] and position-dependent OSA[95–97] also show association to MAS treatment success, although 1 study reported MAS failure in position-dependent OSA,[89] and a few reported resolution of severe OSA on MAS.[6,8,18,89] However having some of these characteristics alone is not enough to ensure a response to MAS treatment in any individual.

Various other clinical prediction tools have been assessed. For example, imaging techniques show relevance to MAS treatment success including cephalometric characteristics (such as short soft palate, short face height, lower hyoid bone position, retroganthic mandible, and long maxilla[91,98–100]), MRI characteristics (such as a low ratio of soft tissue to intramandibular space area, a decrease in tongue length, and an increase in airway volume with MAS[4,101,102]), nasopharyngoscopic characteristics (such as widening of the velopharynx during wakefulness and airway patency during induced-sleep with MAS[67,103,104]).

Velopharyngeal collapse during sleep, identified by flow-volume loops[105] and phrenic nerve stimulation,[106] has also been associated with successful MAS treatment. Higher optimal level of CPAP ($P_{OPTIMAL}$; the nasal pressure at which all respiratory events are corrected) suggests failure of OSA treatment with MAS.[107,108] The optimal advancement position of MAS determined by a remotely controlled mandibular positioner (RCMP) device, which enables for single-night titration of mandibular advancement, can also predict response to MAS treatment.[109–112] Additionally, upper airway closing pressure (P_{CLOSE}; the nasal pressure at which UA collapses) shows significant difference between responders to MAS treatment and nonresponders.[2] Thermoplastic MAS have also been tested to predict response to custom-made MAS.[65]

Nonetheless, the accuracy of these tools to predict OSA response to MAS treatment varies greatly (see **Fig. 2**),[113] and most are inadequate to be considered for clinical practice due to high cost and/or complexity. Comprehensive phenotyping of OSA patients has the potential to identify characteristics that can predict—individually or in combination—OSA response to MAS treatment.

SUMMARY

Although highly efficacious, CPAP effectiveness in OSA treatment is limited by low patient adherence and preference. Although MAS are not as efficacious as CPAP in reducing obstructive respiratory events, patient adherence and preference are greater than CPAP. Additionally, the overall effectiveness of both treatments on general health outcomes, cognitive function, and QOL appears to be equivalent. A key barrier for the implementation of MAS treatment in clinical practice is the interindividual variability in response to MAS treatment. Several prediction tools have been proposed in the literature to enhance patient selection for MAS treatment. However, most of these are inadequate for routine clinical use due to inaccuracy, lack of prospective validation, high cost, and/or complexity. Phenotyping OSA patients comprehensively may reveal patient characteristics that enable the prediction of response to MAS treatment and enhance patient selection and the provision of personalized medicine.

REFERENCES

1. Ramar K, Dort LC, Katz SG, et al. Clinical practice guideline for the treatment of obstructive sleep apnea and snoring with oral appliance therapy: an update for 2015. J Clin Sleep Med 2015;11(7): 773–827.

2. Ng AT, Qian J, Cistulli PA. Oropharyngeal collapse predicts treatment response with oral appliance therapy in obstructive sleep apnea. Sleep 2006; 29(5):666–71.

3. Ryan C, Love L, Peat D, et al. Mandibular advancement oral appliance therapy for obstructive sleep apnoea: effect on awake calibre of the velopharynx. Thorax 1999;54(11):972–7.

4. Chan AS, Sutherland K, Schwab RJ, et al. The effect of mandibular advancement on upper airway structure in obstructive sleep apnoea. Thorax 2010;65(8):726–32.

5. Brown EC, Cheng S, McKenzie DK, et al. Respiratory movement of upper airway tissue in obstructive sleep apnea. Sleep 2013;36(7):1069–76.

6. Petri N, Svanholt P, Solow B, et al. Mandibular advancement appliance for obstructive sleep apnoea: results of a randomised placebo controlled trial using parallel group design. J Sleep Res 2008; 17(2):221–9.

7. Pitsis AJ, Darendeliler MA, Gotsopoulos H, et al. Effect of vertical dimension on efficacy of oral appliance therapy in obstructive sleep apnoea. Am J Respir Crit Care Med 2002;166(6):860–4.

8. Gotsopoulos H, Chen C, Qian J, et al. Oral appliance therapy improves symptoms in obstructive sleep apnea: a randomized controlled trial. Am J Respir Crit Care Med 2002;166(5):743–8.

9. Aarab G, Lobbezoo F, Heymans MW, et al. Long-term follow-up of a randomized controlled trial of oral appliance therapy in obstructive sleep apnea. Respiration 2011;82(2):162–8.

10. Walker-Engstrom ML, Ringqvist I, Vestling O, et al. A prospective randomized study comparing two different degrees of mandibular advancement with a dental appliance in treatment of severe obstructive sleep apnea. Sleep Breath 2003;7(3):119–30.

11. Tegelberg A, Walker-Engstrom ML, Vestling O, et al. Two different degrees of mandibular advancement with a dental appliance in treatment of patients with mild to moderate obstructive sleep apnea. Acta Odontol Scand 2003;61(6):356–62.

12. Bloch KE, Iseli A, Zhang JN, et al. A randomized controlled crossover trial of two oral appliances for sleep apnea treatment. Am J Respir Crit Care Med 2000;162(1):246–51.

13. Blanco J, Zamarron C, Abeleira Pazos MT, et al. Prospective evaluation of an oral appliance in the treatment of obstructive sleep apnea syndrome. Sleep Breath 2005;9(1):20–5.

14. Johnston CD, Gleadhill IC, Cinnamond MJ, et al. Mandibular advancement appliances and obstructive sleep apnoea: a randomized clinical trial. Eur J Orthod 2002;24(3):251–62.

15. O'Sullivan RA, Hillman DR, Mateljan R, et al. Mandibular advancement splint: an appliance to treat snoring and obstructive sleep apnea. Am J Respir Crit Care Med 1995;151(1):194–8.

16. Lettieri CJ, Paolino N, Eliasson AH, et al. Comparison of adjustable and fixed oral appliances for the treatment of obstructive sleep apnea. J Clin Sleep Med 2011;7(5):439–45.

17. Gauthier L, Laberge L, Beaudry M, et al. Efficacy of two mandibular advancement appliances in the management of snoring and mild-moderate sleep apnea: a cross-over randomized study. Sleep Med 2009;10(3):329–36.

18. Mehta A, Qian J, Petocz P, et al. A randomized controlled study of a mandibular advancement splint for obstructive sleep apnea. Am J Respir Crit Care Med 2001;163(6):1457–61.

19. Naismith SL, Winter VR, Hickie IB, et al. Effect of oral appliance therapy on neurobehavioral functioning in obstructive sleep apnea: a randomized controlled trial. J Clin Sleep Med 2005;1(4):374–80.

20. Galic T, Bozic J, Pecotic R, et al. Improvement of cognitive and psychomotor performance in patients with mild to moderate obstructive sleep apnea treated with mandibular advancement device: a prospective 1-year study. J Clin Sleep Med 2016;12(2):177–86.

21. Andren A, Hedberg P, Walker-Engstrom ML, et al. Effects of treatment with oral appliance on 24-h blood pressure in patients with obstructive sleep apnea and hypertension: a randomized clinical trial. Sleep Breath 2013;17(2):705–12.

22. Gotsopoulos H, Kelly JJ, Cistulli PA. Oral appliance therapy reduces blood pressure in obstructive sleep apnea: a randomizeda controlled trial. Sleep 2004;27(5):934–41.

23. Dal-Fabbro C, Garbuio S, D'Almeida V, et al. Mandibular advancement device and CPAP upon cardiovascular parameters in OSA. Sleep Breath 2014;18(4):749–59.

24. Gauthier L, Laberge L, Beaudry M, et al. Mandibular advancement appliances remain effective in lowering respiratory disturbance index for 2.5-4.5 years. Sleep Med 2011;12(9):844–9.

25. Ghazal A, Sorichter S, Jonas I, et al. A randomized prospective long-term study of two oral appliances for sleep apnoea treatment. J Sleep Res 2009; 18(3):321–8.

26. Marklund M. Long-term efficacy of an oral appliance in early treated patients with obstructive sleep apnea. Sleep Breath 2015;20(2):689–94.

27. American Thoracic Society. Indications and standards for use of nasal continuous positive airway

pressure (CPAP) in sleep apnea syndromes. Am J Respir Crit Care Med 1994;150(6 Pt 1):1738–45.

28. Babu AR, Herdegen J, Fogelfeld L, et al. Type 2 diabetes, glycemic control, and continuous positive airway pressure in obstructive sleep apnea. Arch Intern Med 2005;165(4):447–52.

29. Faccenda J, Mackay T, Boon N, et al. Randomized placebo-controlled trial of continuous positive airway pressure on blood pressure in the sleep apnea–hypopnea syndrome. Am J Respir Crit Care Med 2001;163(2):344–8.

30. Engleman HM, Martin SE, Kingshott RN, et al. Randomised placebo controlled trial of daytime function after continuous positive airway pressure (CPAP) therapy for the sleep apnoea/hypopnoea syndrome. Thorax 1998;53(5):341–5.

31. Gay P, Weaver T, Loube D, et al. Evaluation of positive airway pressure treatment for sleep related breathing disorders in adults. Sleep 2006;29(3):381–401.

32. Kribbs NB, Pack AI, Kline LR, et al. Objective measurement of patterns of nasal CPAP use by patients with obstructive sleep apnea. Am Rev Respir Dis 1993;147(4):887–95.

33. Popescu G, Latham M, Allgar V, et al. Continuous positive airway pressure for sleep apnoea/hypopnoea syndrome: usefulness of a 2 week trial to identify factors associated with long term use. Thorax 2001;56(9):727–33.

34. Russo-Magno P, O'Brien A, Panciera T, et al. Compliance with CPAP therapy in older men with obstructive sleep apnea. J Am Geriatr Soc 2001;49(9):1205–11.

35. Chen YF, Hang LW, Huang CS, et al. Polysomnographic predictors of persistent continuous positive airway pressure adherence in patients with moderate and severe obstructive sleep apnea. Kaohsiung J Med Sci 2015;31(2):83–9.

36. Pieters T, Collard P, Aubert G, et al. Acceptance and long-term compliance with nCPAP in patients with obstructive sleep apnoea syndrome. Eur Respir J 1996;9(5):939–44.

37. Collard P, Pieters T, Aubert G, et al. Compliance with nasal CPAP in obstructive sleep apnea patients. Sleep Med Rev 1997;1(1):33–44.

38. Phillips CL, Grunstein RR, Darendeliler MA, et al. Health outcomes of continuous positive airway pressure versus oral appliance treatment for obstructive sleep apnea: a randomized controlled trial. Am J Respir Crit Care Med 2013;187(8):879–87.

39. Doff MH, Hoekema A, Wijkstra PJ, et al. Oral appliance versus continuous positive airway pressure in obstructive sleep apnea syndrome: a 2-year follow-up. Sleep 2013;36(9):1289–96.

40. Barnes M, McEvoy RD, Banks S, et al. Efficacy of positive airway pressure and oral appliance in mild to moderate obstructive sleep apnea. Am J Respir Crit Care Med 2004;170(6):656–64.

41. Engleman HM, McDonald JP, Graham D, et al. Randomized crossover trial of two treatments for sleep apnea/hypopnea syndrome: continuous positive airway pressure and mandibular repositioning splint. Am J Respir Crit Care Med 2002;166(6):855–9.

42. Gagnadoux F, Fleury B, Vielle B, et al. Titrated mandibular advancement versus positive airway pressure for sleep apnoea. Eur Respir J 2009;34(4):914–20.

43. Ferguson KA, Ono T, Lowe AA, et al. A randomized crossover study of an oral appliance vs nasal-continuous positive airway pressure in the treatment of mild-moderate obstructive sleep apnea. Chest 1996;109(5):1269–75.

44. Marklund M, Verbraecken J, Randerath W. Non-CPAP therapies in obstructive sleep apnoea: mandibular advancement device therapy. Eur Respir J 2012;39(5):1241–7.

45. Lam B, Sam K, Mok WY, et al. Randomised study of three non-surgical treatments in mild to moderate obstructive sleep apnoea. Thorax 2007;62(4):354–9.

46. Randerath WJ, Heise M, Hinz R, et al. An individually adjustable oral appliance vs continuous positive airway pressure in mild-to-moderate obstructive sleep apnea syndrome. Chest 2002;122(2):569–75.

47. Li W, Xiao L, Hu J. The comparison of CPAP and oral appliances in treatment of patients with OSA: a systematic review and meta-analysis. Respir Care 2013;58(7):1184–95.

48. Health Quality Ontario. Oral appliances for obstructive sleep apnea: an evidence-based analysis. Ont Health Technol Assess Ser 2009;9(5):1–51.

49. Trzepizur W, Gagnadoux F, Abraham P, et al. Microvascular endothelial function in obstructive sleep apnea: impact of continuous positive airway pressure and mandibular advancement. Sleep Med 2009;10(7):746–52.

50. Tan YK, L'Estrange PR, Luo YM, et al. Mandibular advancement splints and continuous positive airway pressure in patients with obstructive sleep apnoea: a randomized cross-over trial. Eur J Orthod 2002;24(3):239–49.

51. Anandam A, Patil M, Akinnusi M, et al. Cardiovascular mortality in obstructive sleep apnoea treated with continuous positive airway pressure or oral appliance: an observational study. Respirology 2013;18(8):1184–90.

52. Walker-Engstrom ML, Tegelberg A, Wilhelmsson B, et al. 4-year follow-up of treatment with dental appliance or uvulopalatopharyngoplasty in patients with obstructive sleep apnea: a randomized study. Chest 2002;121(3):739–46.

53. Wilhelmsson B, Tegelberg A, Walker-Engstrom ML, et al. A prospective randomized study of a dental appliance compared with uvulopalatopharyngo-plasty in the treatment of obstructive sleep apnoea. Acta Otolaryngol 1999;119(4):503–9.

54. Walker-Engstrom ML, Wilhelmsson B, Tegelberg A, et al. Quality of life assessment of treatment with dental appliance or UPPP in patients with mild to moderate obstructive sleep apnoea: a prospective randomized 1-year follow-up study. J Sleep Res 2000;9(3):303–8.

55. Holty JE, Guilleminault C. Surgical options for the treatment of obstructive sleep apnea. Med Clin North Am 2010;94(3):479–515.

56. Jalbert F, Lacassagne L, Bessard J, et al. Oral ap-pliances or maxillomandibular advancement os-teotomy for severe obstructive sleep apnoea in patients refusing CPAP. Rev Stomatol Chir Maxillo-fac 2012;113(1):19–26.

57. Borel JC, Gakwaya S, Masse JF, et al. Impact of CPAP interface and mandibular advancement de-vice on upper airway mechanical properties as-sessed with phrenic nerve stimulation in sleep apnea patients. Respir Physiol Neurobiol 2012; 183(2):170–6.

58. El-Solh AA, Moitheennazima B, Akinnusi ME, et al. Combined oral appliance and positive airway pres-sure therapy for obstructive sleep apnea: a pilot study. Sleep Breath 2011;15(2):203–8.

59. Xu C, Xie Y, Kang H, et al. Efficacies of using modi-fied oral appliance after uvulopalatopharyngoplasty in the treatment of moderate to severe obstructive sleep apnea hypopnea syndrome. Zhonghua Yi Xue Za Zhi 2015;95(10):761–5 [in Chinese].

60. Han J, Wang B, An Y, et al. Therapeutic effects of oral appliance combined with uvulopalatopharyng-oplasty on obstructive sleep apnea hypopnea syn-drome. Zhonghua Kou Qiang Yi Xue Za Zhi 2014; 49(2):69–72 [in Chinese].

61. Rose E, Staats R, Virchow C, et al. A comparative study of two mandibular advancement appliances for the treatment of obstructive sleep apnoea. Eur J Orthod 2002;24(2):191–8.

62. Lawton HM, Battagel JM, Kotecha B. A comparison of the twin block and herbst mandibular advance-ment splints in the treatment of patients with obstructive sleep apnoea: a prospective study. Eur J Orthod 2005;27(1):82–90.

63. Dort L, Remmers J. A combination appliance for obstructive sleep apnea: the effectiveness of mandibular advancement and tongue retention. J Clin Sleep Med 2012;8(3):265–9.

64. Quinnell TG, Bennett M, Jordan J, et al. A crossover randomised controlled trial of oral mandibular advancement devices for obstructive sleep apnoea-hypopnoea (TOMADO). Thorax 2014;69(10):938–45.

65. Vanderveken OM, Devolder A, Marklund M, et al. Comparison of a custom-made and a thermo-plastic oral appliance for the treatment of mild sleep apnea. Am J Respir Crit Care Med 2008; 178(2):197–202.

66. Kato J, Isono S, Tanaka A, et al. Dose-dependent effects of mandibular advancement on pharyngeal mechanics and nocturnal oxygenation in patients with sleep-disordered breathing. Chest 2000; 117(4):1065–72.

67. Vroegop AV, Vanderveken OM, van de Heyning PH, et al. Effects of vertical opening on pharyngeal di-mensions in patients with obstructive sleep apnoea. Sleep Med 2012;13(3):314–6.

68. Almeida FR, Henrich N, Marra C, et al. Patient preferences and experiences of CPAP and oral appliances for the treatment of obstructive sleep apnea: a qualitative analysis. Sleep Breath 2013; 17(2):659–66.

69. Ferguson KA, Ono T, Lowe AA, et al. A short-term controlled trial of an adjustable oral appliance for the treatment of mild to moderate obstructive sleep apnea. Thorax 1997;52(4):362–8.

70. Lowe AA, Sjoholm TT, Ryan CF, et al. Treatment, airway and compliance effects of a titratable oral appliance. Sleep 2000;23(Suppl 4):S172–8.

71. Inoko Y, Yoshimura K, Kato C, et al. Efficacy and safety of temperature data loggers in measuring compliance with the use of oral appliances. Sleep Biol Rhythms 2009;7(3):188–92.

72. Vanderveken OM, Dieltjens M, Wouters K, et al. Objective measurement of compliance during oral appliance therapy for sleep-disordered breathing. Thorax 2013;68(1):91–6.

73. Dieltjens M, Braem MJ, Vroegop AV, et al. Objec-tively measured vs self-reported compliance dur-ing oral appliance therapy for sleep-disordered breathing. Chest 2013;144(5):1495–502.

74. Bonato RA, Bradley DC. Introducing a novel micro-recorder for the detection of oral appliance compli-ance: dentiTrac. Sleep Diagn Ther 2013;8:5–12.

75. McArdle N, Devereux G, Heidarnejad H, et al. Long-term use of CPAP therapy for sleep apnea/hypopnea syndrome. Am J Respir Crit Care Med 1999;159(4 Pt 1):1108–14.

76. Engleman HM, Wild MR. Improving CPAP use by patients with the sleep apnoea/hypopnoea syn-drome (SAHS). Sleep Med Rev 2003;7(1):81–99.

77. de Almeida FR, Lowe AA, Tsuiki S, et al. Long-term compliance and side effects of oral appliances used for the treatment of snoring and obstructive sleep apnea syndrome. J Clin Sleep Med 2005; 1(2):143–52.

78. Giannasi LC, Almeida FR, Magini M, et al. System-atic assessment of the impact of oral appliance therapy on the temporomandibular joint during

treatment of obstructive sleep apnea: long-term evaluation. Sleep Breath 2009;13(4):375–81.

79. Doff MH, Veldhuis SK, Hoekema A, et al. Long-term oral appliance therapy in obstructive sleep apnea syndrome: a controlled study on temporomandibular side effects. Clin Oral Investig 2012;16(3):689–97.

80. Robertson C, Herbison P, Harkness M. Dental and occlusal changes during mandibular advancement splint therapy in sleep disordered patients. Eur J Orthod 2003;25(4):371–6.

81. Almeida FR, Lowe AA, Sung JO, et al. Long-term sequellae of oral appliance therapy in obstructive sleep apnea patients: part 1. Cephalometric analysis. Am J Orthod Dentofacial Orthop 2006;129(2):195–204.

82. Pliska BT, Nam H, Chen H, et al. Obstructive sleep apnea and mandibular advancement splints: occlusal effects and progression of changes associated with a decade of treatment. J Clin Sleep Med 2014;10(12):1285–91.

83. Doff MH, Finnema KJ, Hoekema A, et al. Long-term oral appliance therapy in obstructive sleep apnea syndrome: a controlled study on dental side effects. Clin Oral Investig 2013;17(2):475–82.

84. Doff MH, Hoekema A, Pruim GJ, et al. Long-term oral-appliance therapy in obstructive sleep apnea: a cephalometric study of craniofacial changes. J Dent 2010;38(12):1010–8.

85. Martinez-Gomis J, Willaert E, Nogues L, et al. Five years of sleep apnea treatment with a mandibular advancement device: side effects and technical complications. Angle Orthod 2010;80(1):30–6.

86. Hammond RJ, Gotsopoulos H, Shen G, et al. A follow-up study of dental and skeletal changes associated with mandibular advancement splint use in obstructive sleep apnea. Am J Orthod Dentofacial Orthop 2007;132(6):806–14.

87. Almeida FR, Lowe AA, Otsuka R, et al. Long-term sequellae of oral appliance therapy in obstructive sleep apnea patients: part 2. Study-model analysis. Am J Orthod Dentofacial Orthop 2006;129(2):205–13.

88. Tsuiki S, Ito E, Isono S, et al. Oropharyngeal crowding and obesity as predictors of oral appliance treatment response to moderate obstructive sleep apnea. Chest 2013;144(2):558–63.

89. Sutherland K, Takaya H, Qian J, et al. Oral appliance treatment response and polysomnographic phenotypes of obstructive sleep apnea. J Clin Sleep Med 2015;11(8):861–8.

90. Suzuki K, Nakata S, Tagaya M, et al. Prediction of oral appliance treatment outcome in obstructive sleep apnoea syndrome: a preliminary study. B-ENT 2014;10(3):185–91.

91. Liu Y, Lowe AA, Fleetham JA, et al. Cephalometric and physiologic predictors of the efficacy of an adjustable oral appliance for treating obstructive sleep apnea. Am J Orthod Dentofacial Orthop 2001;120(6):639–47.

92. Marklund M, Stenlund H, Franklin KA. Mandibular advancement devices in 630 men and women with obstructive sleep apnea and snoring: tolerability and predictors of treatment success. Chest 2004;125(4):1270–8.

93. Hoekema A, Doff MH, de Bont LG, et al. Predictors of obstructive sleep apnea-hypopnea treatment outcome. J Dent Res 2007;86(12):1181–6.

94. Milano F, Billi MC, Marra F, et al. Factors associated with the efficacy of mandibular advancing device treatment in adult OSA patients. Int Orthod 2013;11(3):278–89.

95. Lee CH, Jung HJ, Lee WH, et al. The effect of positional dependency on outcomes of treatment with a mandibular advancement device. Arch Otolaryngol Head Neck Surg 2012;138(5):479–83.

96. Chung JW, Enciso R, Levendowski DJ, et al. Treatment outcomes of mandibular advancement devices in positional and nonpositional OSA patients. Oral Surg Oral Med Oral Pathol Oral Radiol Endod 2010;109(5):724–31.

97. Yoshida K. Influence of sleep posture on response to oral appliance therapy for sleep apnea syndrome. Sleep 2001;24(5):538–44.

98. Shen HL, Wen YW, Chen NH, et al. Craniofacial morphologic predictors of oral appliance outcomes in patients with obstructive sleep apnea. J Am Dent Assoc 2012;143(11):1209–17.

99. Ng AT, Darendeliler MA, Petocz P, et al. Cephalometry and prediction of oral appliance treatment outcome. Sleep Breath 2012;16(1):47–58.

100. Mayer G, Meier-Ewert K. Cephalometric predictors for orthopaedic mandibular advancement in obstructive sleep apnoea. Eur J Orthod 1995;17(1):35–43.

101. Sutherland K, Chan AS, Cistulli PA. Three-dimensional assessment of anatomical balance and oral appliance treatment outcome in obstructive sleep apnoea. Sleep Breath 2016. [Epub ahead of print].

102. Ogawa T, Long J, Sutherland K, et al. Effect of mandibular advancement splint treatment on tongue shape in obstructive sleep apnea. Sleep Breath 2015;19(3):857–63.

103. Johal A, Battagel JM, Kotecha BT. Sleep nasendoscopy: a diagnostic tool for predicting treatment success with mandibular advancement splints in obstructive sleep apnoea. Eur J Orthod 2005;27(6):607–14.

104. Sasao Y, Nohara K, Okuno K, et al. Videoendoscopic diagnosis for predicting the response to oral appliance therapy in severe obstructive sleep apnea. Sleep Breath 2014;18(4):809–15.

105. Chan AS, Lee RW, Srinivasan VK, et al. Use of flow-volume curves to predict oral appliance treatment

outcome in obstructive sleep apnea: a prospective validation study. Sleep Breath 2011;15(2):157–62.

106. Bosshard V, Masse JF, Series F. Prediction of oral appliance efficiency in patients with apnoea using phrenic nerve stimulation while awake. Thorax 2011;66(3):220–5.

107. Sutherland K, Phillips CL, Davies A, et al. CPAP pressure for prediction of oral appliance treatment response in obstructive sleep apnea. J Clin Sleep Med 2014;10(9):943–9.

108. Tsuiki S, Kobayashi M, Namba K, et al. Optimal positive airway pressure predicts oral appliance response to sleep apnoea. Eur Respir J 2010; 35(5):1098–105.

109. Dort LC, Hadjuk E, Remmers JE. Mandibular advancement and obstructive sleep apnoea: a method for determining effective mandibular protrusion. Eur Respir J 2006;27(5):1003–9.

110. Petelle B, Vincent G, Gagnadoux F, et al. One-night mandibular advancement titration for obstructive sleep apnea syndrome: a pilot study. Am J Respir Crit Care Med 2002;165(8):1150–3.

111. Remmers J, Charkhandeh S, Grosse J, et al. Remotely controlled mandibular protrusion during sleep predicts therapeutic success with oral appliances in patients with obstructive sleep apnea. Sleep 2013;36(10):1517–25, 1525A.

112. Tsai WH, Vazquez JC, Oshima T, et al. Remotely controlled mandibular positioner predicts efficacy of oral appliances in sleep apnea. Am J Respir Crit Care Med 2004;170(4):366–70.

113. Okuno K, Pliska BT, Hamoda M, et al. Prediction of oral appliance treatment outcomes in obstructive sleep apnea: a systematic review. Sleep Med Rev 2015;30:25–33.

Residual Daytime Sleepiness in Obstructive Sleep Apnea After Continuous Positive Airway Pressure Optimization

Causes and Management

Julia L. Chapman, BSc, BA, MHSc[a,b,*],
Yasmina Serinel, BSc, MBBS, FRACP[a],
Nathaniel S. Marshall, BSc, BCom, PGDipHealSc, PhD[c],
Ronald R. Grunstein, MBBS, MD, PhD, FRACP[a,b]

KEYWORDS

- Excessive daytime sleepiness • Sleep disorders • Comorbid conditions • CPAP
- Wakefulness promoters • Modafinil • Armodafinil

KEY POINTS

- Excessive daytime sleepiness (EDS) is common in obstructive sleep apnea (OSA) but is also common in the general population.
- The causes of EDS in OSA may not all be related to the OSA, and EDS may remain even with high use of continuous positive airway pressure (CPAP) therapy.
- For these patients, finding and directly treating potential alternative causes of EDS should be considered.
- Modafinil or armodafinil are the only pharmacologic agents indicated for residual sleepiness despite CPAP use in OSA.
- Further research into identifying which patients are vulnerable to the daytime effects of OSA and who is likely to respond best to each treatment is required.

PREVALENCE AND PREDICTORS OF RESIDUAL SLEEPINESS IN OBSTRUCTIVE SLEEP APNEA

A long-standing clinical conundrum in sleep medicine has been patients with obstructive sleep apnea (OSA) who remain excessively sleepy despite effective use of well-fitted continuous positive airway pressure (CPAP) therapy. Residual sleepiness has been estimated to occur in 5% to 55% of CPAP users.[1,2] In a clinical sample that excluded poor CPAP users, the estimated rate of

Disclosure: The authors have received in-kind support in the form of armodafinil and matching placebo from Teva Cephalon for a clinical trial for sleep apnea completed in the last 2 years.
[a] NeuroSleep Centre of Research Excellence, Woolcock Institute of Medical Research, Sleep and Circadian Research Group, University of Sydney, Glebe Point Road, Glebe, Sydney, New South Wales 2050, Australia; [b] Respiratory and Sleep Department, Royal Prince Alfred Hospital, Sydney Local Health District, Missenden Road, Camperdown, Sydney, New South Wales 2050, Australia; [c] Sydney Nursing School, The University of Sydney, M02, Sydney, New South Wales 2006, Australia
* Corresponding author. PO Box M77, Missenden Road, Mallett Street, Sydney, New South Wales 2050, Australia.
E-mail address: Julia.chapman@sydney.edu.au

residual daytime sleepiness was 12%, and when other sleep disorders and major depression were excluded as confounders the remaining prevalence was 6%.[3] However, it is difficult to predict the individuals who will have this residual sleepiness because studies have been small and conflicted.[1,2]

When determining the cause of residual sleepiness in CPAP-treated OSA, it should be remembered that, even in community-based samples, only a very weak association exists between daytime sleepiness and OSA severity.[4] Individuals with mild OSA can have high levels of EDS and individuals with severe OSA may have no symptoms of hypersomnolence.[4] Factors that may contribute to excessive daytime sleepiness (EDS) are shown in **Fig. 1** and outlined in more detail later.

The accepted prevalence of OSA (defined as an apnea hypopnea index [AHI] >5) in middle-aged men is 25% and 15% for women.[5,6] More recent prevalence estimates are as high as 80% for men and 60% for women.[7] At the same time, population-based prevalence estimates of EDS as measured by the Epworth Sleepiness Scale (ESS) are around 15%.[4,8,9] Even if these conditions (OSA and EDS) were completely unrelated, simply multiplying the prevalence of these two conditions together gives an expected coprevalence of around 4% to 20%. The accepted prevalence of sleep apnea syndrome, the combination of OSA and EDS, is between 4% and 12%[5,6,10] EDS is also associated with obesity independent of the effects of OSA.[11] It might therefore be that in individual patients only a portion of their daytime sleepiness symptoms are attributable to sleep apnea. The clinical trial data testing CPAP support this, with mild reductions in daytime sleepiness after controlling for placebo effects.[12,13] EDS may also persist in these patients because of long-term intermittent hypoxia before treatment of OSA, which may lead to irreversible changes in the brain, as has been suggested in mouse models.[14] Studies examining this patient group have found that they tend to have more reduced daytime functioning, fatigue, and poorer general health than those without residual sleepiness.[1,15,16]

This article discusses the prevalence and causes of residual sleepiness in CPAP-treated OSA, provides a diagnostic work-up for clinicians encountering this population, and discusses the treatment of these individuals.

Fatigue or Sleepiness?

Although daytime fatigue and daytime sleepiness are distinct symptoms, they have overlapping

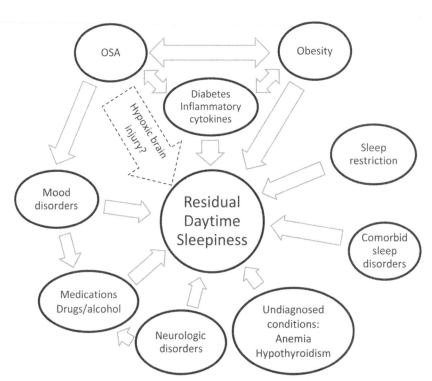

Fig. 1. Factors in ovals are potential contributing factors to the cause of residual daytime sleepiness in OSA. Arrows represent the direction of effects.

features, such as not feeling rested and reduced activity, and this makes the conditions difficult to separate.[17] Fatigue is not associated with a higher propensity for sleep but with a feeling of lethargy and exhaustion and decreased activity, and these are the symptoms that CPAP is designed to alleviate. If these symptoms remain after treatment, there are many potential causes that are beyond the scope of this article. This article focuses primarily on EDS that remains after CPAP treatment, defined as drowsiness, sleep propensity, and decreased alertness that interferes with daily living.

A Distinct Phenotype? Permanent Brain Injury

There is some evidence to show that although EDS does not correlate well with AHI, it may correlate better with other polysomnographic variables, because those patients with OSA with daytime sleepiness had lower minimum oxygen saturation (Spo_2) and lower mean Spo_2.[18] This finding suggests that the daytime sleepiness may be causally related to the hypoxic or hypercapnic conditions experienced overnight. The biological mechanism for this is unknown, but studies in rodent models have shown that long-term intermittent hypoxia can lead to neural damage to brain regions involved with wakefulness.[14,19] There is limited evidence for the causes of this in humans and further research is required. There is some evidence that there are structural brain changes (focused areas of gray-matter volume reductions in hippocampal and frontal structures measured via MRI) that may correlate with sleepiness, memory, attention, and executive function in untreated OSA and may be partially reversed with CPAP.[20]

Because many patients have OSA for many years before seeking treatment, it may be that years of intermittent hypoxia have caused permanent damage to brain regions and this cannot be completely reversed on initiation of CPAP therapy.[1,14,15] Identifying early, targeted treatment of patients at highest risk of developing daytime sleepiness should be the aim for clinical researchers. Better phenotyping and identification techniques are required to determine which patients with OSA would be more prone to permanent damage and would benefit most from early treatment.

MEASUREMENT OF EXCESSIVE DAYTIME SLEEPINESS

As with any condition, residual sleepiness in OSA should be carefully monitored; however, it is not currently possible to adequately measure sleepiness because all available tools have known weaknesses. Subjective measures may not adequately capture the daytime impairment of an individual, and current objective measures may not capture well the sleepiness experienced by the patient. There are as yet no validated biomarkers of sleepiness that can be deployed clinically.

Subjective Measures

Subjective self-reported questionnaires are quick and easy for practicing clinicians to implement, but may not provide the best evidence of patients' sleepiness. The ESS is the most broadly used questionnaire assessing subjective daytime sleepiness in OSA.[21] This single-scale measure is a 24-point questionnaire asking how likely someone is to fall asleep in 8 different situations from 0 (would never doze) to 3 (high chance of dozing). It has been translated into numerous languages and is easy to score and interpret the results. This test has the same problems as any self-reported questionnaire, in that patients may wish to provide answers they think they are expected to give. The Functional Outcomes of Sleep Questionnaire (FOSQ) is still self-reported but attempts to capture some of the dysfunction that comes with sleepiness by asking 30 questions about how daytime sleepiness affects tasks of daily living.[22] The FOSQ is longer and has 5 factor subscales (activity, vigilance, intimacy and sexual relationships, general productivity, and social outcomes), making scoring more complex and time consuming than the shorter and simpler ESS.

Objective Measures

Currently available objective measures are time consuming and expensive and so are not able to be as broadly used as the basic questionnaires. The Maintenance of Wakefulness Test (MWT)[23] and Multiple Sleep Latency Test (MSLT)[24] are commonly used to assess wakefulness and sleepiness, respectively. Both tests involve multiple nap periods throughout the day and measure sleep latency within those periods. These tests are administered within a sleep laboratory setting and require a dedicated sleep technician to monitor the patient throughout the day. Although these tests are often used interchangeably in the literature, they have a key difference I that the MWT asks people to stay awake for as long as they can, and the MSLT assesses how long it takes someone to fall asleep. The MSLT is used primarily in the diagnosis of narcolepsy, in which a quick sleep onset and sleep-onset rapid eye movement sleep periods are used along with clinical history to distinguish this disease.[25] In Australia, a positive

MSLT is required to obtain subsidized medications to treat narcolepsy, so this is often chosen by clinicians in our clinic. The problem with the MSLT is that even healthy people may be able to fall asleep quickly given a comfortable environment,[26] and so a better test of the effects of sleepiness on daytime function may be the MWT, in which people are asked to actively try to stay awake.[27]

To date there is no simple, clinical, validated measure of daytime impairment that may be implemented broadly, and this should be a target of future research (see **Box 2**).

DIAGNOSTIC APPROACH
Optimizing Continuous Positive Airway Pressure

A clinical evaluation of residual sleepiness in CPAP users starts with ensuring that the initial diagnosis of OSA syndrome is correct through history and review of the polysomnogram.[28] Once satisfied, it is imperative to ensure that the patient's CPAP therapy is effective, and that there has been adequate adherence. Assessment of weight gain since the time of diagnosis is crucial. In most cases, a download of the machine may be sufficient to identify ineffective CPAP; for example, by revealing an increased residual AHI ($\geq$10/h) or showing a large leak.[29] Despite an AHI within normal limits, excessive leak may contribute to frequent arousals overnight. The download also provides useful information on the patient's adherence, and may also suggest inadequate sleep duration as a cause of persistent sleepiness. In some cases from our clinic, the download values appear to be within normal limits but there is a clinical suspicion of untreated OSA on history (eg, the patient reports persistent snoring and choking arousals). There is known variability between devices in their ability to detect events.[30] Machine downloads may not always be considered reliable and clinicians may wish to organize an overnight in-laboratory CPAP review study to explore this further.[31,32] A directly observed in-laboratory study can more accurately detect persistent airflow limitation, or even other forms of sleep-disordered breathing such as central sleep apnea that can contribute to daytime sleepiness.[33]

Insufficient Sleep

Poor sleep hygiene and lifestyle is associated with worse daytime sleepiness in patients with untreated mild OSA.[34] This finding has not been specifically investigated in CPAP-using patients with OSA, but insufficient sleep is a common cause of persistent sleepiness in these patients. Careful evaluation of sleep time and wake times should be performed. CPAP downloads may be a good proxy of a patient's sleep opportunity, but may be a poorer measure of sleep duration because a CPAP machine cannot tell whether a patient was asleep or lying awake with the CPAP mask on. Nonetheless, CPAP downloads can be useful in confirming adequate sleep duration in patients using CPAP for long hours. In those with shorter adherence durations (eg, 6 hours), clinicians may wish to organize for the patient to complete sleep diaries or use actigraphy to obtain more objective sleep duration data. Although 6 hours of sleep may be sufficient for some individuals, it can lead to chronic sleep restriction in others.[35]

Ruling Out Concomitant Sleep Disorders

Concomitant sleep disorders such as narcolepsy, idiopathic hypersomnolence (IHS), and restless legs syndrome, can coexist with OSA and should be ruled out.[28,36,37] History taking should review the severity and nature of daytime sleepiness as well as any ancillary features such as sleep paralysis, cataplexy, and hypnagogic and hypnopompic hallucinations. The quantity and duration of naps and whether they are restorative, and the presence or absence of sleep inertia or sleep drunkenness (persistent confusion and cognitive dysfunction on waking) can also help differentiate between narcolepsy and IHS.

Mood Disorders

Mood disorders such as major depression, bipolar type II disorder, or seasonal affective disorder can be associated with hypersomnolence.[38–40] The patient may not yet be formally diagnosed with a mood disorder, hence careful questioning regarding mood, feelings of helplessness and hopelessness, apathy, appetite, or weight changes should be asked because hypersomnolence may be the first clinical clue to the underlying condition. Mood disorders can coexist with OSA or occur years after commencing CPAP, explaining why previously effective CPAP is no longer effective. Clinicians should be aware of the link between OSA and depression because they both may be associated with daytime sleepiness[34] that might be resolved with a combination of antidepressant and CPAP therapy, but this treatment approach has not yet been tested in rigorously designed randomised controlled trials.[41]

Medications or Illicit Drug Use

Many medications and drugs have sedative side effects even when not classically thought of as sedative medications, such as analgesics, antihistamines, anticonvulsants, and certain antidepressants.[42] A careful history should document recently discontinued medications and present intake of all medications, and use of recreational drugs and alcohol.

Neurologic Disorders

A variety of neurologic conditions are associated with hypersomnolence, such as Parkinson disease, myotonic dystrophy, and multiple sclerosis.[43] Careful history taking should include symptoms of anosmia, tremor, bradykinesia, memory loss, muscle weakness, and visual changes. Although rare, a cerebral lesion affecting the arousal centers of the brain can also cause sleepiness. A full neurologic examination should be performed with consideration of cerebral imaging with MRI if appropriate. Pharmacotherapy for some of these disorders (eg, antiepileptics, benzodiazepines) may directly contribute to sleepiness.[42]

Other Uncontrolled or Undiagnosed Medical Conditions

History taking should evaluate the presence of uncontrolled diabetes, hypothyroidism, anemia, and obesity, which can all contribute to feelings of tiredness and sleepiness.[38,44,45] Obesity, diabetes, and OSA are all interrelated and common comorbid conditions that are known to increase the levels of circulating inflammatory cytokines, which may explain the daytime sleepiness in these patients.[46,47]

Unrealistic Expectations

Some individuals report a large symptomatic benefit when first starting CPAP but return a few weeks or months later reporting a reduced benefit with return of hypersomnolence.[28] Around a third of the effect of CPAP may result from a patient's expectation of benefit from the device.[48] Continuing CPAP adherence depends on a complex combination of social, psychological, and biomedical factors.[49] Dysfunction in any of these factors may result in a change in perceived benefit and the loss of this placebo effect. In our clinical experience, discontinuing CPAP for a short period of time allows patients to reexperience their initial symptoms, allowing a subjective comparison with their new baseline. This comparison may lead to an improved perception of the benefit obtained from CPAP.

Investigations

When no clear cause is identified, blood tests may be performed. These tests include full blood count, electrolyte/urea/creatinine levels, liver function tests, iron studies, and thyroid function tests. Chronic viral infections, such as Epstein-Barr virus and other region-specific viruses, should be excluded.[50] In addition, clinicians may consider testing for testosterone levels in men. Low testosterone level is associated with obesity and OSA and can contribute to significant lethargy.[51]

As mentioned, cerebral imaging may be warranted in patients with suspicion of a primary neurologic disorder, or in those with focal neurologic signs.

If these are unremarkable, objective measurement of sleepiness with an overnight diagnostic sleep study on CPAP followed by MSLT should be considered.

MANAGEMENT OF RESIDUAL DAYTIME SLEEPINESS IN OBSTRUCTIVE SLEEP APNEA

After completing the diagnostic work-up and identifying any potential cause for residual sleepiness, clinicians may wish to consider the use of pharmacotherapy in patients with disabling residual symptoms (**Box 1**).

Treat Comorbidities

Treating comorbid depression, diabetes, hypothyroidism, and anemia may assist in reducing residual EDS in patients with OSA. The method for this depends on the individual circumstance and is beyond the scope of this article. Note that follow-up is required in any of these cases and care must be taken when selecting treatments in sleepy patients. For example, treating sleepy, depressed patients with certain antidepressants or anxiolytics may worsen their sleepiness, so caution must be used when selecting appropriate therapies in already sleepy individuals. Our study team has also shown that the use of mirtazapine, a common antidepressant, caused weight gain in patients with OSA, which may worsen OSA.[52]

Box 1
Patient management goals

1. Optimize CPAP therapy

2. Rule out sleep restriction

3. Identify comorbidities/medications that may be contributing to daytime sleepiness and treat accordingly

4. Consider modafinil or armodafinil if sleepiness not otherwise resolved

5. Review patient for worsening/improvement of symptoms via objective tests (eg, MWT)

Treating Sleepiness with Pharmacotherapy

Modafinil and armodafinil

Modafinil and its R-enantiomer armodafinil are nonamphetamine wakefulness promoters.[53,54] Armodafinil is the right enantiomer of racemic modafinil and it is thought to be the more active molecule. Studies comparing the effects of the two drugs have shown that armodafinil has a longer active duration than modafinil.[55]

Mechanism of action The mechanism of action of these medications is unclear, but the best evidence shows that modafinil acts on the dopamine transporter, thus reducing dopamine reuptake and increasing the amount of dopamine in the synapse, but without increasing production of dopamine in the presynapse, as in amphetamines.[56,57] There is also a suggestion from these studies that modafinil works on norepinephrine transporters. The resulting increase in synaptic levels of dopamine and norepinephrine promotes wakefulness through excitatory actions on the ascending arousal pathway beginning in the hypothalamus, and simultaneously prevents sleep by inhibiting sleep-promoting neurons in the ventrolateral preoptic area of the hypothalamus.[58,59]

Because modafinil does not promote the release of these catecholamines from the presynapse, and because it seems to have a dual mode of action on dopamine and norepinephrine transport, there is a reduced propensity for tolerance and addiction than with amphetamines.[60]

Evidence from clinical trials Recently 2 meta-analyses of the clinical trials of modafinil and armodafinil for the treatment of residual sleepiness in CPAP-treated OSA have been reported.[61,62] Our group's meta-analysis showed that in the 10 trials of modafinil or armodafinil for this indication, ESS score improved significantly by 2.2 points compared with placebo (95% confidence interval [CI], 1.5–2.9). The MWT was measured in 8 of these trials and the improvement in sleep onset latency compared with placebo was 3 minutes (95% CI, 2.1–3.8 min).

The Clinical Global Impressions of Change scale (a scale of symptom improvement reported by clinicians at follow-up) showed that 71% of patients on modafinil or armodafinil, compared with 44% on placebo, were at least minimally improved from baseline.[62]

Modafinil/armodafinil tripled the number of adverse events and doubled adverse events leading to withdrawal but did not increase serious adverse events (hospitalizations or death).

Overall, modafinil and armodafinil lead to moderate improvements on objective and subjective measures of daytime sleepiness in patients with OSA with residual sleepiness despite CPAP treatment.

Common side effects The common side effects (occurring in >5% of clinical trial patients) of modafinil and armodafinil are headache, nausea, nervousness, rhinitis, diarrhea, back pain, anxiety, insomnia, dizziness, and dyspepsia.[53,54,62] A more serious, but very uncommon, adverse effect is the development of a severe skin rash (Stevens-Johnson syndrome), which could lead to disability or death. Although clinical trial data showed no clinically significant increase in blood pressure on modafinil/armodafinil compared with placebo,[62] there is a suggestion that hypertension may be increased in some patients on modafinil/armodafinil and blood pressure should be monitored after the initiation of treatment.[53,54]

Clinical application Modafinil is indicated for use in patients with OSA with residual sleepiness despite CPAP treatment in Australia,[63] the United States,[64] and until recently in Europe.[65] Armodafinil is also approved for this indication in the United States[54] and has just been approved in Australia.[66] However, the use of modafinil/armodafinil for this indication has long been a matter of controversy.[67,68] Some clinicians think that it should be available for use in patients in whom other causes of sleepiness have been carefully excluded,[67] which relies on a careful, detailed assessment by the treating physician.[69] Others think that it should not be used because of the side effect profile and the risk of potential harm.[70] In addition, some clinicians argue that monitoring patients on both CPAP and wakefulness promoters would be challenging because these agents could mask uncontrolled OSA.[68]

Amphetamines and Other Sympathomimetics

Low doses of stimulants like amphetamines and methylphenidate may increase arousal, attention, and cognitive enhancement but higher doses lead to mood changes, tolerance, and addiction and can impair cognition. The most common side effects of amphetamines and methylphenidate are blood pressure and heart rate increases and loss of appetite.[60]

Traditional stimulants like amphetamines and methylphenidate are available in generic form and are less expensive than other treatments like modafinil and armodafinil. Although they have long been used in clinical practice and they are still recommended for use in clinical practice guidelines, there is limited high-level randomised controlled trial evidence for their use in any disorder of daytime sleepiness.[71] There are also few studies directly comparing amphetamines with newer agents like modafinil and armodafinil, so the comparative effectiveness of the older agents and the newer ones is unclear.

There is very limited evidence for the use of amphetamines to treat sleepiness in OSA. One study that aimed to augment weight loss in untreated OSA with the amphetaminelike agent phentermine plus topiramate (indicated for weight loss in the United States[72]) showed that there was no difference between treatment and placebo groups in ESS score after 28 weeks of treatment.[73] Amphetamines have the potential risks of tolerance and addiction and so should be used with caution in the treatment of daytime sleepiness.[60]

Caffeine

The effects of caffeine on reducing daytime sleepiness in patients with OSA have not been evaluated via randomised controlled trials. It has been shown that patients with OSA have a higher daily intake of caffeine than those without OSA, perhaps self-medicating for their symptoms of sleepiness.[74] Increased caffeine consumption is associated with increased OSA severity.[75] This caffeine use may reduce cognitive impairment because a study of patients with moderate to severe OSA showed that those who performed best on performance tests were taking around 6 times as much caffeine as those who performed most poorly.[76]

A single-dose trial of caffeine versus modafinil versus placebo in healthy individuals showed that 600 mg of caffeine was comparable with a 200-mg and 400-mg dose of modafinil in maintaining cognitive alertness during 54.5 hours of sleep deprivation.[77] In this single-dose study there were more reported side effects in the caffeine arm than for either dose of modafinil or placebo. The dose of caffeine used was 3 times higher than over-the-counter caffeine tablets and around 6 times higher than a cup of espresso coffee.[77] Long-term effects of this dose of caffeine in a sleep apnea population are yet to be determined, and, given that long-term moderate intake of caffeine increases hypertension and can acutely increase heart rate, it is unlikely to be feasible as a general treatment of sleepiness in OSA.[78,79]

Caffeine is known to have a variable interindividual effects whereby some people are insensitive to the alerting effects of caffeine. This variability has been linked to variations in the adenosine A2A receptor gene but the observation needs to be replicated.[80]

Potential Future Drugs

There is some evidence that proinflammatory cytokines are associated with the pathogenesis of EDS in OSA.[46] A nonrandomized 3-week crossover trial of etanercept, a tumor necrosis factor inhibitor, versus placebo showed a significant reduction in daytime sleepiness measured by MSLT in patients with untreated OSA.[81] While this study did not report any safety data, this drug should not be considered as a suitable treatment of daytime sleepiness in OSA because it requires injection by nursing staff twice a week, it has an immunomodulatory effect, and it is associated with increased risk of serious infections and some malignancies.[82] This medication may not be the answer, but a drug that reduces inflammatory cytokine levels without negative effects may be appropriate for use to treat daytime sleepiness in this population.[81]

The histamine H3 receptor may be a promising drug target for sleep-wake disorders because histaminergic neurons are involved in maintaining wakefulness either directly or via their influence on other wake-regulatory neurotransmitters like gamma-aminobutyric acid and glutamate. There are drugs currently under development for the treatment of narcolepsy, such as pitolisant, a histamine H3 receptor inverse agonist, which reduced daytime sleepiness to the same degree as modafinil and was well tolerated in a small study in narcolepsy.[83] To date, limited data exist from trials in humans for these drugs under development.[84]

Because the orexin/hypocretin system is thought to be responsible for the sleep/wake switch, medications that activate this system may be effective as wakefulness promoters.[84] There are some pharmacologic barriers to this (eg, creating molecules that mimic orexin/hypocretin but are small enough to cross the blood-brain barrier) but there are plans to trial such medications in narcolepsy, which may be followed by other disorders of daytime sleepiness such as patients with residual sleepiness despite CPAP use.[84]

Summary of Pharmacologic Strategies

Amphetamines and methylphenidate are inappropriate for broad use to treat residual sleepiness in CPAP-treated OSA because evidence of efficacy is poor and the potential for side effects and abuse may be higher than with other treatments. Caffeine may be of use in OSA, but the evidence is poor and it seems that side effects from moderate to high doses of caffeine (eg, racing heart rate and hypertension) may not be appropriate in patients with OSA. In addition, because of the availability of caffeine, patients may already be using this if they think it is effective. Reducing the effects of inflammatory cytokines and directly targeting the orexin/hypocretin system seem to be promising treatment targets, but currently there is no feasible option from these classes. At present, the most rigorously tested pharmacologic treatments for EDS are modafinil and armodafinil, but, as with the use of any medication, there is a risk of increased side effects and patients should be monitored carefully.

SUMMARY

Residual EDS despite CPAP treatment is common in OSA. The cause is multifactorial; it may be that a comorbid condition or a combination of comorbid conditions leads to daytime sleepiness that is unlikely to be wholly relieved by CPAP therapy. There is also evidence that long-term intermittent hypoxia may have already led to permanent brain injury by the time patients initiate therapy for their OSA.

The management of residual sleepiness in OSA currently requires an individual approach (see **Box 1**). Because the causes are multifactorial, the treatments must also be multifactorial. An assessment must be made of each individual's comorbid conditions and medications that may contribute to sleepiness. Lifestyle factors that may contribute to sleepiness should be identified, and patients should be educated on the importance of adequate sleep time in their condition.

If sleepiness remains after evaluation of other options, modafinil or armodafinil could be considered to reduce the effects of daytime sleepiness on the activities of daily living.

Periodic reevaluation of residual sleepiness should be conducted to assess for any changes in these symptoms. Ideally a simple, valid, and objective test of sleepiness and daytime functioning that may be broadly implemented will be identified through future research (**Box 2**). Future research should aim to phenotype patients to determine who is likely to have daytime sleepiness despite CPAP use, and target therapies at reducing residual sleepiness in these patients.

Box 2
Future research goals

1. Phenotype patients to determine who is likely to have residual sleepiness and daytime impairment from OSA

2. Develop strategies to implement before the initiation of CPAP to reduce the likelihood of residual sleepiness after initiation of treatment

3. Develop tests of the impact of daytime sleepiness on neurobehavioral performance that may be used diagnostically

---

REFERENCES

1. Gasa M, Tamisier R, Launois SH, et al. Residual sleepiness in sleep apnea patients treated by continuous positive airway pressure. J Sleep Res 2013;22(4):389–97.
2. Koutsourelakis I, Perraki E, Economou NT, et al. Predictors of residual sleepiness in adequately treated obstructive sleep apnoea patients. Eur Respir J 2009;34(3):687–93.
3. Pepin JL, Viot-Blanc V, Escourrou P, et al. Prevalence of residual excessive sleepiness in CPAP-treated sleep apnoea patients: the French multicentre study. Eur Respir J 2009;33(5):1062–7.
4. Gottlieb DJ, Whitney CW, Bonekat WH, et al. Relation of sleepiness to respiratory disturbance index: the Sleep Heart Health Study. Am J Respir Crit Care Med 1999;159(2):502–7.
5. Bearpark H, Elliott L, Grunstein R, et al. Snoring and sleep apnea. A population study in Australian men. Am J Respir Crit Care Med 1995;151(5):1459–65.
6. Young T, Palta M, Dempsey J, et al. The occurrence of sleep-disordered breathing among middle-aged adults. N Engl J Med 1993;328(17):1230–5.
7. Heinzer R, Vat S, Marques-Vidal P, et al. Prevalence of sleep-disordered breathing in the general population: the HypnoLaus study. Lancet Respir Med 2015;3(4):310–8.
8. Bartlett DJ, Marshall NS, Williams A, et al. Sleep health New South Wales: chronic sleep restriction and daytime sleepiness. Intern Med J 2008;38(1):24–31.
9. Gander PH, Marshall NS, Harris R, et al. The Epworth Sleepiness Scale: influence of age, ethnicity, and socioeconomic deprivation. Epworth Sleepiness scores of adults in New Zealand. Sleep 2005;28(2):249–53.
10. Heinzer R, Marti-Soler H, Haba-Rubio J. Prevalence of sleep apnoea syndrome in the middle to old age general population. Lancet Respir Med 2016;4(2):e5–6.
11. Panossian LA, Veasey SC. Daytime sleepiness in obesity: mechanisms beyond obstructive sleep apnea - a review. Sleep 2012;35(5):605–15.
12. Marshall NS, Barnes M, Travier N, et al. Continuous positive airway pressure reduces daytime sleepiness in mild to moderate obstructive sleep apnoea: a meta-analysis. Thorax 2006;61(5):430–4.
13. Giles TL, Lasserson TJ, Smith B, et al. Continuous positive airways pressure for obstructive sleep apnoea in adults. Cochrane Database Syst Rev 2009;(1):CD001106.

14. Veasey SC, Davis CW, Fenik P, et al. Long-term intermittent hypoxia in mice: protracted hypersomnolence with oxidative injury to sleep-wake brain regions. Sleep 2004;27(2):194–201.

15. Vernet C, Redolfi S, Attali V, et al. Residual sleepiness in obstructive sleep apnoea: phenotype and related symptoms. Eur Respir J 2011;38(1):98–105.

16. Vakulin A, Baulk SD, Catcheside PG, et al. Driving simulator performance remains impaired in patients with severe OSA after CPAP treatment. J Clin Sleep Med 2011;7(3):246–53.

17. Pigeon WR, Sateia MJ, Ferguson RJ. Distinguishing between excessive daytime sleepiness and fatigue: toward improved detection and treatment. J Psychosom Res 2003;54(1):61–9.

18. Mediano O, Barceló A, de la Peña M, et al. Daytime sleepiness and polysomnographic variables in sleep apnoea patients. Eur Respir J 2007;30(1): 110–3.

19. Zhan G, Fenik P, Pratico D, et al. Inducible nitric oxide synthase in long-term intermittent hypoxia: hypersomnolence and brain injury. Am J Respir Crit Care Med 2005;171(12):1414–20.

20. Canessa N, Castronovo V, Cappa SF, et al. Obstructive sleep apnea: brain structural changes and neurocognitive function before and after treatment. Am J Respir Crit Care Med 2011;183(10):1419–26.

21. Johns MW. A new method for measuring daytime sleepiness: the Epworth Sleepiness Scale. Sleep 1991;14(6):540–5.

22. Weaver TE, Laizner AM, Evans LK, et al. An instrument to measure functional status outcomes for disorders of excessive sleepiness. Sleep 1997;20(10): 835–43.

23. Mitler MM, Gujavarty KS, Browman CP. Maintenance of wakefulness test: a polysomnographic technique for evaluating treatment efficacy in patients with excessive somnolence. Electroencephalogr Clin Neurophysiol 1982;53(6):658–61.

24. Carskadon MA, Dement WC, Mitler MM, et al. Guidelines for the Multiple Sleep Latency Test (MSLT): a standard measure of sleepiness. Sleep 1987;9(4):519–24.

25. Aldrich MS, Chervin RD, Malow BA. Value of the Multiple Sleep Latency Test (MSLT) for the diagnosis of narcolepsy. Sleep 1997;20(8):620–9.

26. Harrison Y, Bright V, Horne JA. Can normal subjects be motivated to fall asleep faster? Physiol Behav 1996;60(2):681–4.

27. Sangal RB, Thomas L, Mitler MM. Maintenance of wakefulness test and multiple sleep latency test; measurement of different abilities in patients with sleep disorders. Chest 1992;101(4):898–902.

28. Santamaria J, Iranzo A, Ma Montserrat J, et al. Persistent sleepiness in CPAP treated obstructive sleep apnea patients: evaluation and treatment. Sleep Med Rev 2007;11(3):195–207.

29. Freedman N. Positive airway pressure treatment for obstructive sleep apnea. In: Dement KR, editor. Principles and practice of sleep medicine. 6th edition. Philadelphia: Elsevier; 2017. p. 1125–37.

30. Abdenbi F, Chambille B, Escourrou P. Bench testing of auto-adjusting positive airway pressure devices. Eur Respir J 2004;24(4):649–58.

31. Denotti AL, Wong KKH, Dungan GC, et al. Residual sleep-disordered breathing during autotitrating continuous positive airway pressure therapy. Eur Respir J 2012;39(6):1391–7.

32. Rodenstein D. Determination of therapeutic continuous positive airway pressure for obstructive sleep apnea using automatic titration: promises not fulfilled. Chest 2008;133(3):595–7.

33. Epstein LJ, Kristo D, Strollo PJ Jr, et al. Clinical guideline for the evaluation, management and long-term care of obstructive sleep apnea in adults. J Clin Sleep Med 2009;5(3):263–76.

34. Lee SA, Paek JH, Han SH. Sleep hygiene and its association with daytime sleepiness, depressive symptoms, and quality of life in patients with mild obstructive sleep apnea. J Neurol Sci 2015; 359(1–2):445–9.

35. Hirshkowitz M, Whiton K, Albert SM, et al. National Sleep Foundation sleep time duration recommendations: methodology and results summary. Sleep Health 2013;1(1):40–3.

36. Ohayon MM, Roth T. Prevalence of restless legs syndrome and periodic limb movement disorder in the general population. J Psychosom Res 2002;53(1): 547–54.

37. Allen RP, Walters AS, Montplaisir J, et al. Restless legs syndrome prevalence and impact: rest general population study. Arch Intern Med 2005;165(11): 1286–92.

38. Bixler EO, Vgontzas AN, Lin HM, et al. Excessive daytime sleepiness in a general population sample: the role of sleep apnea, age, obesity, diabetes, and depression. J Clin Endocrinol Metab 2005;90(8): 4510–5.

39. Mitchell PB, Wilhelm K, Parker G, et al. The clinical features of bipolar depression: a comparison with matched major depressive disorder patients. J Clin Psychiatry 2001;62(3):212–6.

40. Lam RW, Levitan RD. Pathophysiology of seasonal affective disorder: a review. J Psychiatry Neurosci 2000;25(5):469–80.

41. Harris M, Glozier N, Ratnavadivel R, et al. Obstructive sleep apnea and depression. Sleep Med Rev 2009;13(6):437–44.

42. Steiger A. Sleep and its modulation by substances that affect GABAA receptor function. In: Monti MJ, Pandi-Perumal RS, Möhler H, editors. GABA and sleep: molecular, functional and clinical aspects. Basel (Switzerland): Springer Basel; 2010. p. 121–46.

43. Happe S. Excessive daytime sleepiness and sleep disturbances in patients with neurological diseases: epidemiology and management. Drugs 2003; 63(24):2725–37.

44. Fernandez-Mendoza J, Vgontzas AN, Kritikou I, et al. Natural history of excessive daytime sleepiness: role of obesity, weight loss, depression, and sleep propensity. Sleep 2015;38(3):351–60.

45. Vaidya B, Pearce SHS. Management of hypothyroidism in adults. BMJ 2008;337:a801.

46. Vgontzas AN, Papanicolaou DA, Bixler EO, et al. Sleep apnea and daytime sleepiness and fatigue: relation to visceral obesity, insulin resistance, and hypercytokinemia. J Clin Endocrinol Metab 2000; 85(3):1151–8.

47. Vgontzas AN, Papanicolaou DA, Bixler EO, et al. Elevation of plasma cytokines in disorders of excessive daytime sleepiness: role of sleep disturbance and obesity. J Clin Endocrinol Metab 1997;82(5): 1313–6.

48. Crawford MR, Bartlett DJ, Coughlin SR, et al. The effect of continuous positive airway pressure usage on sleepiness in obstructive sleep apnoea: real effects or expectation of benefit? Thorax 2012; 67(10):920–4.

49. Crawford MR, Espie CA, Bartlett DJ, et al. Integrating psychology and medicine in CPAP adherence – new concepts? Sleep Med Rev 2014;18(2): 123–39.

50. Macsween KF, Johannessen I. Epstein-Barr virus (EBV): infectious mononucleosis and other non-malignant EBV-associated diseases. In: Kaslow AR, Stanberry RL, Le Duc WJ, editors. Viral infections of humans: epidemiology and control. Boston: Springer; 2014. p. 867–96.

51. Liu PY, Caterson ID, Grunstein RR, et al. Androgens, obesity, and sleep-disordered breathing in men. Endocrinol Metab Clin North Am 2007;36(2): 349–63.

52. Marshall NS, Yee BJ, Desai AV, et al. Two randomized placebo-controlled trials to evaluate the efficacy and tolerability of mirtazapine for the treatment of obstructive sleep apnea. Sleep 2008;31(6): 824–31.

53. Nuvigil (armodafinil) medication guide. North Wales (PA): Teva Pharmaceuticals; 2013. Available at: http://www.nuvigil.com/PDF/Medication_Guide.pdf.

54. Provigil (modafinil) medication guide. North Wales (PA): Teva Pharmaceuticals; 2015. Available at: http://www.fda.gov/downloads/Drugs/DrugSafety/UCM231722.pdf.

55. Darwish M, Kirby M, Hellriegel ET, et al. Armodafinil and modafinil have substantially different pharmacokinetic profiles despite having the same terminal half-lives: analysis of data from three randomized, single-dose, pharmacokinetic studies. Clin Drug Investig 2009;29(9):613–23.

56. Spencer TJ, Madras BK, Bonab AA, et al. A positron emission tomography study examining the dopaminergic activity of armodafinil in adults using [11C]altropane and [11C]raclopride. Biol Psychiatry 2010; 68(10):964–70.

57. Madras BK, Xie Z, Lin Z, et al. Modafinil occupies dopamine and norepinephrine transporters in vivo and modulates the transporters and trace amine activity in vitro. J Pharmacol Exp Ther 2006;319(2): 561–9.

58. Mitchell HA, Weinshenker D. Good night and good luck: norepinephrine in sleep pharmacology. Biochem Pharmacol 2010;79(6):801–9.

59. Saper CB, Scammell TE, Lu J. Hypothalamic regulation of sleep and circadian rhythms. Nature 2005; 437(7063):1257–63.

60. Wood S, Sage JR, Shuman T, et al. Psychostimulants and cognition: a continuum of behavioral and cognitive activation. Pharmacol Rev 2014;66(1): 193–221.

61. Sukhal S, Khalid M, Tulaimat A. Effect of wakefulness-promoting agents on sleepiness in patients with sleep apnea treated with CPAP: a meta-analysis. J Clin Sleep Med 2015;11(10):1179–86.

62. Chapman JL, Vakulin A, Hedner J, et al. Modafinil/armodafinil in obstructive sleep apnoea: a systematic review and meta-analysis. Eur Respir J 2016. http://dx.doi.org/10.1183/13993003.01509-2015.

63. Commonwealth of Australia Therapeutic Goods Administration; public Australian register of therapeutic goods summary for modafinil Australia. 2011. Available at: https://www.ebs.tga.gov.au/servlet/xmlmillr6?dbid=ebs/PublicHTML/pdfStore.nsf&docid=82350&agid=(PrintDetailsPublic)&actionid=1. Accessed February 25, 2016.

64. Cephalon Inc. Approved by the US Food and Drug Administration Medication Guide - Provigil (modafinil) tablets. USA: 2010. Available at: http://www.accessdata.fda.gov/drugsatfda_docs/label/2010/020717s030s034s036MedGuide.pdf. Accessed February 25, 2016.

65. European Medicines Agency. Questions and answers on the review of medicines containing modafinil. London (United Kingdom): 2010. Available at: http://www.ema.europa.eu/ema/index.jsp?curl=pages/medicines/human/referrals/Modafinil/human_referral_000236.jsp. Accessed February 22, 2016.

66. Australian Register of Therapeutic Goods ID 226561-NUVIGIL armodafinil 50 mg. 2016. Available at: https://www.tga.gov.au/artg/artg-id-226561. Accessed February 22, 2016.

67. Black J. Pro: modafinil has a role in management of sleep apnea. Am J Respir Crit Care Med 2003; 167(2):105–6. discussion 108.

68. Pollak CP. Con: modafinil has no role in management of sleep apnea. Am J Respir Crit Care Med 2003; 167(2):106–7 [discussion: 107–8].

69. Pack AI. Should a pharmaceutical be approved for the broad indication of excessive sleepiness? Am J Respir Crit Care Med 2003;167(2):109–11.

70. European Medicines Agency. Assessment report for modafinil containing medicinal products. London (United Kingdom): 2011. Available at: http://www.ema. europa.eu/ema/index.jsp?curl=pages/medicines/ human/referrals/Modafinil/human_referral_000236.jsp. Accessed February 22, 2016.

71. Morgenthaler TI, Kapur VK, Brown T, et al. Practice parameters for the treatment of narcolepsy and other hypersomnias of central origin. Sleep 2007; 30(12):1705–11.

72. Phentermine hydrochloride and topiramate extended-release medication guide. California: VIVUS Inc; 2014.

73. Winslow DH, Bowden CH, DiDonato KP, et al. A randomized, double-blind, placebo-controlled study of an oral, extended-release formulation of phentermine/topiramate for the treatment of obstructive sleep apnea in obese adults. Sleep 2012; 35(11):1529–39.

74. Bardwell WA, Ziegler MG, Ancoli-Israel S, et al. Does caffeine confound relationships among adrenergic tone, blood pressure and sleep apnoea? J Sleep Res 2000;9(3):269–72.

75. Aurora RN, Crainiceanu C, Caffo B, et al. Sleep-disordered breathing and caffeine consumption: results of a community-based study. Chest 2012; 142(3):631–8.

76. Norman D, Bardwell WA, Loredo JS, et al. Caffeine intake is independently associated with neuropsychological performance in patients with obstructive sleep apnea. Sleep Breath 2008;12(3):199–205.

77. Wesensten N, Belenky G, Kautz MA, et al. Maintaining alertness and performance during sleep deprivation: modafinil versus caffeine. Psychopharmacology 2002;159(3):238–47.

78. Zhang Z, Hu G, Caballero B, et al. Habitual coffee consumption and risk of hypertension: a systematic review and meta-analysis of prospective observational studies. Am J Clin Nutr 2011;93(6): 1212–9.

79. Noordzij M, Uiterwaal CS, Arends LR, et al. Blood pressure response to chronic intake of coffee and caffeine: a meta-analysis of randomized controlled trials. J Hypertens 2005;23(5): 921–8.

80. Rétey JV, Adam M, Khatami R, et al. A genetic variation in the adenosine A2A receptor gene (ADORA2A) contributes to individual sensitivity to caffeine effects on sleep. Clin Pharmacol Ther 2007;81(5):692–8.

81. Vgontzas AN, Zoumakis E, Lin HM, et al. Marked decrease in sleepiness in patients with sleep apnea by etanercept, a tumor necrosis factor-alpha antagonist. J Clin Endocrinol Metab 2004;89(9): 4409–13.

82. Enbrel (etanercept) prescribing information. Thousand Oaks (CA): Immunex Corporation; 2013.

83. Dauvilliers Y, Bassetti C, Lammers GJ, et al. Pitolisant versus placebo or modafinil in patients with narcolepsy: a double-blind, randomised trial. Lancet Neurol 2013;12(11):1068–75.

84. De la Herran-Arita AK, Garcia-Garcia F. Current and emerging options for the drug treatment of narcolepsy. Drugs 2013;73(16):1771–81.

Disorders of Excessive Daytime Sleepiness Including Narcolepsy and Idiopathic Hypersomnia

Joseph Andrew Berkowski, MD*,
Anita Valanju Shelgikar, MD

KEYWORDS

- Hypersomnolence • Narcolepsy • Idiopathic hypersomnia • Cataplexy
- Excessive daytime sleepiness

KEY POINTS

- Central disorders of hypersomnolence are rare conditions with a poorly understood pathophysiology.
- Clinical history is essential for ruling out secondary causes of hypersomnolence, but the polysomnogram and multiple sleep latency test play critical roles in diagnosis.
- The current focus of treatment is on drugs that promote alertness and, in the case of narcolepsy type 1, those that control cataplexy.

INTRODUCTION

Central disorders of hypersomnolence are less common than secondary causes of daytime sleepiness, such as insufficient sleep and obstructive sleep apnea, but are more likely to present to and be managed within a comprehensive sleep center. The relative infrequency of these disorders and lack of biomarker or highly specific clinical features in many cases make these disorders challenging for even the well-rounded sleep clinician. Particular attention must be paid to identifying mimics or other causes leading to secondary hypersomnolence. The sleep clinician's approach to *rule out* a central disorder of hypersomnolence is equally important as the knowledge of diagnostic criteria to confirm the presence of these disorders.

The 3 main central disorders of hypersomnolence are narcolepsy type 1, narcolepsy type 2, and idiopathic hypersomnia. Recurrent hypersomnia (here used to denote Kleine-Levin syndrome) is extremely rare, though it is addressed in this article. A summary of the characteristics of these conditions is found in **Table 1**.[1–9]

A common challenge in sleep medicine is the meaning and seemingly interchangeable use of English language terms for the ability to fall asleep quickly, both among patients and clinicians, including sleepiness, drowsiness, tiredness, and fatigue, among others. Official medical terminology also poses a challenge. In this article, the terms *hypersomnolence* and *excessive daytime sleepiness* refer to the symptoms of the abnormal tendency or speed at which one enters into a sleep state. Hypersomnia here is defined as the abnormally increased *amount* of sleep time within a 24-hour period. (An exception to this is the use of hypersomnia in the disorder idiopathic hypersomnia.) This distinction is clinically relevant, as

The authors have nothing to disclose.
Michael S. Aldrich Sleep Disorders Laboratory, Department of Neurology, University of Michigan, 1500 East Medical Center Drive, SPC 5845, C728 Med Inn Building, Ann Arbor, MI 48109-5845, USA
* Corresponding author.
E-mail address: andyberk@med.umich.edu

sleep.theclinics.com

Table 1
Characteristics of primary disorders of hypersomnolence

Disorder	Prevalence	Pathogenesis	Clinical Findings	Diagnostic Test Findings
Narcolepsy type 1	25–50 per 100,000 (from multiple studies)	• Hypocretin deficiency • Postinfectious autoimmune	• Hypersomnolence • Cataplexy • Hypnagogic or hypnopompic hallucinations • Sleep paralysis • Dreams during short naps	• <8-min mean sleep onset on MSLT • <5-min mean sleep latency more specific • ≥2 SOREMPs on MSLT and PSG • SOREMP on PSG more specific • Low CSF hypocretin (≤110 pg/mL)
Narcolepsy type 2	20.5 per 100,000 in (Population-based study in Olmsted County, MN by Silber et al[3])	Unknown, may be a syndrome of heterogeneous diseases	• Hypersomnolence • Absence of cataplexy • Sleep paralysis and other features of narcolepsy type 1 may be present but less frequent	• <8-min mean sleep onset on MSLT • ≥2 SOREMPs • Mainly intermediate or normal CSF hypocretin (>110 pg/mL), though small percentage are low but not deficient
Idiopathic hypersomnia	No epidemiologic information based on *ICSD-2* classification (Ohayon[4])	Unknown, may be a syndrome of heterogeneous diseases	• Hypersomnolence • Unrefreshing naps • Sleep inertia	• <8-min mean sleep onset on MSLT • 0–1 SOREMP • Good sleep efficiency on PSG
Recurrent hypersomnia	0.2–1.0 per 100,000 (international estimate by Arnulf et al[5])	Unknown	• Recurrent episodes of several days with severe hypersomnolence • Derealization • Hyperphagia • Hypersexuality • Normal sleep and behavior between episodes	• Electroencephalogram shows background slowing • Hypoperfusion in diencephalon and other cerebral regions on PET

Abbreviations: CSF, cerebrospinal fluid; ICSD-2, *International Classification of Sleep Disorders-2*; MSLT, multiple sleep latency test; PSG, polysomnogram; SOREMP, sleep-onset rapid eye movement periods.

patients with normative total sleep time (lack of hypersomnia) may still have increased propensity to enter the sleep state (hypersomnolence).

This article focuses on the evaluation and management of hypersomnolence. The first portion describes the initial clinical and diagnostic evaluation of a patient who presents with sleepiness. Pharmacologic and nonpharmacologic management, including new treatments on the horizon, and the effects of treatment on these disorders is discussed in the latter part of the article.

PATIENT EVALUATION
Clinical History

A detailed sleep history is paramount, particularly in disorders that are diagnoses of exclusion. **Box 1** contains a list of topics that can be assessed as part of the sleep history.

Diagnostic procedures, such as polysomnography and multiple sleep latency testing, are significant in the overall evaluation but cannot replace the clinical history, which guides the use of further testing. The history should also include discussion of medical conditions that may cause sleepiness, as summarized in **Table 2**.

Subjective questionnaires
Commonly encountered, validated questionnaires can provide some quantitative value to assess the degree of somnolence. These questionnaires include the Epworth Sleepiness Scale, Stanford Sleepiness Scale, and the Karolinska Sleepiness Scale, which are described in **Table 3**.[10–13]

Table 2 Secondary causes of hypersomnolence	
Cause	**Examples**
Sleep-disordered breathing	• Obstructive sleep apnea • Upper airway resistance syndrome • Sleep-related hypoventilation • Central sleep apnea
Drug induced	• Antihistamines • Anticholinergic • Opiates • Benzodiazepines • Antiepileptic • Recreational drugs (eg, heroin, marijuana, barbiturates) • Antipsychotic
Insufficient sleep	• Insomnia disorder • Insufficient sleep syndrome
Circadian rhythm disorders	• Delayed sleep-wake phase • Jet lag • Shift work • Irregular sleep-wake schedule
Psychiatric	• Depression • Bipolar disorder • Somatoform disorders
Other general medical	• Traumatic brain injury • Stroke • Anemia • Hypothyroidism • Hepatic encephalopathy • Obesity hypoventilation syndrome

---

Box 1
Topics for a history of sleepiness

- Sleep onset (bedtime)
- Sleep offset (time getting out of bed)
- Variability on weekends
- Sleep latency
- Total sleep time (including nap time)
- Number and duration of arousals
- Daytime energy level
- Daytime sleepiness
- Refreshing sleep from main sleep period
- Onset of hypersomnolence and progression
- Use of hypnotics and stimulants

Symptoms of Central Disorders of Hypersomnolence

Central disorders of hypersomnolence have many classic features and are distinguishable in part by symptom presentation.

Narcolepsy type 1 is a disorder of hypersomnolence, though not necessarily increased sleep time, with increased dissociation of sleep states.[14,15] The hallmark symptom of narcolepsy type 1 is cataplexy, which is an intrusion into the wake state of the motor atonia generally found in rapid eye movement (stage R) sleep. **Box 2** summarizes the symptoms that can be assessed when evaluating for narcolepsy type 1.[16]

The precise description of the actual cataplexy is essential. It is often helpful to have a second-hand account of the episodes from a companion

Table 3
Description of validated sleepiness scales

Questionnaire	Summary	Advantages	Disadvantages
Epworth	• 8 questions • Rated 0–3 based on chances of dozing in each situation • Sleepiness over recent period (wk/mo) • Score total out of 24	• Daytime situations are easy to comprehend • It has good correlation with MSLT • Scale of sleepiness is cumulative rather than momentary	• Patients sometimes do not encounter the situations listed. • There are multiple questions instead of one.
Stanford	Rating on a 1–7 Likert scale to assess current state of sleepiness	One response	• It represents only momentary level of sleepiness. • There is liberal use of terminology for sleepy or alert feelings.
Karolinska	Rating on a 1–9 Likert scale to assess current state of sleepiness	• One response • Easiest to comprehend	• It represents only momentary level of sleepiness. • Scores <7 may reflect fatigue rather than sleepiness.

Abbreviation: MSLT, multiple sleep latency test.

at the clinic visit, as cataplexy is often apparent to others. Cataplexy is generally triggered by specific positive emotions, including humor, surprise, anger, and giving a quick-witted response.[17] With the onset of the trigger, patients can experience rapid onset of striated muscle atonia from partial and progressive atonia of muscle groups to complete collapse.[14] With incomplete muscle atonia, the most common symptoms experienced are leg weakness including giving out at the knees, jaw dropping, hand weakness, and dysarthria.[17] The atonia can last for a few seconds to a couple of minutes before muscle tone returns.

Mimics of cataplexy include but are not limited to presyncope, atonic seizures, sleep attacks, primary muscle weakness, and imbalance. Exertional activities, stress, fear, and anxiety are more common causes of muscle weakness in patients without true narcolepsy type 1.[17] Because cataplexy is pathognomonic for narcolepsy type 1, a careful history is important to distinguish cataplexy from these other noncataplexy episodes, which can include psychogenic forms of cataplexy in patients with mood or somatoform disorders.[18]

Narcolepsy type 2 (formerly narcolepsy without cataplexy) is a central disorder of hypersomnolence characterized by persistent hypersomnolence and lack of cataplexy. The main distinguishing factor compared with idiopathic hypersomnia is the result of the multiple sleep latency test (MSLT), which is discussed later. Subtle differences exist between the

Box 2
Symptoms in narcolepsy type 1

- Ability to fall asleep quickly
- Cataplexy
- Hypnopompic and hypnagogic hallucinations
- Frequent sleep paralysis
- Dreaming during short naps
- Refreshing short naps
- Sleep attacks
- Arousals during nighttime sleep
- Weight gain at symptom onset
- Onset of symptoms after illness
- Vivid or lucid dreams
- Family history of autoimmune disease
- Vaccination with influenza A or H1N1 before symptoms

symptomatic presentation of narcolepsy type 2 compared with idiopathic hypersomnia, as shown in **Table 4**.[1,8]

Idiopathic hypersomnia is a central disorder of hypersomnolence without cataplexy and other features of stage R intrusions into other sleep and wake states.[1] This disorder may include features of increased 24-hour total sleep time, prolonged and unrefreshing sleep, and sleep inertia. A detailed list of symptoms is included in **Table 4**.

Recurrent hypersomnia is an intermittent disorder of hypersomnolence characterized by brief periods of several days to a few weeks with severe hypersomnolence and increased total sleep time.[1] **Box 3** lists the symptoms that characterize this disorder.[1,5,9]

Physical Examination

The physical examination can be useful, primarily in investigation of noncentral causes of hypersomnolence as detailed in **Table 5**.

The power of observation can reveal signs of somnolence as simple as a patient who dozes off in the waiting area or is snoozing as the clinician enters the room. Subtler signs that can be observed during the history include difficulty with focus, concentration, or attention when answering questions or recalling history. These signs are particularly helpful when they cannot be explained by the patients' medical comorbidities and current medications. For central disorders of hypersomnolence, the clinical history is far more important than the physical examination, which usually will be no different than in the general population. A skilled clinician (or

---

Box 3
Symptoms in recurrent hypersomnia during symptomatic period

- Hypersomnolence
- Very long 24-hour total sleep times
- Hypersexuality
- Feeling of derealization or déjà vu
- Hyperphagia and, less frequently, anorexia
- Personality change
- Poor social interaction
- Episodes last 2 days to a few weeks
- Recurrence is greater than once annually
- Return to normal outside of symptomatic period

Table 4
Symptoms of narcolepsy type 2 and idiopathic hypersomnia

Narcolepsy Type 2	Idiopathic Hypersomnia
• Hypersomnolence	• Hypersomnolence
• Absence of cataplexy	• Absence of cataplexy
• Usually normal total sleep time	• May have increased total sleep time
• Sleep paralysis, hypnagogic hallucinations may be present	• Rare sleep paralysis, hallucinations
	• Sleep inertia (sleep drunkenness)
	• Long, unrefreshing naps

Table 5
Physical examination findings for secondary causes of hypersomnolence

Cause	Physical Examination Findings
Sleep-disordered breathing	• Crowded oropharynx • Retrognathia • Maxillomandibular insufficiency • Obesity • Increased neck circumference
Anemia	• Skin pallor • Conjunctival pallor
Stroke	• Language dysfunction • Hemiparesis • Cranial nerve deficits • Other focal neurologic findings
Hepatic encephalopathy	• Hepatomegaly • Ascites • Scleral icterus • Cognitive impairment
Obesity hypoventilation	• Body mass index >35 kg/m² • Dyspnea at rest • Lack of concentration or attention
Hypothyroidism	• Thyromegaly • Thin or brittle hair • Brittle nails • Edema
Unipolar and bipolar depression	• Anhedonia • Flattened affect • Decreased mood

rather, a skilled comedian) can elicit cataplexy in untreated patients with narcolepsy type 1 by engaging in humor in the clinic and actually observing atonia with emotion from patients. In a rare situation in which severe cataplexy can be elicited, deep tendon reflex testing should demonstrate areflexia with use of a reflex hammer.[19]

Laboratory Testing

General medical testing
Laboratory testing to diagnose central disorders of hypersomnolence is of limited value. A complete blood count and thyroid-stimulating hormone can indicate anemia and hypothyroidism, respectively, which may contribute to patients' experience of sleepiness or fatigue. The urine drug screen is discussed in the section on the MSLT.

Cerebrospinal fluid testing
In narcolepsy type 1, hypocretin deficiency is the pathologic hallmark of this disease; testing for the absence cerebrospinal fluid hypocretin levels can confirm the diagnosis.[1] Although a definitive test in the diagnosis of narcolepsy type 1, the impracticality of the test relegates it to one of last resort. Cerebrospinal fluid analysis for hypocretin is generally reserved for more ambiguous cases in which there is atypical cataplexy, the HLA DQB1*06:02 is positive (see later discussion), and the polysomnogram and MSLT cannot be performed reliably, the results are equivocal, or the circumstances around testing are questionable (discussed in the diagnostic section later).[20,21] Moreover, the authors are not aware of any commercial laboratory that can perform a hypocretin assay currently, as there are only few private university-based laboratories that do perform hypocretin assays in the United States and Europe. This test cannot be performed on a routine basis because of the need to perform lumbar puncture and the lack of a commercial laboratory that can run the assay.

Human leukocyte antibody testing
In patients in which the pretest probability of narcolepsy type 1 is uncertain, serum HLA antibody testing of DQB1*06:02 can be very useful as it has extremely high sensitivity for narcolepsy type 1 and can help to exclude this diagnosis before commencement of polysomnography and MSLT.[20,22] Given the prevalence of approximately 20% in the

general population, a positive result is of little value.[21,22]

Diagnostic Evaluation

Sleep logs
Sleep logs are the patient-maintained documentation of estimated sleep timing and duration. In the most basic format, patients will demarcate a portion of a 24-hour day as sleep time and include sleep onset and offset. Depending on the detail desired, additions to the sleep log may include activities during the day, timing of the use of substances like caffeine, alcohol, nicotine, and so forth. A sample sleep log is shown in **Fig. 1**.

Sleep logs can reveal insufficient sleep duration, circadian rhythm sleep-wake disorder, and inconsistent sleep-wake schedule. Some studies have shown that sleep logs can be nearly as accurate as actigraphy (discussed later) and more accurate in cases of patients with insomnia.[23,24] The *International Classification of Sleep Disorders-3* guidelines recommend 1 week of sleep log documentation before diagnostic polysomnogram and MSLT in the evaluation of hypersomnolence to provide contextual information on the patients' sleep-wake timing and duration.[1]

Actigraphy
Actigraphy uses limb movement as a surrogate measure to estimate sleep-wake time. Actigraphs are wristwatchlike devices that contain accelerometers to measure and record movement. Periods of increased movements are deduced to be wakefulness, whereas times with reduced or absent movement are presumed to be sleep. Studies show agreement rates of total sleep time compared with polysomnography to be 87% to 95%.[25] Actigraphy can be combined with sleep logs for improved accuracy and may also be considered with certain patients (eg, young children, individuals with cognitive impairment) for whom sleep logs may be difficult to maintain.[26] Compared with sleep logs, actigraphy may be more accurate in many situations; but sleep logs are more commonly used because of practicality in clinical practice, largely due to the cost and lack of reimbursement of actigraphy.[23,27]

Polysomnography
A polysomnogram is a diagnostic test of sleep measuring multiple parameters, including electroencephalography (EEG), electrooculography (EOG), electromyography (EMG), electrocardiography,

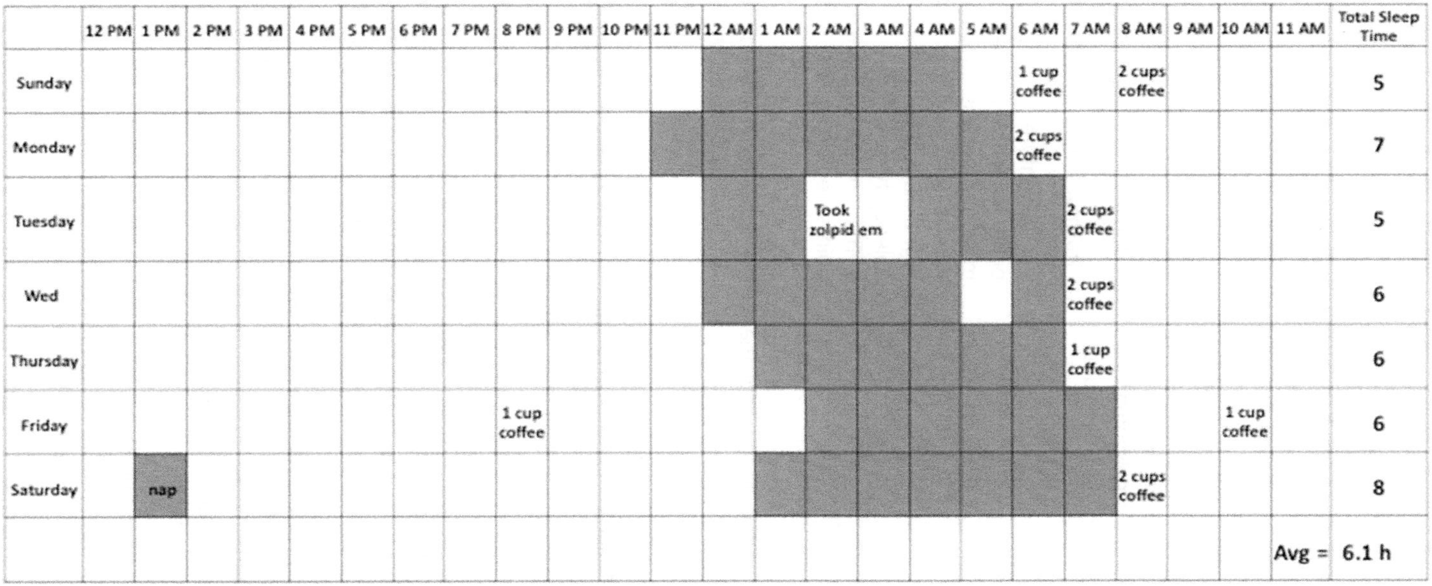

	12 PM	1 PM	2 PM	3 PM	4 PM	5 PM	6 PM	7 PM	8 PM	9 PM	10 PM	11 PM	12 AM	1 AM	2 AM	3 AM	4 AM	5 AM	6 AM	7 AM	8 AM	9 AM	10 AM	11 AM	Total Sleep Time
Sunday													■	■	■	■	■		1 cup coffee		2 cups coffee				5
Monday												■	■	■	■	■	■	■	2 cups coffee						7
Tuesday													■	■	Took zolpidem	■	■	■	■	2 cups coffee					5
Wed													■	■	■	■	■	□	■	2 cups coffee					6
Thursday									1 cup coffee				□	■	■	■	■	■	1 cup coffee						6
Friday														□	■	■	■	■	■	■			1 cup coffee		6
Saturday		nap											■	■	■	■	■	■	■	■	2 cups coffee				8
																									Avg = 6.1 h

Fig. 1. Sample sleep log. Avg, average.

respiratory function, pulse oximetry, and others. It can be used to stage sleep, arousals, respiratory events, limb movements, and so forth. The polysomnogram is the quintessential test of the sleep clinician and plays an essential role in the diagnosis of narcolepsy type 2 and idiopathic hypersomnia.[1] It is part of the diagnostic criteria for narcolepsy type 1; though in the setting of classically described cataplexy, it is more of a confirmation of what is clinically apparent. For central disorders of hypersomnolence, it is frequently used in conjunction with the MSLT. Before the performance of the polysomnogram, many steps must be taken to ensure the validity of the polysomnogram and the ensuing MSLT, which are summarized in **Box 4**.[1,28]

Multiple sleep latency test

The MSLT is crucial to the current diagnosis of narcolepsy type 1, narcolepsy type 2, and idiopathic hypersomnia. It is a tool for evaluation of both unusually short sleep onset during naps (hypersomnolence) and for sleep-onset rapid eye movement (REM) periods occurring within 15 minutes of onset of the sleep state. A summary of the protocol for the MSLT can found in **Box 5**.[28]

Evaluation of the results from the polysomnogram and multiple sleep latency test

The pertinent results from the polysomnogram and MSLT are listed in **Table 1**. Additionally, there are several clinical pearls regarding the results of these tests that are listed in **Box 6**.[1,29]

Miscellaneous tests

There are several other sleep-related tests that may play a small role in the evaluation of central disorders of hypersomnolence. These tests are listed in **Table 6**.[28,30,31]

TREATMENT OF CENTRAL DISORDERS OF HYPERSOMNOLENCE
Pharmacologic Treatment

The current treatment of central disorders of hypersomnolence focuses mainly on agents promoting alertness. Treatments for narcolepsy type 1 also address symptoms of cataplexy. **Fig. 2** illustrates the treatment approach to narcolepsy type 1.[32–52]

The following are additional important points regarding the treatment of narcolepsy type 1:

- Progression of medications should depend on severity of symptoms and side effect profile.

Box 4
Important concepts before polysomnographic testing

- Sleep logs or actigraphy must document consistent duration of sleep along with a consistent sleep-wake pattern for at least 1 week before polysomnography.
- Drugs that affect sleep architecture, including rapid eye movement ([REM] or stage R), and sleep-suppressing medications, including selective-serotonin reuptake, should be discontinued at least 2 weeks or 5 times the drug half-life before testing. A shorter duration or discontinuation before the study can lead to REM rebound and false-positive sleep-onset REM periods.
- If the sleep logs or actigraphy demonstrate a circadian rhythm variation, such as delayed sleep-wake phase, this may require alteration of the timing of the polysomnogram and MLST to accommodate the variation in circadian timing.
- Use of substances that influence sleepiness, such as sedatives, nicotine, caffeine, and illicit drugs, should be obtained. For an ideal study, these should be discontinued 2 weeks before the polysomnogram; but if impractical or unreasonable (eg, smoking cessation), documentation of usage informs the clinical interpretation of test results.
- Urine drug screen should be used to screen for certain illegal drugs and prescription medications on the morning of the MSLT; more detailed testing with gas chromatography can be considered on a case-by-case basis. The urine drug screen is frequently performed following the polysomnogram and before the MSLT to help identify other factors that may influence test results.
- Comorbid sleep-disordered breathing, if present, should be optimally treated before diagnostic testing to quantify daytime sleepiness.

Box 5
Summary of protocol of multiple sleep latency test

- The test consists of 5 naps, 2 hours apart, beginning 1.5 to 3.0 hours after sleep offset.

- Patients have 20 minutes to enter a sleep state and, if entered, have 15 additional minutes until the nap is ended to determine the presence of a SOREMP and to mitigate the effect of one nap on the results from each subsequent nap.

- The test generally uses EEG, EOG, and chin EMG markers to determine wake and sleep staging. In between, patients must remain awake, traditionally doing nonexertional activities, such as watching television or reading a book. This requirement is by convention as many arguments can be made for and against this regarding the effects of natural and artificial light and normal daytime activity versus sedentary activity and their effects on sleep and circadian rhythms.

- Primary in performance of the polysomnogram before the MSLT is the confirmation that another sleep disorder, in particular significant sleep-disordered breathing, is not present to affect patients' sleep quality, symptoms, and the outcome of a forthcoming MSLT.

- In patients with previously diagnosed sleep-disordered breathing, patients may undergo polysomnography with the patients' home therapy, such as nasal positive airway pressure; the sleep study should confirm good sleep quality for that sleep period.

- The patients' use of substances of dependence, such as caffeine, should be avoided; nicotine should not be used within 30 minutes of a nap session.

- However, withdrawal from such substances due to abrupt cessation may also influence the results.

- In a variation of normal testing, timing of MSLT may be adjusted to suit the natural sleep onset and offset of patients seen in the sleep log, so that patients obtain sufficient sleep duration on the polysomnogram and the MSLT is performed during the natural daytime of patients.

Abbreviation: SOREMP, sleep-onset REM period.

For example, many patients without disabling cataplexy may be well controlled on a mild stimulant, such as caffeine or modafinil, without the need for amphetamines or sodium oxybate.

- Atomoxetine may be helpful as it has a dual function as a mild stimulant with some anticataplectic properties.[37]

- Although the original purpose of sodium oxybate was to eliminate cataplexy, the sleep-consolidating effects may improve daytime alertness as well.[50–52]

Narcolepsy type 2 and idiopathic hypersomnia lack cataplexy; therefore, selective serotonin reuptake inhibitors or serotonin-norepinephrine

Box 6
Clinical pearls of polysomnogram and MSLT results

- Polysomnography can reveal whether the presence of sleep-disordered breathing is a factor in patients' clinical symptoms.

- Evaluation of sleep architecture can be helpful in revealing other sleep disorders or the presence of drugs. For example, in a narcolepsy type 1 evaluation, a significant latency to from sleep onset to first stage R epoch may be inconsistent with this diagnosis or suggest an REM-suppressant agent.

- Marked sleep fragmentation can suggest another underlying condition, anywhere from a neurodegenerative disorder (including in combination with REM without atonia) to insomnia disorder.

- If the mean sleep latency for idiopathic hypersomnia is greater than 8 minutes, then 660 minutes or more of total sleep time on the preceding polysomnogram or averaged in the sleep logs can be used as a surrogate.

- The test-retest unreliability of the MSLT has been well documented, and failure to determine pretest probability based on a good clinical history can lead to inaccurate results.

Table 6
Miscellaneous tests for hypersomnolence

Test	Description	Role in Hypersomnolence
Maintenance of wakefulness	• It is similar in diagnostic setup to MSLT but patients sit upright in bed. • Patients try to remain awake with eyes open for 4 sessions of 40 min. • Sleep latency, if any, is determined.	• It is not useful in diagnosis because it is a test of avoiding sleep, not the degree of somnolence. • It has a role in evaluating efficacy of therapeutics for hypersomnolence.
Psychomotor vigilance task	• It is a test of attention and alertness. • Patients must press a button when a light flashes. • The number of missed lights and false pushes are used to determine vigilance.	• Performance in central disorders of hypersomnolence is worse than in patients with hypersomnolence due to insufficient sleep. • Theoretically, it could be used to assess efficacy in therapeutics for hypersomnolence.
PET	• It is a scan that measures glucose metabolism in regions of the brain. • Patients with recurrent hypersomnia have hypermetabolism in certain regions during asymptomatic period and additional regions with hypermetabolism and hypometabolism during symptomatic period.	• It is impractical because of rarity of disorder, lack of access and reimbursement to PET scanners, and unlikelihood of obtaining scan during a symptomatic period. • The lack of patient numbers studied by this technique makes the test unlikely to aid in diagnosis currently.

reuptake inhibitors may not be specifically helpful. Symptomatically, these patients benefit most from stimulant medications, though there is some evidence for improved daytime alertness with sleep consolidation from sodium oxybate as well.[53,54] Treatment of hypersomnolence is an active area of research, and investigational therapeutics are included in **Table 7**.[14,55–58]

For recurrent hypersomnia, a Cochrane Review in 2013 found that there were no placebo-controlled, blinded studies for treatment.[59]

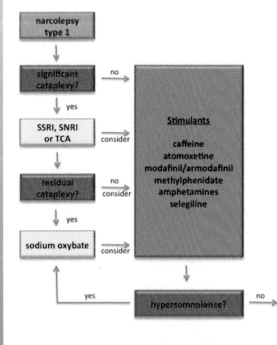

Fig. 2. Treatment flowchart for narcolepsy type 1. SNRI, serotonin-norepinephrine reuptake inhibitor; SSRI, selective-serotonin reuptake inhibitor; TCA, tricyclic antidepressant.

Table 7
Investigational therapeutics for hypersomnolence

Agent	Mechanism of Action
Clarithromycin	GABA-A receptor antagonist
Flumazenil	GABA-A receptor antagonist
Tiprolisant	Histamine receptor 3 inverse agonist/antagonist
Hypocretin analogues	Bind to hypocretin receptors

Abbreviation: GABA, γ-aminobutyric acid.

Case series have shown that strong stimulants improve hypersomnolence during these periods but antidepressants and mood stabilizers have no effect on psychiatric symptoms.[9] There may be some evidence for lithium; but randomized trials are needed, and the data are not convincing.[9]

Medication Side Effects

With central disorders of hypersomnolence requiring lifelong medical management, monitoring for drug side effects is as important as determining treatment efficacy. **Table 8** summarizes the medications used in these conditions and key adverse effects.[16,35,37,38,41–45,49,53,55]

Alternative Therapies

Not unique to central disorders of hypersomnolence are the effects of nonpharmacologic approaches to combat somnolence. Some of the alternatives to medications that improve hypersomnolence are listed in **Box 7**.[60–65]

Table 8
Medication adverse effects

Medication	Adverse Effects	Medication	Adverse Effects
Modafinil/ armodafinil	• Headache • Dizziness • Nervousness • Anxiety • Decreased efficacy of oral contraceptives	Sodium oxybate	• Nausea • Enuresis • Amnesia • Respiratory suppression • Hypertension (from large sodium load) • Increase in parasomnia • Increase effects of other sedatives
Amphetamines	• Headache • Anorexia • Insomnia • Anxiety • Tremor • Cardiac arrhythmia	Clarithromycin	• GI intolerance • Tolerance • Disruption of GI microbiome • Antimicrobial resistance • Arrhythmia
Selegiline	• Orthostatic hypotension • Decrease systolic blood pressure • GI intolerance • Weight loss	SSRIs/SNRIs	• Nausea • Xerostomia • Dizziness • Urinary hesitancy • Anorgasmia • Decreased libido
Caffeine	• Anxiety • Tremor • Dependence	Flumazenil	• Seizure • Respiratory depression
Atomoxetine	• GI intolerance • Anorexia • Menstrual irregularity • Decreased libido • Xerostomia	—	—

Abbreviations: GI, gastrointestinal; SNRI, serotonin-norepinephrine reuptake inhibitor; SSRI, selective serotonin reuptake inhibitor.

Box 7
Alternative therapies for hypersomnolence

- A regular sleep-wake wake schedule, specifically a fixed sleep offset, can firmly establish a 24-hour sleep-wake cycle and eliminate somnolence due to interference with the endogenous circadian rhythm.
- Brief, scheduled napping can restore alertness and has been shown to be efficacious in narcolepsy type 1 when combined with regulation of sleep habits.
- Natural sunlight or high-intensity, blue-wave spectrum light therapy both in the first hour after sleep offset and at midday can promote wakefulness.
- Weight loss can help to reverse some of the effects of hypersomnolence in obesity.
- Patients with narcolepsy type 1 often learn to modulate emotions, such as humor, in order to reduce cataplexy.
- Support groups and social media can help provide social support for patients and families. These communities can quickly disseminate new breakthroughs in diagnosis and treatment, particularly those individuals without regular access to a comprehensive sleep center.

SUMMARY AND FUTURE CONSIDERATIONS

Central disorders of hypersomnolence are life-long conditions with the primary symptom of excessive daytime sleepiness. Because of the rarity of these disorders and general lack of bio-markers or specific tests, misdiagnosis is common. The comprehensive sleep clinician must take a meticulous history; though the polysom-nogram and MSLT have a critical role in diag-nosis, they cannot stand independently from the complete clinical picture. The mainstay of treatment currently involves the use of stimulants and, in narcolepsy type 1, anticataplectic agents; but future drug discovery may focus on reduc-tion of somnolence rather than an increase in alertness. Certainly advancement in elucidating the pathogenesis of these disorders will help guide therapeutics that address the causes and not only the symptoms. Additionally, narcolepsy type 2 and idiopathic hypersomnia are diag-nosed based on findings on the MSLT. Defining what these entities actually are—whether a spectrum of disease, two unique disorders, or even a heterogeneous combination of pathol-ogies that lead to a symptomatic phenotype—will be crucial to the diagnosis and treatment in the future.

REFERENCES

1. American Academy of Sleep Medicine. International classification of sleep disorders. 3rd edition: diag-nostic and coding manual. Chicago: American Academy of Sleep Medicine; 2014.
2. Longstreth WT Jr, Koepsell TD, Ton TG, et al. The epidemiology of narcolepsy. Sleep 2007;30(1):13–26.
3. Silber MH, Krahn LE, Olson EJ, et al. The epidemiology of narcolepsy in Olmsted County, Minnesota: a population-based study. Sleep 2002;25(2):197–202.
4. Ohayon MM. From wakefulness to excessive sleep-iness: what we know and still need to know. Sleep Med Rev 2008;12(2):129–41.
5. Arnulf I, Lin L, Gadoth N, et al. Kleine–Levin syn-drome: a systematic study of 108 patients. Ann Neu-rol 2008;63(4):482–93.
6. Huang YS, Guilleminault C, Kao PF, et al. SPECT findings in the Kleine-Levin syndrome. Sleep 2005;28(8):955–60.
7. Oka Y, Inoue Y, Kanbayashi T, et al. Narcolepsy without cataplexy: 2 subtypes based on CSF hypocretin-1/orexin-A findings. Sleep 2006;29(11):1439–43.
8. Ali M, Auger RR, Slocumb NL, et al. Idiopathic hy-persomnia: clinical features and response to treat-ment. J Clin Sleep Med 2009;5(6):562–8.
9. Arnulf I, Zeitzer JM, File J, et al. Kleine-Levin syndrome: a systematic review of 186 cases in the literature. Brain 2005;128(Pt 12):2763–76.
10. Johns MW. A new method for measuring daytime sleepiness: the Epworth sleepiness scale. Sleep 1991;14(6):540–5.
11. Hoddes E, Zarcone V, Smythe H, et al. Quantification of sleepiness: a new approach. Psychophysiology 1973;10(4):431–6.
12. Akerstedt T, Gillberg M. Subjective and objective sleepiness in the active individual. Int J Neurosci 1990;52(1–2):29–37.
13. Fulke P, Vaughan S. Sleep deprivation. Hauppauge (NY): Nova Science Publishers, Inc; 2009.
14. Dauvilliers Y, Arnulf I, Mignot E. Narcolepsy with cataplexy. Lancet (London, England) 2007;369(9560):499–511.
15. Broughton R, Dunham W, Newman J, et al. Ambulatory 24 hour sleep-wake monitoring in

narcolepsy-cataplexy compared to matched controls. Electroencephalogr Clin Neurophysiol 1988; 70(6):473–81.

16. Aran A, Einen M, Lin L, et al. Clinical and therapeutic aspects of childhood narcolepsy-cataplexy: a retrospective study of 51 children. Sleep 2010;33(11): 1457–64.

17. Anic-Labat S, Guilleminault C, Kraemer HC, et al. Validation of a cataplexy questionnaire in 983 sleep-disorders patients. Sleep 1999;22(1):77–87.

18. Rohit Shankar VJ, Matthew Walker AZ. Pseudocataplexy and transient functional paralysis: a spectrum of psychogenic motor disorder. J Neuropsychiatry Clin Neurosci 2010;22(4):445–50.

19. Guilleminault C, Wilson RA, Dement WC. A study on cataplexy. Arch Neurol 1974;31(4):255–61.

20. Mignot E, Lammers G, Ripley B, et al. The role of cerebrospinal fluid hypocretin measurement in the diagnosis of narcolepsy and other hypersomnias. Arch Neurol 2002;59(10):1553–62.

21. Kawai M, O'Hara R, Einen M, et al. Narcolepsy in African Americans. Sleep 2015;38(11):1673–81.

22. Mignot E, Hayduk R, Black J, et al. HLA DQB1*0602 is associated with cataplexy in 509 narcoleptic patients. Sleep 1997;20(11):1012–20.

23. Lockley SW, Skene DJ, Arendt J. Comparison between subjective and actigraphic measurement of sleep and sleep rhythms. J Sleep Res 1999;8(3): 175–83.

24. Hauri PJ, Wisbey J. Wrist actigraphy in insomnia. Sleep 1992;15(4):293–301.

25. Sadeh A, Hauri PJ, Kripke DF, et al. The role of actigraphy in the evaluation of sleep disorders. Sleep 1995;18(4):288–302.

26. Kushida CA, Chang A, Gadkary C, et al. Comparison of actigraphic, polysomnographic, and subjective assessment of sleep parameters in sleep-disordered patients. Sleep Med 2001;2(5): 389–96.

27. Auger RR, Varghese R, Silber MH, et al. Total sleep time obtained from actigraphy versus sleep logs in an academic sleep center and impact on further sleep testing. Nat Sci Sleep 2013;5:125–31.

28. Littner MR, Kushida C, Wise M, et al. Practice parameters for clinical use of the multiple sleep latency test and the maintenance of wakefulness test. Sleep 2005;28(1):113–21.

29. Trotti LM, Staab BA, Rye DB. Test-retest reliability of the multiple sleep latency test in narcolepsy without cataplexy and idiopathic hypersomnia. J Clin Sleep Med 2013;9(8):789–95.

30. Thomann J, Baumann CR, Landolt H-P, et al. Psychomotor vigilance task demonstrates impaired vigilance in disorders with excessive daytime sleepiness. J Clin Sleep Med 2014;10(9):1019–24.

31. Dauvilliers Y, Bayard S, Lopez R, et al. Widespread hypermetabolism in symptomatic and asymptomatic episodes in Kleine-Levin syndrome. PLoS One 2014; 9(4):e93813.

32. Billiard M. Narcolepsy: current treatment options and future approaches. Neuropsychiatr Dis Treat 2008;4(3):557–66.

33. Akimoto H, Honda Y, Takahashi Y. Pharmacotherapy in narcolepsy. Dis Nerv Syst 1960;21:704–6.

34. Nishino S, Mignot E. Pharmacological aspects of human and canine narcolepsy. Prog Neurobiol 1997; 52(1):27–78.

35. Schachter M, Parkes JD. Fluvoxamine and clomipramine in the treatment of cataplexy. J Neurol Neurosurg Psychiatry 1980;43(2):171–4.

36. Guilleminault C, Mancuso J, Salva MA, et al. Viloxazine hydrochloride in narcolepsy: a preliminary report. Sleep 1986;9(1 Pt 2):275–9.

37. Niederhofer H. Atomoxetine also effective in patients suffering from narcolepsy? Sleep 2005;28(9):1189.

38. Smith M, Parkes JD, Dhalitz M. Venlafaxine in the treatment of the narcoleptic syndrome. J Sleep Res 1996;5(Suppl 1):217.

39. Billiard M, Besset A, Montplaisir J, et al. Modafinil: a double-blind multicentric study. Sleep 1994;17(8 Suppl):S107–12.

40. Randomized trial of modafinil for the treatment of pathological somnolence in narcolepsy. US Modafinil in Narcolepsy Multicenter Study Group. Ann Neurol 1998;43(1):88–97.

41. Randomized trial of modafinil as a treatment for the excessive daytime somnolence of narcolepsy: US Modafinil in Narcolepsy Multicenter Study Group. Neurology 2000;54(5):1166–75.

42. Mitler MM, Aldrich MS, Koob GF, et al. Narcolepsy and its treatment with stimulants. ASDA standards of practice. Sleep 1994;17(4):352–71.

43. Harsh JR, Hayduk R, Rosenberg R, et al. The efficacy and safety of armodafinil as treatment for adults with excessive sleepiness associated with narcolepsy. Curr Med Res Opin 2006;22(4): 761–74.

44. Guilleminault C. Amphetamines and narcolepsy: use of the Stanford database. Sleep 1993;16(3): 199–201.

45. Mayer G, Ewert Meier K, Hephata K. Selegiline hydrochloride treatment in narcolepsy. A double-blind, placebo-controlled study. Clin Neuropharmacol 1995;18(4):306–19.

46. A randomized, double blind, placebo-controlled multicenter trial comparing the effects of three doses of orally administered sodium oxybate with placebo for the treatment of narcolepsy. Sleep 2002;25(1):42–9.

47. A 12-month, open-label, multicenter extension trial of orally administered sodium oxybate for the treatment of narcolepsy. Sleep 2003;26(1):31–5.

48. U.S. Xyrem Multicenter Study Group. Sodium oxybate demonstrates long-term efficacy for the

treatment of cataplexy in patients with narcolepsy. Sleep Med 2004;5(2):119–23.

49. Xyrem International Study Group. Further evidence supporting the use of sodium oxybate for the treatment of cataplexy: a double-blind, placebo-controlled study in 228 patients. Sleep Med 2005; 6(5):415–21.

50. Black J, Houghton WC. Sodium oxybate improves excessive daytime sleepiness in narcolepsy. Sleep 2006;29(7):939–46.

51. Pardi D, Black J. Gamma-hydroxybutyrate/sodium oxybate: neurobiology, and impact on sleep and wakefulness. CNS Drugs 2006;20(12):993–1018.

52. Black J, Pardi D, Hornfeldt CS, et al. The nightly use of sodium oxybate is associated with a reduction in nocturnal sleep disruption: a double-blind, placebo-controlled study in patients with narcolepsy. J Clin Sleep Med 2010;6(6):596–602.

53. Morgenthaler TI, Kapur VK, Brown T, et al. Practice parameters for the treatment of narcolepsy and other hypersomnias of central origin. Sleep 2007; 30(12):1705–11.

54. Mignot EJM. A practical guide to the therapy of narcolepsy and hypersomnia syndromes. Neurotherapeutics 2012;9(4):739–52.

55. Trotti LM, Saini P, Freeman AA, et al. Improvement in daytime sleepiness with clarithromycin in patients with GABA-related hypersomnia: clinical experience. J Psychopharmacol (Oxford, England) 2013; 28(7):697–702.

56. Rye DB, Bliwise DL, Parker K, et al. Modulation of vigilance in the primary hypersomnias by endogenous enhancement of GABAA receptors. Sci Transl Med 2012;4(161):161ra151.

57. Dauvilliers Y, Bassetti C, Lammers GJ, et al. Pitolisant versus placebo or modafinil in patients with narcolepsy: a double-blind, randomised trial. Lancet Neurol 2013;12(11):1068–75.

58. Leu-Semenescu S, Nittur N, Golmard JL, et al. Effects of pitolisant, a histamine H3 inverse agonist, in drug-resistant idiopathic and symptomatic hypersomnia: a chart review. Sleep Med 2014; 15(6):681–7.

59. Oliveira MM, Conti C, Prado GF. Pharmacological treatment for Kleine-Levin syndrome. Cochrane Database Syst Rev 2013;8:CD006685.

60. Rogers AE, Aldrich MS, Lin X. A comparison of three different sleep schedules for reducing daytime sleepiness in narcolepsy. Sleep 2001;24(4):385–91.

61. Broughton RJ, Billiard M. The behavioral management of narcolepsy. In: Bassetti CL, Billiard M, Mignot E, editors. Narcolepsy and hypersomnia. New York: Informa Healthcare; 2007. p. 497–512.

62. Beaven CM, Ekstrom J. A comparison of blue light and caffeine effects on cognitive function and alertness in humans. PLoS One 2013;8(10):e76707.

63. Fernandez-Mendoza J, Vgontzas AN, Kritikou I, et al. Natural history of excessive daytime sleepiness: role of obesity, weight loss, depression, and sleep propensity. Sleep 2015;38(3):351–60.

64. de Zambotti M, Pizza F, Covassin N, et al. Facing emotions in narcolepsy with cataplexy: haemodynamic and behavioural responses during emotional stimulation. J Sleep Res 2014;23(4):432–40.

65. Goswami M. Quality of life and psychosocial issues in narcolepsy: implications for management. In: Goswami M, Thorpy MJ, Pandi-Perumal SR, editors. Narcolepsy: a clinical guide. 2nd edition. Cham (Switzerland): Springer International Publishing; 2016. p. 195–215.

Diagnosis and Treatment of Insomnia Comorbid with Obstructive Sleep Apnea

Leon Lack, PhD*, Alexander Sweetman, BPsych(Hons)

KEYWORDS

- OSA • Comorbid insomnia • PAP therapy • PAP adherence • CBTi • Nondrug insomnia treatment

KEY POINTS

- The prevalence of insomnia comorbid with obstructive sleep apnea (OSA) is high.
- Comorbid insomnia-OSA is a severe sleep disorder and reduces positive airway pressure treatment acceptance and adherence.
- Drug treatment of comorbid insomnia is not recommended.
- Cognitive behavior therapy for insomnia is effective and durable and promises to improve comorbid patient outcomes in sleep medicine clinics.
- Clinics should include diagnosis and treatment of comorbid insomnia in their normal operation.

INTRODUCTION

Insomnia and obstructive sleep apnea (OSA) are the 2 most common sleep disorders. Clinically significant insomnia is indicated by difficulties getting to sleep, staying asleep, or waking prematurely and not being able to get back to sleep, as well as daytime symptoms of fatigue, irritability, and reported cognitive impairments. It is not usually indicated by self-reported sleepiness.[1] It is typically more common in women.

OSA is usually associated with clinical symptoms of heavy snoring and choking while asleep, excessive daytime sleepiness, and being overweight and male.[2] Its diagnosis is confirmed with a nighttime sleep study or polysomnography (PSG) measuring respiration and blood gases showing sleep-disordered breathing.

Perhaps because of the differences in the conceptualizations of these 2 common sleep disorders and presumed demographic differences, there seems to have been little recognition in the past of their overlap or comorbidity. Despite the early detection, in 1973, of comorbid insomnia with sleep apnea by Guilleminault and colleagues,[3] there was little follow-up investigation of its prevalence or clinical implications until about the turn of the century when, in 2001, Krakow and colleagues[4] found about 50% of clinically diagnosed OSA patients also had significant insomnia symptoms. Subsequent studies have confirmed this high rate of comorbidity with a range of about 30% to 70% of sleep apnea patients in sleep disorder clinics also showing insomnia.[5]

This revelation has very important implications for the almost all sleep medicine clinics around the world that are largely devoted to the diagnosis and treatment of sleep apnea. Many of them do not have diagnostic resources available for the detection of insomnia (eg, Insomnia Severity Index [ISI] questionnaire, sleep diary, measures of daytime fatigue without sleepiness). Furthermore, very few sleep clinics seem to have clinicians available (eg, sleep psychologists) to treat insomnia with best-practice cognitive behavior therapy for insomnia (CBTi).

School of Psychology, Flinders University of South Australia, Adelaide, South Australia, Australia
* Corresponding author. School of Psychology, Flinders University of South Australia, GPO Box 2100, Adelaide 5001, South Australia, Australia.
E-mail address: Leon.lack@flinders.edu.au

Sleep Med Clin 11 (2016) 379–388
http://dx.doi.org/10.1016/j.jsmc.2016.05.006

There is now considerable evidence that OSA patients with comorbid insomnia are less likely to adhere to the most common OSA treatment, positive airway pressure (PAP).[6–10] Therefore, not only is the insomnia likely to remain covert in this sleep clinic population but, if it is discovered, options for effective insomnia-treatments may be limited and the OSA is less likely to be adequately treated. Thus, this often unrecognized and undertreated comorbid insomnia represents a significant deficiency in the potential effectiveness of sleep medicine clinics around the world.

CONSEQUENCES OF COMORBID INSOMNIA/OSA

In general, it seems that the morbidity of the comorbid patients is greater than those experiencing a single disorder.[11,12] Not surprisingly, comorbid patients also experience greater daytime and quality of life impairments, and psychiatric symptoms, than those with either disorder alone.[4,5,13–16] It seems that the comorbid patients generally experience the additive detrimental effects from both disorders manifested in their sleep symptoms, as well as daytime impairments. Therefore, these prevalent groups of comorbid insomnia-OSA patients generally are more severely sleep disordered and suffer greater daytime consequences. They require and deserve accurate diagnosis and adequate treatment.

MUTUAL INTERACTIONS BETWEEN OBSTRUCTIVE SLEEP APNEA AND INSOMNIA

The high prevalence of comorbid insomnia in patients presenting with OSA at sleep medicine clinics suggests the 2 are certainly not mutually exclusive, nor even independent of each other. The population prevalence of clinical insomnia of 5% to 10%, and the prevalence of insomnia sleep symptoms of 15% to 25%, is considerably below the 30% to 70% prevalence in the OSA population previously mentioned.[5] This suggests that the presence of insomnia can exacerbate or contribute to the development of OSA, that OSA can contribute to the development of insomnia, or that insomnia and OSA are engaged in a reciprocal relationship whereby each disorder exacerbates the other. For example, the chronic hyperarousal, which is suggested to underlie chronic insomnia,[17] may prolong the transition between wake and sustained sleep, and generally lighten the stages of sleep, thereby increasing the amount of the sleep period vulnerable to apneic events and increasing the apnea-hypopnea index (AHI).[18]

Alternatively, OSA may also lead to insomnia symptoms in some patients. Repetitive respiratory events and postapneic awakenings occurring during sleep-wake transitions may be perceived as periods of continued wakefulness. It is common for insomnia patients to misperceive prior sleep as wakefulness and overestimate their time spent awake during the sleep period.[19] With repeated nights of perceived sleep onset difficulties, worry and frustration are likely, and may trigger sympathetic nervous system (SNS) and hypothalamic-pituitary-adrenal (HPA) axis activation. Following repetitive association of the bedroom environment, the time of night, and the desire to fall asleep with sympathetic activation, this physiologic activation response can become conditioned to those always present cues and underlie the development of psychophysiological or conditioned insomnia. This same process may also underlie the development of conditioned sleep maintenance insomnia or early morning awakening insomnia in which it takes a long time to get back to sleep following a nighttime awakening or a complete failure to reinitiate sleep, respectively.

This purported causal mechanism linking OSA and insomnia would suggest that, although OSA may have been the primary cause of the perceived difficulty getting to sleep, the insomnia response at the beginning of the sleep period would, with enough associations, become independent and self-sustaining. In that case, the attempt to treat the OSA with PAP would most likely eliminate the apneic events at sleep onset but not eliminate the well-established insomnia arousal response. Thus, the long sleep onset latencies are likely to continue, the perceived efficacy of PAP likely to be questioned, and adherence to PAP be diminished.[10]

Alternatively, putting aside the possibility of conditioned insomnia, the sleep onset difficulty may be considered entirely secondary to the OSA and disappear with the effective use of PAP treatment. This latter view may have been predominant in sleep medicine clinics in the past and contributed to the curious but inappropriate lack of attention to the possible role of insomnia in the OSA population. If there were some complaints of insomnia, they were considered secondary to the OSA and would ameliorate with PAP therapy.

However, PAP therapy is often suboptimal due to poor adherence and insomnia is a significant impediment to adherence.[6,7,9] Therefore, a better appreciation of the possible development of conditioned insomnia in the OSA population and a better understanding of its underlying mechanism by sleep physicians may well improve the effectiveness of sleep disorder treatments and help to sustain the important role sleep medicine clinics play in improving the health and well-being of the populations they serve.

SHOULD INSOMNIA COMORBID WITH OBSTRUCTIVE SLEEP APNEA BE TREATED?

If the insomnia symptoms in the OSA clinical population are entirely secondary to the OSA, there would be no purpose in expending any resources to treat the insomnia directly. Treatment as usual would be at least equally effective with the comorbid patients as with the patients without insomnia symptoms. Indeed, if the insomnia symptoms, as well as those accruing from OSA alone, were alleviated with PAP therapy, the comorbid patients would experience greater improvements in health and well-being than those with OSA alone, controlling, of course, between groups for OSA severity.

On the other hand, if insomnia exists independently of the OSA (eg, precursor to OSA or conditioned insomnia developed from initial OSA), the separate treatment of the insomnia would be an independent benefit because it would increase PAP compliance, make treatment of the OSA more effective, and generally result in better health outcomes. These possibilities are, of course, not mutually exclusive and may be present to varying degrees. In other words, comorbid patients are likely to vary in the extent to which they have developed an entrenched conditioned insomnia. Given the findings of reduced PAP compliance in the comorbid population, it is most likely that conditioned insomnia exists in at least a cohort of these patients. Indeed, it seems most likely that different comorbid phenotypes exist defined by the extent of independent conditioned insomnia. Presently, ongoing research projects testing the efficacy of insomnia treatment in this comorbid population should be able to identify different phenotypes based on their response to insomnia treatment and PAP adherence.[20,21]

If it is assumed that some independent conditioned insomnia does exist in the comorbid population, then insomnia treatment would be indicated. It would address the insomnia symptoms, as well as possibly improve OSA treatment by removing an impediment to PAP adherence. However, an initial question to be addressed is whether the insomnia comorbid with OSA can be effectively treated. If it is entirely secondary to the OSA, the best-practice CBTi is unlikely to be effective.

The existence of some conditioned insomnia, however, should be ameliorated with CBTi. Even so, CBTi usually involves some degree of sleep restriction in the first few weeks of its application, resulting in at least a period (1–3 weeks) of increased sleepiness and entailing a potential risk.[22] For the comorbid population more likely to be experiencing initially higher levels of daytime sleepiness (Epworth Sleepiness Score [ESS] of 8–10) than those suffering insomnia alone (ESS of 4–6), the risk may be unacceptable. With regard the question about whether CBTi can effectively treat insomnia in this population, a 2011 clinical CBTi study by Lack and colleagues[23] examined the relative effectiveness of CBTi in those referred for the treatment of their insomnia. The improvements in sleep and measures of daytime functioning were comparable between the group with insomnia alone and in those referred for insomnia treatment but having mild to severe covert comorbid OSA. Although the moderate to severe OSA patients had an initially higher ESS of 7 compared with 5.5 in the insomnia alone group, their ESS actually decreased through the treatment program. An additional recent study by Fung and colleagues[24] also examined the effectiveness of CBTi in a population of older-aged veterans. Of the 134 participants, 95 were found to have mild to moderate sleep apnea (AHI$\geq$5–<15), and showed similar improvements in measures of sleep and sleep quality, compared with subjects without sleep apnea. Whether the comorbid insomnia in patients referred to sleep medicine clinics with suspected OSA (rather than insomnia) would improve as effectively remains to be determined.

DIAGNOSIS OF INSOMNIA COMORBID WITH OBSTRUCTIVE SLEEP APNEA

An appropriate diagnosis enables the most appropriate choice of therapy. In the case of diagnosing insomnia comorbid with OSA, the aim is to identify those apparently comorbid patients who would benefit most from the treatment of their insomnia symptoms.

The identification of the presence of both OSA and insomnia rests primarily on the measures of nighttime sleep. As briefly previously discussed, diagnosis of OSA usually follows the path of indicative clinical symptoms leading to a confirmatory PSG recording and meeting the sleep disordered breathing criteria specified by the of the *International Classification of Sleep Disorders*, 3rd edition (ICSD-3).[1] The sleep symptoms that indicate insomnia are initial difficulty getting to sleep, difficulty maintaining sleep evidenced by many or long awakenings, and waking earlier than desired and being unable to return to sleep in the morning.

Satisfying these criteria for insomnia comorbid with OSA to a minimum level of confidence can make use of a retrospective questionnaire about these symptoms. For example, the ISI has been compared with clinical diagnoses and been shown to be a reliable and valid measure of perceived insomnia severity.[25] The first 3 questions on the ISI have the patient rank the severity of these 3 sleep symptoms on a 5-point scale from none to very severe, scored 0 to 4. The remaining 4 questions deal with the patient's estimate of impact on their lives and degree of worry about their sleep problem. Because it is likely that these latter questions about daytime impact are common to both OSA and insomnia, a focus on the first 3 questions may help to differentiate the presence of insomnia separate from OSA.[26] A minimum score from the first 3 questions of 4 or 5 or a minimum score of 3 (severe) on at least 1 of the items will ensure that the patient reports adequate severity of 1 of these insomnia sleep symptoms.

Preferably, or in addition to the ISI, the completion of at least 1 week of a sleep-wake diary is highly recommended. The patient is to complete the diary on arising each morning to capture the experience of the just completed sleep period. This has the advantage of more accurate and less biased recall than retrospective questionnaires. It can also capture the variability of sleep from night to night, give feedback to patients that a good recovery sleep usually occurs following 1 or 2 bad sleeps,[27] and serve as a sleep monitor to guide treatment and give feedback of progress. As well as documentation of bedtimes, arising times, and total time in bed (TIB), the diaries provide estimates of sleep onset latency (SOL), number of awakenings, amount of wake time after initial sleep onset, and total sleep time (TST). An important monitor of sleep quality, sleep efficiency (SE), can then be calculated as the percentage of TIB estimated to be asleep and is calculated as SE = (TST/TIB) × 100. Commonly used criteria for insomnia derived from the sleep diary are average SOL greater than 30 minutes, average wake time after initial sleep onset greater than 45 minutes, or SE less than 75%. Alternatively, and more in line with the variability of sleep and the ICSD-3 criteria,[1] this criteria would have to occur at least 3 times per week and be present for at least 3 months to qualify as chronic insomnia.

The diagnosis of insomnia requires the report of significant daytime impairment despite adequate opportunity to sleep.[1] However, daytime impairments are also a diagnostic criteria for OSA. The listing of possible daytime impairments for both disorders includes many in common. Thus, the reliance on daytime symptoms to identify the presence of a separate insomnia disorder can be problematic.

Nevertheless, some daytime symptoms are more common to insomnia, whereas others are more prominent in OSA, and these distinctions may be used to confirm the presence of an independent component of insomnia in comorbid cases. The main daytime symptom reported in chronic insomnia is fatigue that reduces with effective treatment of the insomnia.[28] Conversely, the symptom of excessive daytime sleepiness (eg, ESS>10) is uncommon.[28,29] OSA alone without comorbid insomnia typically presents with excessive daytime sleepiness that reduces with effective treatment of the OSA.[30] However, fatigue and lack of energy are also commonly reported with OSA and decrease with effective treatment.[30] In comorbid cases, the daytime symptoms of both conditions are expected, including raised levels of sleepiness and fatigue.

However, not all comorbid cases will show elevations of all daytime symptoms. In particular, a patient presenting with high fatigue but low subjective sleepiness (eg, ESS<6) could be more confidently identified as having comorbid insomnia likely to be independent of OSA. The dominant model of severe chronic insomnia is that of chronic hyperarousal[17] and accounts for the reduced TST and SE but also increased hypervigilance (reduced sleepiness). This implies chronic activation of the SNS and HPA axis and results in feelings of physical or mental exhaustion and fatigue.

Although reduced sleepiness is generally true in chronic insomnia (mean ESS ≤5), some patients report elevated daytime sleepiness, particularly in the hour or 2 before bed. However, this sleepiness often evaporates in bed and is replaced by racing thoughts, worry, or frustration and is associated with extended SOL. This would be a case in which the arousal is not chronic but more confined to the bed environment and attempt to sleep. It arises from an arousal or activation response conditioned to the cues of the bed, time of night, and attempt to sleep, as detailed previously, with the suggestion that the presence of multiple respiratory events at the transition to sleep and postapneic awakenings are perceived as an extended time taken to fall asleep. This perceived sleep onset delay and inferred reduced TST is seen as a mild threat to well-being the following day. The result is a triggering of the fight-or-flight response or SNS activation and further delay of sleep onset. Multiple associations of these bedtime cues with this response results in a conditioned or learned response, and the response being automatically triggered by the cues.

The presence of this conditioned insomnia response is suggested when sleepiness disappears in bed but was prominent earlier when not attempting to sleep (eg, while watching television). It is also suggested when the patient reports sleeping better in a different room of the house, other location (eg, motels, camping), or in other circumstances (eg, being recorded with PSG). Many insomnia patients report sleeping as well or better than normal in the presence of all the attachments required for full PSG recording, an experience that good sleepers almost never report. In some patients, a strong cue for the insomnia response is the desire or mental attempt to sleep. The technique of paradoxic intentions[31] is based on changing this attempt to sleep to the attempt to stay awake across the night. When a patient reports improved sleep when attempting to stay awake, it suggests the presence of insomnia response conditioned to the attempt or desire to sleep.

In summary, the documented difficulties initiating or maintaining sleep are the main criteria for diagnosing insomnia as a comorbidity to OSA. The presence of these difficulties, despite less sleep than normal and the disruption to sleep caused by a comorbid OSA, strongly suggests the presence of a conditioned insomnia response that is unlikely to ameliorate with PAP therapy alone. The diagnosis of insomnia is strengthened by daytime symptoms of reported fatigue but without sleepiness, the typical result of chronic hyperarousal of chronic insomnia. Others, who do report elevated daytime sleepiness but whose beforebed sleepiness then is replaced by an alert, agitated mind after retiring to bed, are likely to have a more specific arousal response to the bed environment and attempt to sleep. These cases are also appropriate targets for treatment of the insomnia.

TREATMENT OF INSOMNIA COMORBID WITH OBSTRUCTIVE SLEEP APNEA

Diagnosis of insomnia in general practice almost always results in a prescription for hypnotic drugs after a standard-length consultation.[32] Whether those comorbid patients referred to sleep medicine clinics, discovered to have insomnia, are as likely to receive pharmacotherapy for their insomnia is yet to be investigated. Future research should investigate the fate of those OSA patients with discovered comorbid insomnia. Do they get a prescription for hypnotics from a sleep physician, are they given sleep hygiene instructions, and/or do they get referred back to their general practitioner for hypnotics? It is very unlikely they will receive best-practice CBTi from a sleep psychologist because of the relative dearth of these specialists in sleep medicine clinics. Earlier studies recommended against the use of benzodiazepines with OSA patients due to their muscle relaxant and AHI exacerbating tendency.[33] Newer benzodiazepine receptor agonists show little or no effect on AHI but whether their use enhances PAP compliance and final therapeutic outcome is still uncertain.[34]

However, pharmacotherapy for insomnia has many disadvantages. Although it can provide some symptomatic relief of the insomnia symptoms while being used, it does not address the causes of the insomnia (eg, conditioned insomnia) so that discontinuation usually results in a loss of benefit at best,[35] and some rebound or intensified insomnia at worst.[36] Although rebound insomnia is more likely with discontinuation of short-acting benzodiazepines,[37] longer acting hypnotics can result in carryover daytime sedation effects, slowed reactions, and memory impairment.[38] Nighttime fugue or amnesic experiences have also been documented with the benzodiazepine receptor agonists.[39] There is also some evidence of increased mortality risk and cancer incidence with the use of hypnotic drugs.[40]

Probably the greatest disadvantage of hypnotic medications is that of dependency and the difficulty of discontinuation. Because most hypnotics are sedating and anxiolytic to some extent, withdrawal usually results in the opposite effect (ie, very poor sleep combined with mild anxiety and agitation). The aversiveness of withdrawal can motivate abstainers to resume medicating.[41] This may not be seen as a great disadvantage by sleep physicians hoping to improve PAP compliance for the potentially long-term use of PAP therapy. However, the range of adverse side-effects, the unknown long-term health consequences, and simply the long-term cost of prolonged sedative use should encourage sleep physicians to seek alternative treatments for the comorbid insomnia.

The good news is that very effective nondrug therapies exist. The plural, therapies, is used purposely because insomnia is usually multifactorial in its causes and thus best-practice therapy usually includes many components. Some different phenotypes of insomnia have already been identified (eg, delayed or advanced sleep patterns) and appropriate nondrug therapies have been shown to be effective in treating these types.[42] The more generic term now used to indicate this combination of different therapeutic elements is cognitive/behavior therapy for insomnia (CBTi). The most consistently effective element is a behavioral component that addresses the learned or conditioned insomnia response in chronic insomnia. The cognitive elements recognize that humans are complex thinking or cognitive beings whose attitudes and beliefs can determine response to events or situations. Therefore, addressing potentially maladaptive cognitive elements can help ameliorate detrimental physiologic and behavioral responses. CBTi has been shown to be more effective in the long term than pharmacotherapy, without the adverse side effects.[43] It has the advantage that its benefits last well beyond the treatment period and that patients can take over the control of therapy if relapse occurs at some future time.

BEHAVIORAL THERAPIES

A broadly accepted learning model offers a theoretic explanation for the development of chronic hyperarousal, sleep disturbance, and daytime impairments of chronic insomnia.[44] If insomnia is maintained by maladaptive learning, falling asleep quickly could be relearned using these same principles by changing behavior and establishing new associations. The 2 most applied behavior change therapies are stimulus control therapy (SCT)[44] and bed period or sleep restriction therapy (SRT).[45]

SCT is the most widely studied and endorsed single-component treatment method.[44] Its instructions are

1. Do not have a predetermined bedtime, go to bed only when sleepy
2. Get out of bed if not asleep within 15 minutes
3. Repeat 1 and 2 until a rapid sleep occurs
4. Maintain the same wake-up time regardless of sleep length
5. Do not nap during the day.

These instructions aim to reassociate the bed environment with sleep and reverse the conditioned insomnia. Adjunct suggestions include eliminating from the bedroom environment other behaviors incompatible with sleep (eg, using electronic screen devices, eating, arguments with bed partner, worrying about losing sleep). Although SCT is considered effective for both sleep onset and sleep maintenance insomnia, it is mostly used when initial sleep onset problems are predominant.

If sleep maintenance problems are predominant (excessive periods awake and excessive TIB), SRT is most commonly indicated. As its name implies, it consists of restricting TIB (eg, later bedtime and/or earlier out of bed in the morning) to equate with the average amount of reported TST over a week of sleep diary. SE (percent of TIB asleep) is monitored weekly before and during treatment. Over 1 to 2 weeks of SRT, sleep typically becomes more consolidated and SE increases. When it rises to greater than 85% and when sleepiness, usually apparent in the hour or 2 before the later bedtime, becomes difficult to resist, TIB can then be extended in small increments (eg, 30 minutes per week) as long as SE is maintained at greater than 85%.

After the initial period of sleep restriction, the subsequent extension of TIB is typically associated with reported improvements in daytime functioning and feelings of greater energy. SRT has moderate guideline support for its efficacy and recent strong clinical research support.[46,47] The assumed mechanism of action is the eventual conditioning of a rapid sleep onset and/or return to sleep, reducing the learned hyperarousal of chronic insomnia.

EFFECTIVENESS OF BEHAVIORAL THERAPIES

Although the 2 behavioral therapies have different instructions, they share common features that directly address the major cause perpetuating the chronic insomnia. Both therapies reduce TIB and prohibit napping. They effectively reduce TST over the first few weeks of therapy and increase homeostatic sleep drive, or sleep pressure, and reduce both chronic hyperarousal and time awake in bed. They effectively reassociate the bedroom environment and intention of falling asleep with rapid sleep onsets, thus reversing the previously learned insomnia response.

Although the behavioral therapies have strong empirical support for their effectiveness from randomized control trials, their effectiveness in clinical practice is less well documented. The therapies present some challenges of implementation.[46] Their administration is typically associated with a lag in treatment response (3–4 weeks), some early treatment daytime sleepiness,[22] and difficulties with treatment compliance. Compliance is necessary for successful treatment but is often suboptimal, very likely arising from the difficulty in changing lifestyle habits at home and the discomfort associated with sleep loss in the early weeks of the treatment. Furthermore, therapy instructions are counterintuitive to the typical patient's tendency to extend TIB in the attempt (usually futile) to gain extra sleep. Therefore, it can be useful to help the patient find alternative activities outside of bed and reassure them of the relatively benign effects of temporarily reduced sleep time.

The temporary increase of daytime sleepiness typical of the behavior therapies may be particularly problematic for the comorbid patients reporting elevated daytime sleepiness (eg, ESS>10) before treatment. Even a temporary increase of daytime sleepiness in these patients may pose an unacceptable increased health risk (eg, from a vehicle accident). The general administration guideline for SRT therapy is to restrict TIB to the reported average nightly TST as reported in their sleep diary before treatment with 5 hours TIB considered an absolute minimum regardless of reported sleep. It has been known since 1976 that chronic insomnia patients, in retrospective questionnaires and diaries, tend to underestimate their objective sleep.[48] It seems that underestimation of TST also occurs in comorbid patients but less so than in those with insomnia alone.[11] Nevertheless, it would be prudent in the administration of SRT to err on the generous side in establishing the initial TIB instructions.

For these patients referred to sleep medicine clinics and found to have comorbid insomnia and OSA, they will have had objective TST measured in their diagnostic PSG. If a sleep diary is also completed by the patient, it can indicate the degree of underestimation of objective sleep for that night. By extrapolation it would be possible to estimate the objective total sleep during the week of sleep diary evidence and provide a more confident starting point for instructed TIB in the first week of SRT.

Alternatively, the initial TIB can start with the present TIB of the patient and then be reduced by 30 minutes each week until SE reaches the target 85% level, after which it can then be relaxed again until daytime symptoms subside. In either case, the daytime sleepiness levels should be monitored with weekly ESS measures and patients should be warned of possible increases in daytime sleepiness. For those patients already indicating excessive daytime sleepiness, it would be unwise to try to implement these 2 behavioral therapies. In these cases, sleep hygiene measures, including regularization of bed period, elimination of daytime napping, and moderation of caffeine and alcohol, may be the only available alternatives.

There is also the possibility that comorbid patients who report excessive daytime sleepiness with few clinical signs of conditioned insomnia are a phenotype whose insomnia sleep symptoms are not conditioned but are generated by the OSA. In these cases, PAP treatment may be all that is required, ameliorating both the OSA and insomnia. Randomized clinical trials of combined treatments for these comorbid patients presently in progress may, in the near future, provide answers to these questions.[20,21]

Because of the potential risk of increased sleepiness from the 2 behavioral therapies in those comorbid patients with pre-existing excessive daytime sleepiness, alternative behavioral therapies could be considered. A novel behavior therapy, intensive sleep retraining (ISR), has more recently been proposed and evaluated for its effectiveness.[49] ISR is a laboratory-based procedure that has been shown to be as effective as SCT for the treatment of chronic insomnia, and when combined with SCT it is more effective than either therapy alone.[50] ISR combines total sleep deprivation with many opportunities to fall asleep (every 30 minutes across a 24-hour period). As soon as sleep is attained, the patient is awoken to continue the sleep deprivation and maintain high sleep drive. This guarantees rapid sleep onsets (<5 minutes) for most sleep attempts across the 24-hour laboratory period. It essentially condenses the experience of several weeks of SCT into a single 24-hour period. A major disadvantage of ISR is the cost of the laboratory procedure and limited access. There is the potential, however, for translating the treatment to the home environment[51] with the use of new EEG technology and even iPhone apps (eg, http://www.sleeponq.com/). Because ISR can confine the patient safely to the laboratory or home environment for the period of treatment until a full recovery sleep the following night, it promises to be a safer and very effective treatment of insomnia in those comorbid patients with pre-existing high levels of sleepiness.

COGNITIVE ELEMENTS AND THERAPY

The other broad element to CBTi, apart from the behavior therapies, is that of the cognitive elements and therapy. Inaccurate and maladaptive cognitions, perceptions, and beliefs can contribute to insomnia and, therefore, be a target for therapy. The strength of these beliefs should be assessed at the start of therapy with the brief version of the Dysfunctional Beliefs and Attitudes about Sleep (DBAS-16) questionnaire.[52,53] If one believes that normal sleep is a deep unbroken valley of unconsciousness, as most apparently do,[54] then experiencing nighttime awakenings can be disturbing. Sleep education about the cyclic nature of sleep can change this belief to recognize that nighttime awakenings, particularly in the older population, should be considered a normal part of the sleep period, thus reducing their perceived threat and consequent SNS activation.

If a patient strongly holds the belief that a bad night of sleep will produce serious daytime impairments, then taking longer to get to sleep or get back to sleep after an awakening will be a perceived threat that intensifies the longer the wakefulness continues. This will trigger an increasingly strong SNS activation, prolonging wakefulness and strengthening the learned component of the insomnia. Cognitive therapy identifies the patient's strongly held maladaptive beliefs and attempts to reduce the strength of belief through more accurate information, or experiments to test the validity of those beliefs. Because comorbid patients will have a PSG recording of their objective sleep, this can be used in conjunction with their sleep diary to examine possible underestimations of their total sleep and ameliorate some of their worry about their perceived sleep deficiency.

In the attempt to cope with the adversity of insomnia, patients may indulge in safety behaviors that exacerbate the insomnia, such as spending more TIB attempting to gain more sleep. Other safety behaviors used to protect against the effects of a night of poor sleep may be to cancel appointments or obligations the following day. This action, of course, inadvertently increases the possible threat of poor sleep by magnifying the negative consequences. Cognitive therapy can improve understanding of how these coping behaviors are maladaptive and can redirect patients to more helpful behaviors. Cognitive therapy has proven to be as effective in the long term as behavioral therapies when used as a stand-alone treatment.[55] The combination of behavioral and cognitive procedures, known as CBTi, was more effective than either alone and had an excellent responder rate (67%) that was maintained at 6 months post-treatment.[55] These results support the notion that chronic insomnia is typically multifactorial and is thus best treated with a multicomponent therapy.

SUMMARY ABOUT THE TREATMENT OF INSOMNIA COMORBID WITH OBSTRUCTIVE SLEEP APNEA

- It is suggested that the efficacy of CBTi could be further improved by identifying the contributing factors or phenotype of a patient's insomnia and customizing the therapy appropriate for that patient. This is particularly important in the diagnosis and treatment of insomnia in comorbid patients.
- Those patients with pre-existing excessive daytime sleepiness and without clear signs of conditioned insomnia not only may be refractory to CBTi but may be put at increased risk with the use of SCT or SRT behavior therapies. It is still possible that novel behavior therapies or cognitive therapy may be effective for their insomnia treatment, but these are questions yet to be investigated.

- It seems likely that a significant number of the comorbid patients referred to sleep medicine clinics have an insomnia disorder (eg, conditioned insomnia, mistimed body clock) that can effectively be treated with nondrug (eg, CBTi) therapies. There is some evidence for this from patients with occult comorbid OSA in clinical patients referred for insomnia treatment.[24,25] However, this question is presently being investigated in comorbid patients referred for suspected OSA and remains to be confirmed.

TREATMENT OF INSOMNIA BEFORE OR DURING POSITIVE AIRWAY PRESSURE THERAPY?

Another main treatment question relates to the timing of insomnia treatment in relation to the timing of PAP treatment. If it is the case that the presence of insomnia reduces acceptance and adherence to PAP treatment, it would be logical to reduce the insomnia disorder before the introduction of PAP treatment. Apart from very severe OSA and excessive daytime sleepiness that may require immediate PAP treatment, the typical timing of consultations and procedures in sleep medicine clinics probably allows time after the initial diagnostic PSG for at least a short course of CBTi before PAP titration or the introduction of PAP therapy. A short 4-week CBTi course has been shown to be effective for chronic insomnia.[47] Whether it is effective for the comorbid patients is presently under investigation.[20,21] However, CBTi started concurrently with PAP therapy may be as effective, or more so than CBTi before PAP therapy, at least for those comorbid patients who do not reject PAP outright because of their comorbid insomnia. Again, answers to these questions should be emerging in 2017 to 2018 from ongoing clinical trials.[20,21]

RECOMMENDATIONS FOR SLEEP MEDICINE CLINICS

1. Be attentive to the presence of comorbid insomnia in the OSA diagnosed population. It is highly prevalent (30%–70%), contributes to PAP rejection and low adherence rates, and diminishes overall treatment effectiveness and health outcomes.
2. Adopt procedures and measures to identify comorbid insomnia, including the ISI questionnaire, a week of sleep-wake diary, and measures of daytime impairment separate from sleepiness that are more specific to insomnia (eg, daytime fatigue).[29]

3. Consider treating the insomnia before or concurrent with PAP or other OSA therapy with the best-practice nondrug CBTi administered in group or individual treatment sessions by a sleep psychologist possessing CBTi skills and trained in sleep and sleep disorders. It would be additionally advantageous to integrate such a therapist into the clinic's operation (eg, cross-referrals, participation in case conferences) to create a more multidisciplinary, more comprehensive, and more effective sleep medicine clinic.

REFERENCES

1. American Academy of Sleep Medicine. International classification of sleep disorders. 3rd edition. Darien (IL): American Academy of Sleep Medicine; 2014.
2. Young T, Skaturd J, Peppard PE. Risk factors for obstructive sleep apnea in adults. J Am Med Assoc 2004;291(16):2013–6.
3. Guilleminault C, Eldridge FL, Dement WC. Insomnia with sleep apnea: a new syndrome. Science 1973; 181(4102):856–8.
4. Krakow B, Melendrez D, Ferreira E, et al. Prevalence of insomnia symptoms in patients with sleep-disordered breathing. Chest 2001;120(6):1923–9.
5. Sweetman A, Lack LC, Catcheside PG, et al. Developing a successful treatment for co-morbid insomnia and sleep apnea. Sleep Medicine Reviews, in press. http://dx.doi.org/10.1016/j.smrv.2016.04.004.
6. Wallace DM, Vargas SS, Schwartz SJ, et al. Determinants of continuous positive airway pressure adherence in a sleep clinic cohort of South Florida Hispanic veterans. Sleep Breath 2013;17(1):351–63.
7. Wickwire EM, Smith MT, Birnbaum S, et al. Sleep maintenance insomnia complaints predict poor CPAP adherence: a clinical case series. Sleep Med 2010;11(8):772–6.
8. Wickwire EM, Schumacher JA, Richert AC, et al. Combined insomnia and poor CPAP compliance: a case study and discussion. Clin Case Stud 2008; 7(4):267–86.
9. Pieh C, Bach M, Popp R, et al. Insomnia symptoms influence CPAP compliance. Sleep Breath 2012; 17(1):99–104.
10. Smith SS, Dunn N, Douglas J, et al. Sleep onset insomnia is associated with reduced adherence to CPAP therapy. Sleep Biol Rhythms 2009;7:A74.
11. Bianchi M, Williams KL, McKinney S, et al. The subjective-objective mismatch in sleep perception among those with insomnia and sleep apnea. J Sleep Res 2013;22(5):557–68.
12. Li Z, Li Y, Yang L, et al. Characterization of obstructive sleep apnea in patients with insomnia across gender and age. Sleep Breath 2015;19(2):723–7.
13. Ong JC, Crawford MR. Insomnia and obstructive sleep apnea. Sleep Med Clin 2013;8(3):289–98.
14. Goonerante NS, Gehrman PR, Nkwuo E, et al. Consequences of comorbid insomnia symptoms and sleep-related breathing disorder in elderly subjects. Arch Intern Med 2006;166(16):1732–8.
15. Smith S, Sullivan K, Hopkins W, et al. Frequency of insomnia report in patients with obstructive sleep apnoea hypopnea syndrome (OSAHS). Sleep Med 2004;5(5):449–56.
16. Björnsdóttir E, Janson C, Gíslason T, et al. Insomnia in untreated sleep apnea patients compared to controls. J Sleep Res 2012;22(2):131–8.
17. Bonnet MH, Arand DL. Hyperarousal and insomnia: state of the science. Sleep Med Rev 2010;14:9–15.
18. Ratnavadivel R, Chau N, Stadler D, et al. Marked reduction in obstructive sleep apnea severity in slow wave sleep. J Clin Sleep Med 2009;5(6): 519–24.
19. Mercer JD, Bootzin RR, Lack L. Insomniacs' perception of wake instead of sleep. Sleep 2002; 25(5):559–66.
20. Crawford MR, Turner AD, Wyatt JK, et al. Evaluating the treatment of obstructive sleep apnea comorbid with insomnia disorder using an incomplete factorial design. Contemp Clin Trials 2016;47:146–52.
21. Australian New Zealand Clinical Trials Registry. Available at: https://www.anzctr.org.au/Trial/Registration/TrialReview.aspx?id=365184&isReview=true.
22. Kyle SD, Miller CB, Rogers Z, et al. Sleep restriction therapy for insomnia is associated with reduced objective total sleep time, increased daytime somnolence, and objectively-impaired vigilance: implications for the clinical management of insomnia disorder. Sleep 2014;37(2):229–37.
23. Lack LC, Hunter M, Gradisar M, et al. Is the treatment of insomnia impaired when OSA is also present? Sleep 2011;34(Abstract Suppl):A174.
24. Fung CH, Martin JL, Josephson K, et al. Efficacy of cognitive behavioral therapy for insomnia in older adults with occult sleep-disordered breathing. Psychosom Med 2016;78(5):629–39.
25. Bastien CH, Vallières A, Morin CM. Validation of the Insomnia Severity Index as an outcome measure for insomnia research. Sleep Med 2001;2(4):297–307.
26. Glidewell RN, Renn BN, Roby E, et al. Predictors and patterns of insomnia symptoms in OSA before and after PAP therapy. Sleep Med 2014;15(8):899–905.
27. Perlis ML, Zee J, Swinkels C, et al. The incidence and temporal patterning of insomnia: a second study. J Sleep Res 2014;23(5):499–507.
28. Gradisar M, Lack L, Harris J, et al. The Flinders Fatigue Scale: preliminary psychometric properties and clinical sensitivity of a new scale for measuring daytime fatigue associated with insomnia. J Clin Sleep Med 2007;3(7):722–8.
29. Lichstein KL, Means MK, Noe SL, et al. Fatigue and sleep disorders. Behav Res Ther 1997;35(8): 733–40.

30. Chotinaiwattarakul W, O'Brien LM, Fan L, et al. Fatigue, tiredness, and lack of entegy improve with treatment for OSA. J Clin Sleep Med 2009;5(3):222–7.

31. Chesson AL, Anderson WM, Littner M, et al. Practice parameters for the nonpharmacologic treatment of chronic insomnia: an American Academy of Sleep Medicine report. Sleep 1999;22(8):1128–33.

32. Charles J, Harrison C, Britt H. Insomnia. Aust Fam Physician 2009;38(5):284.

33. Guilleminault C. Benzodiazepines, breathing, and sleep. Am J Med 1990;88(3A):25S–8S.

34. Luyster FS, Buysse DJ, Strollo PJ. Comorbid insomnia and obstructive sleep apnea: challenges for clinical practice and research. J Clin Sleep Med 2010;6(2):196–204.

35. Roehrs TA, Randall S, Harris E, et al. Twelve months of nightly zolpidem does not lead to dose escalation: a prospective placebo-controlled study. Sleep 2011;34(2):207–12.

36. Kales A, Scharf MB, Kales JD. Rebound insomnia: a new clinical syndrome. Science 1978;201(4360):1039–41.

37. Soldatos CR, Dikeos DG, Whitehead A. Tolerance and rebound insomnia with rapidly eliminated hypnotics: a meta-analysis of sleep laboratory studies. Int Clin Psychopharmacol 1999;14(5):287–303.

38. Puustinen J, Lahteenmaki R, Polo-Kantola P, et al. Effect of withdrawal from long-term use of temazepam, zopiclone or zolpidem as hypnotic agents on cognition in older adults. Eur J Clin Pharmacol 2014;70(3):319–29.

39. Morgenthaler TI, Silber MH. Amnestic sleep-related eating disorder associated with zolpidem. Sleep Med 2002;3(4):323–7.

40. Kripke DF. Possibility that certain hypnotics might cause cancer in skin. J Sleep Res 2008;17(3):245–50.

41. Hohagen F, Rink K, Kappler C, et al. Prevalence and treatment of insomnia in general practice. A longitudinal study. Eur Arch Psychiatry Clin Neurosci 1993;242(6):329–36.

42. Lovato N, Lack L. The role of bright light therapy in managing insomnia. Sleep Med Clin 2013;8(3):351–9.

43. Morin CM, Colecchi C, Stone J, et al. Behavioral and pharmacological therapies for late-life insomnia: a randomized controlled trial. J Am Med Assoc 1999;281:991–9.

44. Bootzin RR, Epstein DR. Understanding and treating insomnia. Annu Rev Clin Psychol 2011;7:435–58.

45. Spielman AJ, Saskin P, Thorpy MJ. Treatment of chronic insomnia by restriction of time in bed. Sleep 1987;10(1):45–56.

46. Kyle SD, Morgan K, Spiegelhalder K, et al. No pain, no gain: an exploratory within-subjects mixed-methods evaluation of the patient experience of sleep restriction therapy (SRT) for insomnia. Sleep Med 2011;12(8):735–47.

47. Lovato N, Lack L, Wright H, et al. Evaluation of a brief treatment program of cognitive behavior therapy for insomnia in older adults. Sleep 2014;37:117–26.

48. Carskadon MA, Dement WC, Mitler MM, et al. Self-reports versus sleep laboratory findings in 122 drug-free subjects with complaints of chronic insomnia. Am J Psychiatry 1976;133(12):1382–8.

49. Harris J, Lack L, Wright H, et al. Intensive sleep retraining treatment for chronic primary insomnia: a preliminary investigation. J Sleep Res 2007;16:276–84.

50. Harris J, Lack L, Kemp K, et al. A randomized controlled trial of intensive sleep retraining (ISR): a brief conditioning treatment for chronic insomnia. Sleep 2012;35(1):49–60.

51. Spielman AJ, Glovinsky PB. What a difference a day makes. Sleep 2012;35(1):11–2.

52. Morin CM, Vallières A, Ivers H. Dysfunctional Beliefs and Attitudes about Sleep (DBAS): validation of a brief version (DBAS-16). Sleep 2007;30(11):1547–54.

53. Carney CE, Edinger JD, Morin CM, et al. Examining maladaptive beliefs about sleep across insomnia patient groups. J Psychosom Res 2010;68(1):57–65.

54. Bruck D, Dolan CL, Lack LC. Beliefs about the 'shape' and continuity of healthy sleep as a function of age. J Psychosom Res 2015;78(1):39–44.

55. Harvey AG, Bélanger L, Talbot L, et al. Comparative efficacy of behavior therapy, cognitive therapy, and cognitive behavior therapy for chronic insomnia: a randomized controlled trial. J Consult Clin Psychol 2014;82(4):670–83.

Diagnosis, Cause, and Treatment Approaches for Delayed Sleep-Wake Phase Disorder

Michelle Magee, PhD[a,c,*,1], Emily M. Marbas, BA[b,1],
Kenneth P. Wright Jr, PhD[b],
Shantha M.W. Rajaratnam, PhD[a,c,d,e],
Josiane L. Broussard, PhD[b]

KEYWORDS

- Delayed sleep phase • Circadian rhythms • Homeostat • Melatonin • Phototherapy • Delayed sleep
- Bright light • Circadian phase

KEY POINTS

- Delayed sleep-wake phase disorder (DSWPD) is a circadian rhythm sleep disorder associated with misalignment of the circadian pacemaker and the desired sleep-wake cycle, and manifests as delayed sleep-wake timing relative to societal norms.
- Approximately 10% of patients with chronic insomnia are reported to have DSWPD, suggesting the requirement of strict diagnostic criteria to differentiate DSWPD from sleep onset insomnia.
- Current treatment options have short-term efficacy, but relapse to a delayed sleep time is likely to occur if patients are noncompliant.
- Diagnosis and evaluation of treatment outcomes are typically based on subjective patient reports, but may be improved with the incorporation of an objective circadian measure.
- Future research should examine the efficacy of combined treatment approaches for DSWPD.

INTRODUCTION

Circadian rhythms are endogenous, entrainable biological rhythms with an approximate oscillation of 24 hours. Circadian rhythms regulate aspects of biology and appropriately time behavior to coordinate physiologic functions with specific times of day or night.

Circadian misalignment is defined as an altered or inappropriate relationship between sleep-wake timing relative to internal circadian timing. During

Disclosure Statement: See last page of article.
[a] Cooperative Research Centre for Alertness, Safety and Productivity, School of Psychological Sciences, Monash University, BASE Facility, Ground Level 264 Ferntree Gully Road, Notting Hill, Victoria 3168, Australia; [b] Sleep and Chronobiology Laboratory, Department of Integrative Physiology, University of Colorado, 1725 Pleasant Street, Clare Small 114, Boulder, CO 80309-0354, USA; [c] Monash Institute of Cognitive and Clinical Neurosciences, Monash University, 18 Innovation Walk, Wellington Road, Clayton, Victoria 3800, Australia; [d] Division of Sleep and Circadian Disorders, Departments of Medicine and Neurology, Brigham and Women's Hospital, 75 Francis Street, Boston, MA 02115, USA; [e] Division of Sleep Medicine, Harvard Medical School, 25 Shattuck Street, Boston, MA 02115, USA
[1] These authors equally contributed to the article.
* Corresponding author. Be Active Sleep and Eat (BASE) Facility, Monash Institute of Cognitive and Clinical Neurosciences, School of Psychological Sciences, Monash University, Ground Level, 264 Ferntree Gully Road, Notting Hill, Victoria 3168, Australia.
E-mail address: michelle.magee@monash.edu

Sleep Med Clin 11 (2016) 389–401
http://dx.doi.org/10.1016/j.jsmc.2016.05.004
1556-407X/16/$ – see front matter © 2016 Elsevier Inc. All rights reserved.

circadian misalignment, sleep is often attempted at an internal circadian time when the clock is strongly promoting wakefulness. It is important to note that insufficient sleep is an extrinsic factor that can also lead to a degree of circadian misalignment.[1]

Circadian misalignment leads to impaired cognition[2,3] and disturbed sleep,[3,4] and is associated with negative health consequences.[5–7] Circadian misalignment occurs in response to alterations in light-dark and/or wake-sleep schedules, such as in shift work and jet lag, as well as in circadian rhythm sleep-wake disorders[8] (CRSWDs). Shift work and jet lag disorders are considered extrinsic CRSWDs. In contrast, other CRSWDs are intrinsic in origin and include irregular sleep-wake rhythm disorder, non–24-hour sleep-wake disorder, advanced sleep-wake phase disorder, delayed sleep-wake phase disorder (DSWPD), and CRSWD not otherwise specified.[8] However, regardless of origin, CRSWDs are associated with difficulty maintaining normal work/life/social schedules and typically result in significant impairments in daytime function and overall quality of life.

This article focuses on the specific diagnosis, cause, and treatment approaches for DSWPD.

CLASSIFICATION OF DELAYED SLEEP-WAKE PHASE DISORDER

The *International Classification of Sleep Disorders, 3rd Edition* (ICSD-3), defines DSWPD as having the following criteria: "(a) there is a significant delay in the phase of the major sleep episode in relation to the desired or required sleep time and wake-up time, as evidenced by a chronic or recurrent complaint by the patient or a caregiver of inability to fall asleep and difficulty awakening at a desired or required clock time; (b) the symptoms are present for at least three months; (c) when patients are allowed to choose their ad libitum schedule, they will exhibit improved sleep quality and duration for age and maintain a delayed phase of the 24-h sleep-wake pattern; (d) sleep log and, whenever possible, actigraphy monitoring for at least seven days (preferably 14 days) demonstrate a delay in the timing of the habitual sleep period. Both work/school days and free days must be included within this monitoring; and (e) the sleep disturbance is not better explained by another current sleep disorder, medical or neurological disorder, mental disorder, medication use, or substance use disorder"[8] **(Fig. 1)**.

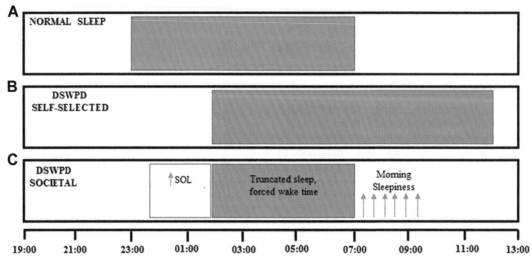

Fig. 1. The timing of sleep episodes in normal sleepers (*A*), individuals with DSWPD when given the opportunity to self-select sleep-wake timing (*B*), and individuals with DSWPD when sleep is truncated because of the need to wake up for school or work activities during the daytime (*C*). Comparisons of sleep episodes in normal sleepers and patients with DSWPD differ in the timing of bedtimes and wake times. Here, the blue bar (*A*) represents the timing of sleep in a normal sleeper with a duration of approximately 8 hours. Compared with patients who have DSWPD under self-selected times (*B*), individuals have a delayed sleep and wake time (represented by the blue bar) and may have extended sleep duration. In contrast, in situations in which patients with DSWPD have daytime commitments (*C*), patients may attempt an earlier (required) sleep time, resulting in a longer sleep onset latency (SOL). In addition, the sleep episode is truncated in the morning to meet daytime commitments and the level of sleepiness is increased.

In addition, the current volume of the *Diagnostic and Statistical Manual of Mental Disorders, 5th Edition* (DSM-5), adds that 3 criteria must be met for a diagnosis of DSWPD: "(1) the characteristic misalignment of sleep, in conjunction with (2) excessive sleepiness or insomnia and (3) significant daytime impairment in social, occupational or other important areas of functioning."[9] As noted in the ICSD-3, individuals with DSWPD may show excessive sleep inertia (extreme difficulty awakening and confusion) in the morning as a result of curtailed sleep time and forced awakening during a circadian phase of high sleep propensity. Individuals with DSWPD may have increased rates of mental disturbances, such as DSM-5 axis I disorders or symptoms (eg, mood disorders or depressive symptoms). Attempts to cope with the inability to fall asleep earlier may result in the development of insomnia symptoms. Individuals may use alcohol, sedatives, hypnotics, or stimulant substances to alleviate symptoms of insomnia and excessive sleepiness, thereby perpetuating the underlying sleep disorder.[8] Further, a recent study by Reid and colleagues[10] suggests that patients with DSWPD have a high rate of comorbidity with social phobias and obsessive-compulsive disorder.

Prevalence of DSWPD is estimated to range from 0.13% to 10% of the population.[11–14] Findings from a study in adolescents suggest a higher prevalence of DSWPD in male patients.[15] In contrast, findings from an epidemiologic study reported no evidence of sex differences,[14] whereas another found an increased prevalence of DSWPD in female patients.[16] However, on average, males have been reported to have later chronotypes than females,[17] which is important to consider when examining potential sex differences in DSWPD prevalence. In addition, adolescence is associated with a shift toward later chronotypes,[17] which may play a role in the suggested increase in DSWPD prevalence in this age group (as reviewed in Ref.[18]).

Clinically, patients with DSWPD complain of delayed bedtimes more than 2 hours later than conventional or socially acceptable timing[8] and difficulty awakening at the desired or necessary time in the morning to fulfil social or occupational obligations. When not obliged to maintain a strict schedule, the patients sleep normally but at a delayed clock time.[8]

PATIENT EVALUATION OVERVIEW
Diagnostic Issues

Differing interpretations of diagnostic criteria and the similarity of DSWPD symptoms to other disorders presents clinicians with challenges in the accurate diagnosis of DSWPD. Although individuals with DSWPD have delays in their habitual sleep timing, other factors, such as depression or poor sleep hygiene, can contribute to sleep abnormalities that present similarly to DSWPD.[19] Diagnosing DSWPD in adolescents also presents challenges, because this period of development is associated with many changes in sleep/wake timing.[20] As noted above, many adolescents show symptoms similar to those of DSWPD, such as difficulty waking up in the morning[21] and a significant delay in sleep and wake times on the weekends compared with weekdays, with some studies suggesting a delay of up to 3 hours.[22]

In addition, up to 10% of insomnia cases have been suggested to be misdiagnosed as DSWPD[8,23] due to the presence of sleep initiation problems and some overlap between the diagnostic criteria. In contrast to patients with insomnia, patients with DSWPD have few problems with sleep initiation and maintenance when able to self-select their sleep schedule.[8] In addition, patients with DSWPD may experience excessive sleepiness in the morning when wakefulness occurs before their preferred wake time. Therefore, considerations must be made to distinguish DSWPD from other disorders that involve excessive sleepiness. Patients with other disorders often do not have the pronounced delay in sleep timing associated with DSWPD, and their sleep and sleepiness problems do not dissipate with self-selected sleep schedules.[8] With these considerations in mind when diagnosing DSWPD, it is essential to follow ICSD and DSM criteria, as well as to use all available assessment tools.

Current Assessment Tools

There is a spectrum of assessment tools that can be used for the diagnosis and study of DSWPD. Each tool has its own strengths and weaknesses, and is used to identify the extent to which patients' symptoms match set DSWPD criteria. These measures include both subjective and objective assessments, and are often used in conjunction to provide a more comprehensive view of the patient's sleep habits, duration, and quality (**Table 1**).

Sleep logs

Sleep logs or diaries allow patients to track their habitual sleep and wake times. The logs document several sleep parameters, such as when lights are turned out, when the patient gets into bed, how long it takes for the patient to fall asleep (sleep onset latency [SOL]), time spent awake after sleep onset (wake after sleep onset [WASO]), and wake

Table 1
Current assessment tools used to diagnose or study DSWPD

Tool	Uses	Limitations
Sleep logs	Documents habitual sleep-wake schedule over time (eg, 2 wk), and characterizes sleep-wake disturbances	• Self-reported
Actigraphy	Uses watch-like device to record activity levels and potentially also ambient light exposure. Often used in conjunction with sleep logs to verify self-reported sleep and wake times	• Cost • Decreased reliability for SOL and WASO
Morningness-eveningness questionnaire	Self-assessment of patient's behavioral preference for the timing of sleep-wakefulness and activities during the day	• Does not provide direct assessment of habitual sleep-wake timing or sleep disturbances
DLMO	Repeated collection of blood or saliva samples in the evening hours, under dim light conditions, can be used to determine the timing of the onset of the endogenous melatonin rhythm. Useful in confirming circadian misalignment and for determining treatment outcome	• Cost • Staff training required • Environmental controls (dim light conditions) • Patient burden

Abbreviations: DLMO, dim light melatonin onset; SOL, sleep onset latency; WASO, wake after sleep onset.

time in the morning.[24] In addition, logs can also include areas to document when caffeine, alcohol, sleep aids, or other medications are ingested in order to gain a more comprehensive understanding of factors influencing the patient's sleep-wake timing. ICSD-3 guidelines recommend at least 14 days of sleep log documentation, preferably verified by actigraphy with concurrent light exposure measurement, when diagnosing DSWPD.[8]

Actigraphy

Actigraphy is a method of monitoring activity and light exposure levels through the use of a small device, typically worn on the patient's wrist. Since its introduction in 1991, actigraphy monitoring has become widely used and accepted as a reliable and valid measure of sleep-wake activity.[25] In conjunction with sleep diaries, the ICSD-3 recommends the use of actigraphy to document habitual sleep episodes in DSWPD. Issues have been noted in the past with the accuracy of actigraphy monitors to detect SOL and WASO (reviewed in Ref.[25]), therefore actigraphy data are often used in conjunction with sleep log data to verify estimation of SOL and WASO.

Morningness-eveningness questionnaires

Since first introduced by Horne and Ostberg[26] in 1975, the 19-question Morning-Eveningness Questionnaire (MEQ) has been used by sleep researchers and physicians to assess an individual's preference for earlier or later wakefulness. Those with a higher score on the MEQ is associated with a preferences for earlier rise and bedtimes (morning types), as well as significantly earlier peaks in body temperature and other markers of circadian phase, as compared with a lower score on the MEQ (evening types).[26] Studies in both healthy sleepers and DSWPD populations show a negative correlation between MEQ score and circadian phase.[27,28] Patients with DSWPD are considered extreme evening types, whereas not all evening types experience the disruption to everyday life typically observed in individuals with DSWPD.[8] MEQ score is therefore informative to the diagnosis of DSWPD, but should be used in conjunction with other, more direct assessment methods.

Circadian phase markers

Several hormones circulate throughout the body in a predictable, circadian-dependent manner, and can be used as reliable markers of the endogenous circadian pacemaker. Melatonin rhythm is most commonly assessed by determining the onset of nocturnal endogenous secretion, defined as dim light melatonin onset (DLMO). Melatonin levels can be easily assessed from saliva or plasma samples, showing high specificity and sensitivity.[29] When an individual is normally entrained and obtains sufficient sleep, melatonin levels typically increase before habitual bedtime, peak during the sleep episode, and decrease to low levels near habitual wake time.[30]

Although the relationship between sleep and melatonin levels has been extensively researched in healthy individuals, less was known about the association in those with DSWPD until recently. In 2008, a study conducted by Rahman and colleagues[19] tested the specificity and sensitivity of DLMO as a reliable marker of circadian phase in individuals with DSWPD. Individuals with DSWPD showed a delay in DLMO, corresponding with a delay in circadian phase. Clinical sensitivity and specificity of DLMO in those with DSWPD were 90.3% and 83.0%, respectively, suggesting that DLMO may be an effective method of differentiating between DSWPD and other sleep disorders.[31] Demonstrating an objective delay in circadian timing is not currently a criterion for DSWPD diagnosis according to the ICSD-3, however, clinicians are recommended to use DLMO assessment to confirm the delayed circadian phase.[8]

CAUSE

Mechanisms that may contribute to the cause of DSWPD can be classed into 3 categories: physiologic, behavioral, and genetic (**Fig. 2**).

Physiologic

Delay in timing of circadian rhythm
A significant delay in circadian phase is an underlying cause of DSWPD.[11] Circadian phase delays of between 2 and 6 hours have been reported in individuals with DSWPD compared with healthy sleepers.[23,32–34] This delay coincides with a delay in the wake maintenance zone, giving rise to increased alertness at the patient's desired bedtime,[18,35] thus precipitating difficulty initiating sleep at the desired bedtime.

Longer circadian period (tau)
The suprachiasmatic nucleus of the anterior hypothalamus coordinates circadian, ~24-hour rhythmicity[36–38] and is synchronized by the light/dark cycle. Circadian period length is on average ~24.15 hours in healthy adults.[39,40] Longer periods are associated with sleep onset difficulties, delayed timing of circadian phase,[41] and evening preference,[28] all of which are defining characteristics of DSWPD. A longer period in DSWPD may promote a continual tendency to delay the circadian system along with the sleep-wake cycle. It has therefore been hypothesized that circadian period is longer in patients with DSWPD.[42] This difference in period has been shown in in vitro and in vivo studies[41,43]; however, in clinical cases, evidence is limited. To our knowledge, only 2 studies have investigated period length in a DSWPD clinical population. The first study showed in 1 patient with DSWPD a longer tau (25.4 hours) compared with the 3 healthy sleepers (24.2 hours). Micic and colleagues[44] replicated this study showing a longer period in patients with DSWPD (n = 6; 24.9 hours) compared with healthy controls (n = 7; 24.5 hours).

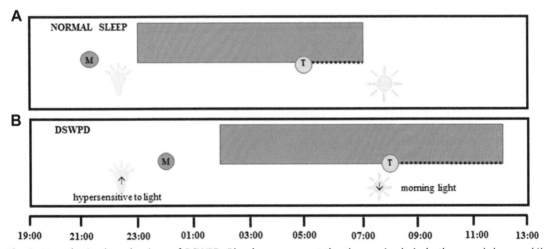

Fig. 2. Hypothesized mechanisms of DSWPD. Blue bars represent the sleep episode in both normal sleepers (*A*) and individuals with DSWPD (*B*). Timing of DLMO is represented by the blue circle labeled M, whereas minimum core body temperature (CBT$_{min}$) is represented by the blue circle labeled T. In an individual with DSWPD (*B*), DLMO occurs later than in a normal sleeper (*A*) and is potentially influenced by hypersensitivity to evening light, increased evening light exposure, and decreased morning light exposure. A delay in the phase of the circadian pacemaker and sleep-wake timing has been reported in patients with DSWPD, manifesting as a longer interval between CBT$_{min}$ and sleep offset time, compared with normal sleepers (*A*).

Phase relationships between circadian phase and sleep timing

The relationship between the endogenous circadian pacemaker and sleep timing of an individual defines the phase angle of entrainment and is thought to play an important role in the cause of DSWPD. It is well established that the circadian response to light depends on circadian timed light exposure, as described by the phase response curve (PRC) to light.[45]

However, in DSWPD there are significant differences in the CBT minimum (CBT_{min}) relative to sleep timing,[33,46] in which a longer interval between the temperature minimum and sleep offset was reported compared with controls. In healthy sleepers, the temperature minimum during sleep occurs ~2 hours before sleep offset, whereas in DSWPD the temperature minimum has been reported to occur ~4 hours before sleep offset.[23,33,46,47] In contrast, no significant differences in the timing of the DLMO relative to sleep onset[48,49] and offset[49] times have been reported between DSWPD and controls unclear whether there is a longer interval between CBT_{min} and sleep offset in DSWPD and further investigations are warranted under controlled constant routine conditions.

Hypersensitivity to light

Clinical characteristics of DSWPD have been hypothesized to manifest from reduced morning light exposure.[50,51] In addition, patients with DSWPD may have hypersensitivity to evening light exposure, when individuals are most sensitive to a circadian phase delay. Out of a clinical population of 322 individuals with CRSWDs (of whom 83.5% had DSWPD), 47% reported subjective sensitivity to light compared with 19.6% of healthy sleepers.[52]

In one study published investigating the potential hypersensitivity to evening light exposure in DSWPD, patients with DSWPD and controls were exposed to 1000 lux of light 2 hours before the peak in melatonin secretion, and showed a greater suppression in melatonin production in patients with DSWPD (71%) compared with healthy sleepers (56%).[53] Most recently, in a preliminary study by Cain and colleagues[54] in which participants were exposed to regular room light (200 lux) for 3 hours before habitual bedtime, greater melatonin suppression was observed in patients with DSWPD (n = 4) compared with controls (n = 5) (unpublished abstract). With a paucity of research within this area, future investigations are required to understand whether hypersensitivity to evening light perpetuates clinical characteristics of DSWPD.

Decreased buildup of homeostatic sleep drive

Sleep is not only regulated by the circadian pacemaker, but also by the sleep homeostat (the drive to sleep, which increases with time awake and dissipates with sleep). Pubescence is a time that coincides with a decline in the rate of accumulation of sleep pressure[55] and concurrently is a period in which DSWPD symptoms are likely to emerge. Based on this association, dysregulation of the homeostatic sleep process may be an underlying mechanism that contributes to later sleep onset times in patients with DSWPD. As shown by Uchiyama and colleagues,[56,57] sleep propensity during wake differs between patients with DSWPD and controls following sleep restriction, with patients with DSWPD accumulating homeostatic sleep drive at a slower rate compared with controls.

In combination with slower homeostatic sleep drive accumulation, it has also been theorized that DSWPD symptoms may be influenced by slower dissipation of sleep pressure. Studies have reported that patients with DSWPD have longer habitual total sleep times compared with normal sleepers.[56,57] In addition, polysomnography studies show reduced sleep efficiency, increased total sleep time, and reduction in the amount and percentage of slow wave sleep (a marker of accumulated sleep pressure) in patients with DSWPD compared with healthy controls.[58] However, the diagnostic criteria indicate that patients with DSWPD have normal sleep architecture based on polysomnography when allowed to self-select sleep-wake schedules.[8,59,60] Future work should investigate the extent to which altered homeostatic sleep regulation plays a causal role in DSWPD.

Behavioral Modulation of Light Exposure

Electronic device use is becoming increasingly prevalent in modern society and electronic screen use before sleep can contribute to poor sleep quality.[61] This screen light may exacerbate possible underlying causes (ie, hypersensitivity to light) in a DSWPD population. A proposed mechanism for technology's negative impact on sleep is an individual's exposure to bright light.[61] In particular, Chellappa and colleagues[62] shown that 2-hour blue-enriched (446–483 nm) light exposure in men suppresses salivary melatonin secretion, resulting in faster response times in tasks assessing sustained attention. More recently, Chang and colleagues[63] investigated the use of electronic devices before bed and found that the use of an e-reader in the hours before bedtime suppressed levels of melatonin secretion, increased SOL, and increased subjective morning sleepiness levels. Late night light exposure may therefore be an environmental contributor to DSWPD.

Genetic

Quantitative genetic studies have shown genetic influence on a variety of sleep disorders, with current research focusing on circadian genes such as Period (Per) given their role in the regulation of the circadian pacemaker and sleep behaviors.[64] Per genes are thought to contribute to individual differences in sleep timing by affecting circadian rhythmicity, as shown in animal models.[65–67] In humans, the coding region of the Per3 gene shows a length polymorphism that is significantly associated with morning and evening preference,[68,69] in which the shorter (4-repeat) allele is associated with eveningness. In addition, the Per3 4-repeat allele is more prevalent in a DSWPD population (0.88) compared with the 5-repeat allele (0.12).[68] Others have also shown a higher incidence of alterations in arylalkylamine N-acetyltransferase[70] and human leukocyte antigen DR1[71] and decreased frequency of the N408 allele in the casein kinase I epsilon (ckiε) gene (phosphorylates CLOCK proteins) in patients with DSWPD relative to controls. DSWPD may also be associated with polymorphisms in Per1[72] and Per2[73] genes, given the prevalence of these gene polymorphisms in individuals with extreme evening preference.

TREATMENT OPTIONS

Current DSWPD treatment options place emphasis on advancing circadian and sleep timing in order to increase sleep duration and improve daytime functioning[74]; however, treatment regimens vary in efficacy. Chronotherapeutic, chronobiotic, photic, and other treatment approaches to DSWPD are summarized in **Table 2** and **Fig. 3**.

Chronotherapeutic Treatment

Prescribed sleep scheduling is used to correct a delay in bed and wake times. First described by Czeisler and colleagues,[42] prescribed sleep scheduling involves delaying an individual's sleep episode incrementally to further delay the patient's bedtime until reaching the desired bedtime (**Fig. 3**B). Once reached, the patient is asked to rigorously maintain the new sleep-wake schedule. Although studies in adolescents with subclinical DSWPD[75] and case reports have shown positive results,[42] there are currently no published controlled trials that have shown efficacy for this

Table 2
Current treatment approaches to DSWPD

Treatment	Methodology	Limitations
Chronotherapeutic	Prescribed sleep scheduling: changing the timing of sleep onset to progressively delay until it matches desired bedtime	• Difficult to implement • Interferes with daytime activities while progressively delaying • Relapse rate high • No controlled trials to support efficacy
Photic	Morning bright light therapy	• Ideally, should measure circadian phase before treatment to optimize phase advance • Patient compliance: difficulty waking patient to achieve light exposure • No standard guidelines for dose and timing
Chronobiotic	Administration of melatonin or melatonin agonists	• No standard guidelines on dose and timing • Determination of circadian phase required • Relapse rate high[97]
Other	Influence of environmental factors: controlling extrinsic factors that may exacerbate DSWPD symptoms (technology use, sleep hygiene, caffeine intake, exercise close to bedtime)	• Compliance for limiting technology use in the bedroom

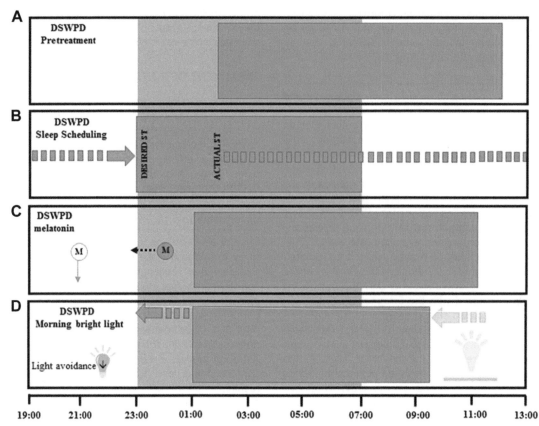

Fig. 3. Treatment principles in DSWPD. Blue bars represent the sleep episode under different treatment approaches. Grey shading represents timing of the desired sleep-wake episode (23:00–07:00). Treatment principles in DSWPD: (*A*) prior to implementing treatment, DSPWD patients demonstrate a delay in bedtime and wake times, (*B*) sleep scheduling, (*C*) administration of melatonin (*open circle*), and (*D*) morning bright light exposure. For sleep scheduling (*B*), patients are advised to delay their habitual bedtime incrementally until they reach their desired bedtime. The administration of melatonin (*C*, open circle labeled M) is recommended 2 to 4 hours before DLMO (blue circle labeled M) to induce a maximal phase advance. Morning bright light therapy (*D*) involves administering light shortly after CBT_{min} to adjust timing of the circadian pacemaker and subsequently advance sleep timing. Light avoidance in the evening is also recommended along with morning bright light therapy.

treatment approach.[76] Findings from one study indicate that prescribed sleep scheduling is associated with high relapse rates,[77] whereas another reports the development of free-running CRSWDs in a patient with DSWPD after the sleep scheduling intervention.[78]

Chronobiotic Treatment

Chronobiotic treatments for DSWPD are based on the principle of phase shifting an individual's circadian pacemaker through use of exogenous melatonin or melatonin agonists. Current chronobiotic treatments are listed below.

Melatonin
It is widely accepted that exogenous melatonin functions as a chronobiotic drug, also with soporific properties.[79] Melatonin administration 2 to

4 hours before DLMO induces a maximal phase advance (**Fig. 3**C), whereas melatonin administration 12 to 15 hours after DLMO or up to 4 hours after waking is reported to induce maximal phase delays.[80] A meta-analysis conducted in 2010 by Geijlswijk and colleagues[81] investigating the efficacy of melatonin for DSWPD indicated that, compared with placebo, melatonin treatment advances endogenous melatonin onset by, on average, 1.18 hours, decreases SOL by 23 minutes, and advances sleep onset by 0.67 hours. Although this meta-analysis did not take dosage of melatonin into consideration, others have shown that a small dose of 0.3 to 0.5 mg is as effective as 3 mg for advancing sleep onset.[80,82]

Melatonin receptor agonists
Melatonin receptor agonists such as ramelteon and tasimelteon are known to induce phase shifts

of the circadian pacemaker, suggesting efficacy in the treatment of several CRSWDs.[83–85] However, the role of these melatonin agonists in DSWPD is yet to be tested. The demonstrated phase-shifting and sleep-promoting effects strongly suggest that the melatonin agonists may be efficacious in the treatment of DSWPD. Tasimelteon now has US Food and Drug Administration approval for use in the treatment of non–24-hour sleep-wake rhythm disorder at a 20 mg dose, taken before bedtime.

Photic Treatment

Photic therapy is used to adjust the timing of the circadian pacemaker via morning bright light exposure. The magnitude of response depends on the timing, intensity, duration, and wavelength of the lighting administered.[51,86,87] In order to achieve optimal phase advance, timing should be based on the light PRC in humans.[45,88–90] According to the light PRC, light has a maximum phase advancing effect when administered shortly after the CBT_{min}.[45] Optimal timing of light can be difficult to estimate based on habitual sleep-wake timing, because of the large degree of interindividual variability in the timing of CBT_{min} relative to the sleep-wake cycle. Circadian phase assessment is therefore recommended before photic treatment to ensure optimal treatment outcomes.[31]

When administered between 6:00 and 9:00 AM, bright light therapy (2500 lux, 2 hours) resulted in a 2-hour advance of DLMO, reduced SOL, advanced sleep onset time, and improved daytime alertness in patients with DSWPD.[91] In conjunction with prescribed morning phototherapy, evening light avoidance is crucial to avoid exacerbating the natural tendency to phase delay (**Fig. 3**D). More recently, studies have investigated different wavelengths for treatment of DSWPD and found that administration of early-morning blue light (light-emitting diodes, 470-nm peak wavelength, irradiance = 65 $\mu W/cm^2$) advanced timing of endogenous melatonin and wake time, but did not change sleep onset times.[87]

Other Treatments

Extrinsic environmental factors, such as poor sleep hygiene (eg, the use of electronic devices in bed), diet, exercise timing,[92] and stimulant use,[93,94] can exacerbate DSWPD symptoms. Patient education about behavioral practices that promote better sleep habits may improve patient outcomes (**Fig. 3**).[93,95]

Evaluation of treatment options

Current treatment regimens for DSWPD focus on advancing the circadian pacemaker. Chronotherapeutic, chronobiotic, photic, and other treatment practices all provide short-term efficacy but long-term efficacy data are limited. A combined treatment approach, with ongoing monitoring and coaching, may be required to optimize treatment outcomes and minimize relapse. In addition, accurate determination of circadian phase before treatment may improve efficacy through optimized timing of treatment and assessment of treatment outcomes.

SUMMARY

DSWPD is a circadian rhythm sleep disorder that should be differentiated from sleep onset insomnia. According to the ISCD-3, sleep diaries and wrist actigraphy (when available) are relied on to document the consistent pattern of delayed sleep onset and waking (when sleep is unrestricted), in order to confirm a DSWPD diagnosis in clinical practice. Circadian phase markers are not routinely assessed, but should be considered. Treatment of DSWPD has mainly focused on advancing the circadian pacemaker. Maintaining this phase advance is challenging and a relapse in the delay is probable.[96,97] Combined treatment approaches using pharmacotherapy and phototherapy along with circadian phase assessments may improve the efficacy of treatment and may provide a more successful long-term result for individuals with DSWPD. Given the lack of research investigating the efficacy of combined therapies tailored to individual circadian phases, future work is warranted.

DISCLOSURE STATEMENT

M. Magee and E. Marbas report no conflicts of interest. K.P. Wright, Jr, reports grants from National Institutes of Health and the Office of Naval Research and Philips Inc, and personal fees from the American College of Chest Physicians, The Obesity Society, the Obesity Medicine Association, and Torvec, Inc during the preparation of this work. He has also served as a consultant for Takeda Pharmaceuticals North America. S.W.M. Rajaratnam has served as a consultant through his institution to Vanda Pharmaceuticals, Philips Respironics, EdanSafe, The Australian Workers' Union, National Transport Commission, and Transport Accident Commission, and has through his institution received research grants and/or unrestricted educational grants from Vanda Pharmaceuticals, Takeda Pharmaceuticals North America, Philips Lighting, Philips Respironics, Cephalon, and ResMed Foundation, and reimbursements for conference travel expenses from Vanda Pharmaceuticals. His institution has received equipment donations or other support from Optalert, Compumedics, and Tyco Healthcare. He has also served as an expert witness and/or consultant to shift work organizations. S.W.M. Rajaratnam also serves as a program leader in the Cooperative Research Centre for Alertness, Safety and Productivity. J.L. Broussard reports no conflicts of interest.

REFERENCES

1. Markwald RR, Melanson EL, Smith MR, et al. Impact of insufficient sleep on total daily energy expenditure, food intake, and weight gain. Proc Natl Acad Sci U S A 2013;110(14):5695–700.

2. Wright KP, Hull JT, Czeisler CA. Relationship between alertness, performance, and body temperature in humans. Am J Physiol Regul Integr Comp Physiol 2002;283(6):R1370–7.

3. Wright KP Jr, Hull JT, Hughes RJ, et al. Sleep and wakefulness out of phase with internal biological time impairs learning in humans. J Cogn Neurosci 2006;18(4):508–21.

4. McHill AW, Melanson EL, Higgins J, et al. Impact of circadian misalignment on energy metabolism during simulated nightshift work. Proc Natl Acad Sci U S A 2014;111(48):17302–7.

5. Morris CJ, Yang JN, Garcia JI, et al. Endogenous circadian system and circadian misalignment impact glucose tolerance via separate mechanisms in humans. Proc Natl Acad Sci U S A 2015;112(17): E2225–34.

6. Scheer FA, Hilton MF, Mantzoros CS, et al. Adverse metabolic and cardiovascular consequences of circadian misalignment. Proc Natl Acad Sci U S A 2009;106(11):4453–8.

7. Buxton OM, Cain SW, O'Connor SP, et al. Adverse metabolic consequences in humans of prolonged sleep restriction combined with circadian disruption. Sci Transl Med 2012;4(129):129ra143.

8. The International Classification of Sleep Disorders. Diagnostic and coding manual. 3rd edition. Westchester (IL): American Academy of Sleep Medicine; 2014.

9. Diagnostic and statistical manual of mental disorders. 5th edition. Arlington (VA): American Psychiatric Association; 2013.

10. Reid KJ, Jaksa AA, Eisengart JB, et al. Systematic evaluation of Axis-I DSM diagnoses in delayed sleep phase disorder and evening-type circadian preference. Sleep Med 2012;13(9):1171–7.

11. Weitzman ED, Czeisler CA, Coleman RM, et al. Delayed sleep phase syndrome. A chronobiological disorder with sleep-onset insomnia. Arch Gen Psychiatry 1981;38(7):737–46.

12. Paine SJ, Fink J, Gander PH, et al. Identifying advanced and delayed sleep phase disorders in the general population: a national survey of New Zealand adults. Chronobiol Int 2014;31(5):627–36.

13. Schrader H, Bovim G, Sand T. The prevalence of delayed and advanced sleep phase syndromes. J Sleep Res 1993;2(1):51–5.

14. Saxvig IW, Pallesen S, Wilhelmsen-Langeland A, et al. Prevalence and correlates of delayed sleep phase in high school students. Sleep Med 2012; 13(2):193–9.

15. Thorpy MJ, Korman E, Spielman AJ, et al. Delayed sleep phase syndrome in adolescents. J Adolesc Health Care 1988;9(1):22–7.

16. Sivertsen B, Pallesen S, Stormark KM, et al. Delayed sleep phase syndrome in adolescents: prevalence and correlates in a large population based study. BMC Public Health 2013;13:1163.

17. Roenneberg T, Kuehnle T, Pramstaller PP, et al. A marker for the end of adolescence. Curr Biol 2004;14(24):R1038–9.

18. Micic G, Lovato N, Gradisar M, et al. The etiology of delayed sleep phase disorder. Sleep Med Rev 2016; 27:29–38.

19. Rahman SA, Kayumov L, Tchmoutina EA, et al. Clinical efficacy of dim light melatonin onset testing in diagnosing delayed sleep phase syndrome. Sleep Med 2009;10(5):549–55.

20. Crowley SJ, Acebo C, Carskadon MA. Sleep, circadian rhythms, and delayed phase in adolescence. Sleep Med 2007;8(6):602–12.

21. Carskadon MA. Patterns of sleep and sleepiness in adolescents. Pediatrician 1990;17(1):5–12.

22. Roenneberg T, Wirz-Justice A, Merrow M. Life between clocks: daily temporal patterns of human chronotypes. J Biol Rhythms 2003;18(1):80–90.

23. Watanabe T, Kajimura N, Kato M, et al. Sleep and circadian rhythm disturbances in patients with delayed sleep phase syndrome. Sleep 2003;26(6): 657–61.

24. Lack LC, Wright HR, Bootzin RR. Delayed sleep-phase disorder. Sleep Med Clin 2009;4(2):229–39.

25. Sadeh A. The role and validity of actigraphy in sleep medicine: an update. Sleep Med Rev 2011;15(4): 259–67.

26. Horne JA, Ostberg O. A self-assessment questionnaire to determine morningness-eveningness in human circadian rhythms. Int J Chronobiol 1976;4(2): 97–110.

27. Liu X, Uchiyama M, Shibui K, et al. Diurnal preference, sleep habits, circadian sleep propensity and melatonin rhythm in healthy human subjects. Neurosci Lett 2000;280(3):199–202.

28. Duffy JF, Rimmer DW, Czeisler CA. Association of intrinsic circadian period with morningness-eveningness, usual wake time, and circadian phase. Behav Neurosci 2001;115(4):895–9.

29. Lewy AJ, Sack RL. The dim light melatonin onset as a marker for orcadian phase position. Chronobiol Int 1989;6(1):93–102.

30. Arendt J. Melatonin and human rhythms. Chronobiol Int 2006;23(1–2):21–37.

31. Keijzer H, Smits MG, Duffy JF, et al. Why the dim light melatonin onset (DLMO) should be measured before treatment of patients with circadian rhythm sleep disorders. Sleep Med Rev 2014;18(4):333–9.

32. Oren DA, Turner EH, Wehr TA. Abnormal circadian rhythms of plasma melatonin and body temperature in the delayed sleep phase syndrome. J Neurol Neurosurg Psychiatry 1995;58(3):379.

33. Ozaki S, Uchiyama M, Shirakawa S, et al. Prolonged interval from body temperature nadir to sleep offset in patients with delayed sleep phase syndrome. Sleep 1996;19(1):36–40.

34. Shibui K, Uchiyama M, Okawa M. Melatonin rhythms in delayed sleep phase syndrome. J Biol Rhythms 1999;14(1):72–6.

35. Regestein QR, Monk TH. Delayed sleep phase syndrome: a review of its clinical aspects. Am J Psychiatry 1995;152(4):602–8.

36. Schwartz WJ, Busis NA, Hedley-Whyte ET. A discrete lesion of ventral hypothalamus and optic chiasm that disturbed the daily temperature rhythm. J Neurol 1986;233(1):1–4.

37. Eastman CI, Mistlberger RE, Rechtschaffen A. Suprachiasmatic nuclei lesions eliminate circadian temperature and sleep rhythms in the rat. Physiol Behav 1984;32(3):357–68.

38. Cohen RA, Albers HE. Disruption of human circadian and cognitive regulation following a discrete hypothalamic lesion: a case study. Neurology 1991;41(5):726–9.

39. Czeisler CA, Duffy JF, Shanahan TL, et al. Stability, precision, and near-24-hour period of the human circadian pacemaker. Science 1999;284(5423):2177–81.

40. Duffy JF, Cain SW, Chang AM, et al. Sex difference in the near-24-hour intrinsic period of the human circadian timing system. Proc Natl Acad Sci U S A 2011;108(Suppl 3):15602–8.

41. Lazar AS, Santhi N, Hasan S, et al. Circadian period and the timing of melatonin onset in men and women: predictors of sleep during the weekend and in the laboratory. J Sleep Res 2013;22(2):155–9.

42. Czeisler CA, Richardson GS, Coleman RM, et al. Chronotherapy: resetting the circadian clocks of patients with delayed sleep phase insomnia. Sleep 1981;4(1):1–21.

43. Hasan S, Santhi N, Lazar AS, et al. Assessment of circadian rhythms in humans: comparison of real-time fibroblast reporter imaging with plasma melatonin. FASEB J 2012;26(6):2414–23.

44. Micic G, de Bruyn A, Lovato N, et al. The endogenous circadian temperature period length (tau) in delayed sleep phase disorder compared to good sleepers. J Sleep Res 2013;22(6):617–24.

45. Minors DS, Waterhouse JM, Wirz-Justice A. A human phase-response curve to light. Neurosci Lett 1991;133(1):36–40.

46. Ozaki N, Iwata T, Itoh A, et al. Body temperature monitoring in subjects with delayed sleep phase syndrome. Neuropsychobiology 1988;20(4):174–7.

47. Uchiyama M, Okawa M, Shibui K, et al. Altered phase relation between sleep timing and core body temperature rhythm in delayed sleep phase syndrome and non-24-hour sleep-wake syndrome in humans. Neurosci Lett 2000;294(2):101–4.

48. Micic G, Lovato N, Gradisar M, et al. Nocturnal melatonin profiles in patients with delayed sleep-wake phase disorder and control sleepers. J Biol Rhythms 2015;30(5):437–48.

49. Chang AM, Reid KJ, Gourineni R, et al. Sleep timing and circadian phase in delayed sleep phase syndrome. J Biol Rhythms 2009;24(4):313–21.

50. Dijk DJ, Visscher CA, Bloem GM, et al. Reduction of human sleep duration after bright light exposure in the morning. Neurosci Lett 1987;73(2):181–6.

51. Rosenthal NE, Joseph-Vanderpool JR, Levendosky AA, et al. Phase-shifting effects of bright morning light as treatment for delayed sleep phase syndrome. Sleep 1990;13(4):354–61.

52. Dagan Y, Eisenstein M. Circadian rhythm sleep disorders: toward a more precise definition and diagnosis. Chronobiol Int 1999;16(2):213–22.

53. Aoki H, Ozeki Y, Yamada N. Hypersensitivity of melatonin suppression in response to light in patients with delayed sleep phase syndrome. Chronobiol Int 2001;18(2):263–71.

54. Cain SW, Stanghi J, McConchie O, et al. Hypersensitivity of the circadian system to light in Delayed Sleep Phase Disorder. Paper presented at: Society for Research on Biological Rhythms. Montana, June 14–18, 2013.

55. Campbell IG, Feinberg I. Longitudinal trajectories of non-rapid eye movement delta and theta EEG as indicators of adolescent brain maturation. Proc Natl Acad Sci U S A 2009;106(13):5177–80.

56. Uchiyama M, Okawa M, Shibui K, et al. Poor recovery sleep after sleep deprivation in delayed sleep phase syndrome. Psychiatry Clin Neurosci 1999;53(2):195–7.

57. Uchiyama M, Okawa M, Shibui K, et al. Poor compensatory function for sleep loss as a pathogenic factor in patients with delayed sleep phase syndrome. Sleep 2000;23(4):553–8.

58. Watanabe T, Kato M, Sekimoto M, et al. Polysomnography and body temperature changes by phototherapy in a delayed sleep phase syndrome case. Psychiatry Clin Neurosci 1998;52(2):255–6.

59. Saxvig IW, Wilhelmsen-Langeland A, Pallesen S, et al. Objective measures of sleep and dim light melatonin onset in adolescents and young adults with delayed sleep phase disorder compared to healthy controls. J Sleep Res 2013;22(4):365–72.

60. Sack RL, Auckley D, Auger RR, et al. Circadian rhythm sleep disorders: part II, advanced sleep phase disorder, delayed sleep phase disorder, free-running disorder, and irregular sleep-wake rhythm. An American Academy of Sleep Medicine review. Sleep 2007;30(11):1484–501.

61. Cain N, Gradisar M. Electronic media use and sleep in school-aged children and adolescents: a review. Sleep Med 2010;11(8):735–42.

62. Chellappa SL, Steiner R, Blattner P, et al. Non-visual effects of light on melatonin, alertness and cognitive performance: can blue-enriched light keep us alert? PLoS One 2011;6(1):e16429.

63. Chang AM, Aeschbach D, Duffy JF, et al. Evening use of light-emitting eReaders negatively affects sleep, circadian timing, and next-morning alertness. Proc Natl Acad Sci U S A 2015;112(4):1232–7.

64. Franken P, Dijk DJ. Circadian clock genes and sleep homeostasis. Eur J Neurosci 2009;29(9):1820–9.

65. Shiromani PJ, Xu M, Winston EM, et al. Sleep rhythmicity and homeostasis in mice with targeted disruption of mPeriod genes. Am J Physiol Regul Integr Comp Physiol 2004;287(1):R47–57.

66. King DP, Takahashi JS. Molecular genetics of circadian rhythms in mammals. Annu Rev Neurosci 2000; 23:713–42.

67. Takahashi JS. Molecular neurobiology and genetics of circadian rhythms in mammals. Annu Rev Neurosci 1995;18:531–53.

68. Archer SN, Carpen JD, Gibson M, et al. Polymorphism in the PER3 promoter associates with diurnal preference and delayed sleep phase disorder. Sleep 2010;33(5):695–701.

69. Archer SN, Robilliard DL, Skene DJ, et al. A length polymorphism in the circadian clock gene Per3 is linked to delayed sleep phase syndrome and extreme diurnal preference. Sleep 2003;26(4): 413–5.

70. Hohjoh H, Takasu M, Shishikura K, et al. Significant association of the arylalkylamine N-acetyltransferase (AA-NAT) gene with delayed sleep phase syndrome. Neurogenetics 2003;4(3):151–3.

71. Hohjoh H, Takahashi Y, Hatta Y, et al. Possible association of human leucocyte antigen DR1 with delayed sleep phase syndrome. Psychiatry Clin Neurosci 1999;53(4):527–9.

72. Carpen JD, von Schantz M, Smits M, et al. A silent polymorphism in the PER1 gene associates with extreme diurnal preference in humans. J Hum Genet 2006;51(12):1122–5.

73. Carpen JD, Archer SN, Skene DJ, et al. A single-nucleotide polymorphism in the 5'-untranslated region of the hPER2 gene is associated with diurnal preference. J Sleep Res 2005;14(3): 293–7.

74. Auger RR, Burgess HJ, Emens JS, et al. Clinical practice guideline for the treatment of intrinsic circadian rhythm sleep-wake disorders: advanced sleep-wake phase disorder (ASWPD), delayed sleep-wake phase disorder (DSWPD), non-24-hour sleep-wake rhythm disorder (N24SWD), and irregular sleep-wake rhythm disorder (ISWRD). An update for 2015: an American Academy of Sleep Medicine clinical practice guideline. J Clin Sleep Med 2015; 11(10):1199–236.

75. Sharkey KM, Carskadon MA, Figueiro MG, et al. Effects of an advanced sleep schedule and morning short wavelength light exposure on circadian phase in young adults with late sleep schedules. Sleep Med 2011;12(7):685–92.

76. Morgenthaler TI, Lee-Chiong T, Alessi C, et al. Practice parameters for the clinical evaluation and treatment of circadian rhythm sleep disorders. An American Academy of Sleep Medicine report. Sleep 2007;30(11):1445–59.

77. Wyatt JK. Circadian rhythm sleep disorders. Pediatr Clin North Am 2011;58(3):621.

78. Oren DA, Wehr TA. Hypernyctohemeral syndrome after chronotherapy for delayed sleep phase syndrome. N Engl J Med 1992;327(24):1762.

79. Wirz-Justice A, Armstrong SM. Melatonin: nature's soporific? J Sleep Res 1996;5(2):137–41.

80. Burgess HJ, Revell VL, Molina TA, et al. Human phase response curves to three days of daily melatonin: 0.5 mg versus 3.0 mg. J Clin Endocrinol Metab 2010;95(7):3325–31.

81. van Geijlswijk IM, Korzilius HP, Smits MG. The use of exogenous melatonin in delayed sleep phase disorder: a meta-analysis. Sleep 2010;33(12):1605–14.

82. Mundey K, Benloucif S, Harsanyi K, et al. Phase-dependent treatment of delayed sleep phase syndrome with melatonin. Sleep 2005;28(10):1271–8.

83. Suhner A, Schlagenhauf P, Johnson R, et al. Comparative study to determine the optimal melatonin dosage form for the alleviation of jet lag. Chronobiol Int 1998;15(6):655–66.

84. Lockley SW, Dressman MA, Licamele L, et al. Tasimelteon for non-24-hour sleep-wake disorder in totally blind people (SET and RESET): two multicentre, randomised, double-masked, placebo-controlled phase 3 trials. Lancet 2015;386(10005): 1754–64.

85. Dodson ER, Zee PC. Therapeutics for circadian rhythm sleep disorders. Sleep Med Clin 2010;5(4): 701–15.

86. Wilhelmsen-Langeland A, Saxvig IW, Pallesen S, et al. A randomized controlled trial with bright light and melatonin for the treatment of delayed sleep phase disorder: effects on subjective and objective sleepiness and cognitive function. J Biol Rhythms 2013;28(5):306–21.

87. Lack L, Bramwell T, Wright H, et al. Morning blue light can advance the melatonin rhythm in mild delayed sleep phase syndrome. Sleep Biol Rhythms 2007;5(1):78–80.

88. Czeisler CA, Kronauer RE, Allan JS, et al. Bright light induction of strong (type 0) resetting of the human circadian pacemaker. Science 1989;244(4910): 1328–33.

89. Khalsa SB, Jewett ME, Cajochen C, et al. A phase response curve to single bright light pulses in human subjects. J Physiol 2003;549(Pt 3):945–52.

90. St Hilaire MA, Gooley JJ, Khalsa SB, et al. Human phase response curve to a 1 h pulse of bright white light. J Physiol 2012;590(13):3035–45.

91. Saxvig IW, Wilhelmsen-Langeland A, Pallesen S, et al. A randomized controlled trial with bright light and melatonin for delayed sleep phase disorder: effects on subjective and objective sleep. Chronobiol Int 2014;31(1):72–86.

92. Baehr EK, Eastman CI, Revelle W, et al. Circadian phase-shifting effects of nocturnal exercise in older compared with young adults. Am J Physiol Regul Integr Comp Physiol 2003;284(6):R1542–50.

93. Gradisar M, Crowley SJ. Delayed sleep phase disorder in youth. Curr Opin Psychiatry 2013;26(6): 580–5.

94. Burke TM, Markwald RR, McHill AW, et al. Effects of caffeine on the human circadian clock in vivo and in vitro. Sci Transl Med 2015;7(305):305ra146.

95. Bartlett DJ, Biggs SN, Armstrong SM. Circadian rhythm disorders among adolescents: assessment and treatment options. Med J Aust 2013;199(8): 16–20.

96. Ito A, Ando K, Hayakawa T, et al. Long-term course of adult patients with delayed sleep phase syndrome. Jpn J Psychiatry Neurol 1993;47(3): 563–7.

97. Dagan Y, Yovel I, Hallis D, et al. Evaluating the role of melatonin in the long-term treatment of delayed sleep phase syndrome (DSPS). Chronobiol Int 1998;15(2):181–90.

Printed and bound by CPI Group (UK) Ltd, Croydon, CR0 4YY

16/10/2024

01774869-0001